T0198252

Infection Prevention and Control in Healthcare, Part II: Management of Infections

Editors

KEITH S. KAYE
SORABH DHAR

INFECTIOUS DISEASE CLINICS OF NORTH AMERICA

www.id.theclinics.com

Consulting Editor
HELEN W. BOUCHER

December 2021 • Volume 35 • Number 4

ELSEVIER

1600 John F. Kennedy Boulevard • Suite 1800 • Philadelphia, Pennsylvania, 19103-2899.
http://www.theclinics.com

INFECTIOUS DISEASE CLINICS OF NORTH AMERICA Volume 35, Number 4
December 2021 ISSN 0891–5520, ISBN-13: 978-0-323-81369-3

Editor: Kerry Holland
Developmental Editor: Hannah Almira Lopez

Infectious Disease Clinics of North America (ISSN 0891–5520) is published in March, June, September, and December by Elsevier Inc., 360 Park Avenue South, New York, NY 10010-1710. Periodicals postage paid at New York, NY and additional mailing offices. Subscription prices are $347.00 per year for US individuals, $922.00 per year for US institutions, $100.00 per year for US students, $396.00 per year for Canadian individuals, $973.00 per year for Canadian institutions, $432.00 per year for international individuals, $973.00 per year for international institutions, $100.00 per year for Canadian students, and $200.00 per year for international students. To receive student rate, orders must be accompanied by name of affiliated institution, date of term, and the *signature* of program/residency coordinator on institution letterhead. Orders will be billed at individual rate until proof of status is received. Foreign air speed delivery is included in all *Clinics* subscription prices. All prices are subject to change without notice. **POSTMASTER**: Send address changes to *Infectious Disease Clinics of North America*, Elsevier Health Sciences Division, Subcription Customer Service, 3251 Riverport Lane, Maryland Heights, MO 63043. **Customer Service: 1-800-654-2452 (US). From outside of the US and Canada, call 1-314-447-8871. Fax: 1-314-447-8029. E-mail: JournalsCustomerService-usa@elsevier.com (print support) or JournalsOnlineSupport-usa@elsevier.com (online support).**

Infectious Disease Clinics of North America is also published in Spanish by Editorial Inter-Médica, Junin 917, 1er A 1113, Buenos Aires, Argentina.

Reprints. For copies of 100 or more, of articles in this publication, please contact the Commercial Reprints Department, Elsevier Inc., 360 Park Avenue South, New York, New York 10010-1710. Tel. 212-633-3874, Fax: 212-633-3820, E-mail: reprints@elsevier.com.

Infectious Disease Clinics of North America is covered in *MEDLINE/PubMed (Index Medicus), Current Contents/Clinical Medicine, Science Citation Alert, SCISEARCH,* and *Research Alert.*

Contributors

CONSULTING EDITOR

HELEN W. BOUCHER, MD, FIDSA, FACP
Director, Infectious Diseases Fellowship Program, Division of Geographic Medicine and Infectious Diseases, Tufts Medical Center, Associate Professor of Medicine, Tufts University School of Medicine, Boston, Massachusetts, USA

EDITORS

KEITH S. KAYE, MD, MPH
Chief, Division of Allergy, Immunology and Infectious Diseases, Professor of Medicine, Robert Wood Johnson Medical School, New Brunswick, New Jersey, USA

SORABH DHAR, MD
Associate Professor of Medicine, Division of Infectious Diseases, Wayne State University School of Medicine, Medical Director of Infection Prevention, Hospital Epidemiology, and Antimicrobial Stewardship, John D. Dingell VA Medical Center, Harper University Hospital, Detroit, Michigan, USA

AUTHORS

GEORGE J. ALANGADEN, MD
Clinical Professor of Medicine, Wayne State University, Division of Infectious Diseases, Henry Ford Hospital, Detroit, Michigan, USA

DEVERICK J. ANDERSON, MD, MPH
Professor of Medicine, Division of Infectious Diseases and International Health, Department of Medicine, Duke University, Division of Infectious Diseases, Duke Center for Antimicrobial Stewardship and Infection Prevention, Duke University School of Medicine, Durham, North Carolina, USA

DAVID B. BANACH, MD, MPH, MS
Associate Professor of Medicine, Department of Medicine, University of Connecticut School of Medicine, Farmington, Connecticut, USA

GAUD CATHO, MD
Infectious Diseases Physician, Infection Control Programme, Faculty of Medicine, University of Geneva Hospitals, Geneva, Switzerland

KELLY A. CAWCUTT, MD, MS
Division of Infectious Diseases, University of Nebraska Medical Center, Omaha, Nebraska, USA

CAROL E. CHENOWETH, MD
Professor, Division of Infectious Diseases, Department of Internal Medicine, University of Michigan Medical School, University Hospital, Ann Arbor, Michigan, USA

TEENA CHOPRA, MD, MPH
Professor, Infectious Diseases, Wayne State University/Detroit Medical Center, Detroit, Michigan, USA

NOELLE COCOROS, DSc, MPH
Department of Population Medicine, Harvard Medical School, Harvard Pilgrim Health Care Institute, Boston, Massachusetts, USA

CASEY E. GODSHALL, MD
Assistant Professor, Department of Medicine, University of Connecticut, Farmington, Connecticut, USA

STEPHAN HARBARTH, MD, MS
Professor, Hospital Epidemiologist, Infection Control Programme, Faculty of Medicine, University of Geneva Hospitals, Geneva, Switzerland

BENEDIKT D. HUTTNER, MD, MS
Infectious Diseases Physician, Division of Infectious Diseases, University of Geneva Hospitals, Geneva, Switzerland; Assistant Professor, Faculty of Medicine, University of Geneva, Geneva, Switzerland

SEEMA JOSHI, MD
Division of Infectious Diseases, Henry Ford Hospital, Detroit, Michigan, USA

MICHAEL KLOMPAS, MD, MPH
Department of Population Medicine, Harvard Medical School, Harvard Pilgrim Health Care Institute, Department of Medicine, Brigham and Women's Hospital, Boston, Massachusetts, USA

AMAR KRISHNA, MD
Hospitalist, Internal Medicine, Norther Light AR Gould Hospital, Presque Isle, Maine, USA

ANDIE S. LEE, MBBS, DTM&H, MSc
Infectious Diseases Physician and Microbiologist, Departments of Infectious Diseases and Microbiology, Royal Prince Alfred Hospital, Clinical Senior Lecturer, Faculty of Medicine, University of Sydney, Sydney, New South Wales, Australia

DROR MARCHAIM, MD
Sackler School of Medicine, Tel-Aviv University, Tel-Aviv, Israel; Division of Infectious Diseases, Shamir (Assaf Harofeh) Medical Center, Zerifin, Israel

JOHN P. MILLS, MD
Division of Infectious Diseases, University of Michigan Medical School, Ann Arbor, Michigan, USA

SARAH R. PERLOFF, DO
Associate Chair, Department of Medicine, Program Director, Infectious Disease Fellowship Program, Associate Program Director, Internal Medicine Residency Program, Einstein Medical Center, Assistant Clinical Professor of Medicine, Sidney Kimmel Medical College of Thomas Jefferson University, Philadelphia, Pennsylvania, USA

JOSHUA G. PETRIE, PhD
Research Assistant Professor, Department of Epidemiology, University of Michigan School of Public Health, Ann Arbor, Michigan, USA

MARK E. RUPP, MD
Division of Infectious Diseases, University of Nebraska Medical Center, Omaha, Nebraska, USA

JESSICA SEIDELMAN, MD, MPH
Assistant Professor, Division of Infectious Diseases and International Health, Department of Medicine, Duke University, Division of Infectious Diseases, Duke Center for Antimicrobial Stewardship and Infection Prevention, Duke University School of Medicine, Durham, North Carolina, USA

LAURA M. SELBY, DO
Division of Infectious Diseases, University of Nebraska Medical Center, Omaha, Nebraska, USA

ANITA SHALLAL, MD
Division of Infectious Diseases, Henry Ford Hospital, Detroit, Michigan, USA

GEEHAN SULEYMAN, MD, MLS (ASCP)
Clinical Assistant Professor, Wayne State University, Medical Director of Infection Prevention and Control, Henry Ford Hospital, Detroit, Michigan, USA

NEERAJA SWAMINATHAN, MD
Department of Medicine, Einstein Medical Center, Philadelphia, Pennsylvania, USA

THOMAS R. TALBOT, MD, MPH, FSHCA, FIDSA
Professor of Medicine, Division of Infectious Diseases, Department of Medicine, Vanderbilt University School of Medicine, Nashville, Tennessee, USA

JEREMY WEINBERGER, MD
Department of Population Medicine, Harvard Medical School, Harvard Pilgrim Health Care Institute, Department of Medicine, Brigham and Women's Hospital, Division of Pulmonary, Critical Care, and Sleep Medicine, Tufts Medical Center, Boston, Massachusetts, USA

MARCUS ZERVOS, MD
Division Head, Professor of Medicine, Assistant Dean of Global Affairs, Division of Infectious Diseases, Henry Ford Hospital, Wayne State University, Detroit, Michigan, USA

JERRY M. ZUCKERMAN, MD
Vice President, Infection Prevention and Control, Department of Patient Safety and Quality, Hackensack Meridian Health, Edison, New Jersey, USA; Assistant Professor of Medicine, Hackensack Meridian School of Medicine, Nutley, New Jersey, USA

Contents

Preface: Infection Prevention and Control in Health Care, Part II: Management of Infections　　　　xiii

Keith S. Kaye and Sorabh Dhar

Prevention of Central-Line Associated Bloodstream Infections: 2021 Update　　　　841

Laura M. Selby, Mark E. Rupp, and Kelly A. Cawcutt

> Despite a large volume of research in prevention, central line–associated bloodstream infections and catheter-related bloodstream infections continue to cause significant morbidity, mortality, and increased health care costs. Strategies in prevention, including decision about catheter placement, insertion bundles, adherence to standard of care guidelines, and technologic innovations, shown to decrease rates of catheter-related bloodstream infections and central line-associated bloodstream infections are described in this update. The coronavirus disease 2019 pandemic has resulted in increased health care–acquired infections, including central line-associated bloodstream infections.

Urinary Tract Infections: 2021 Update　　　　857

Carol E. Chenoweth

> Catheter-associated urinary tract infection (CAUTI) remains one of the most prevalent, but preventable, health care–associated infections and predominantly occurs in patients with indwelling urinary catheters. Duration of urinary catheterization is the most important modifiable risk factor for development of CAUTI. Alternatives to indwelling catheters should be considered in appropriate patients. If indwelling catheterization is necessary, proper aseptic practices for catheter insertion and maintenance and use of a closed catheter collection system are essential for preventing CAUTI. The use of intervention bundles and collaboratives helps in the effective implementation of CAUTI prevention measures.

Ventilator-Associated Events: Epidemiology, Risk Factors, and Prevention　　　　871

Jeremy Weinberger, Noelle Cocoros, and Michael Klompas

> The Centers for Disease Control and Prevention shifted the focus of safety surveillance in mechanically ventilated patients from ventilator-associated pneumonia to ventilator-associated events in 2013 to increase the objectivity and reproducibility of surveillance and to encourage quality improvement programs to focus on preventing a broader array of complications. Ventilator-associated events are associated with a doubling of the risk of dying. Prospective studies have found that minimizing sedation, increasing spontaneous awakening and breathing trials, and conservative fluid management can decrease event rates and the duration of ventilation. Multifaceted interventions to enhance these practices can decrease ventilator-associated event rates.

Surgical Site Infections 901

Jessica Seidelman and Deverick J. Anderson

> Surgical site infections (SSIs) are among the most common and most costly health care–associated infections, leading to adverse patient outcomes and death. Wound contamination occurs with each incision, but proven strategies exist to decrease the risk of SSI. In particular, improved adherence to evidence-based preventive measures related to appropriate antimicrobial prophylaxis can decrease the rate of SSI. Aggressive surgical debridement and effective antimicrobial therapy are needed to optimize the treatment of SSI.

Methicillin-Resistant *Staphylococcus aureus*: An Update on Prevention and Control in Acute Care Settings 931

Andie S. Lee, Benedikt D. Huttner, Gaud Catho, and Stephan Harbarth

> Methicillin-resistant *Staphylococcus aureus* (MRSA) is a leading cause of health-care–associated infections. Controversies regarding the effectiveness of various control strategies have contributed to varying approaches to MRSA control. However, new evidence from large-scale studies has emerged, particularly concerning screening and decolonization. Importantly, implementation and outcomes of control measures in practice are not only influenced by scientific evidence, but also economic, administrative, and political factors, as demonstrated by decreasing MRSA rates in a number of countries after concerted and coordinated efforts at a national level. Flexibility to adapt measures based on local epidemiology and resources is essential for successful MRSA control.

Vancomycin-Resistant Enterococci: Epidemiology, Infection Prevention, and Control 953

Seema Joshi, Anita Shallal, and Marcus Zervos

> Vancomycin-resistant enterococcus (VRE) is a pathogen of growing concern due to increasing development of antibiotic resistance, increasing length of hospitalizations and excess mortality. The utility of some infection control practices are debatable, as newer developments in infection prevention strategies continued to be discovered. This article summarizes the significance of VRE and VRE transmission, along with highlighting key changes in infection control practices within the past 5 years.

Multidrug-Resistant Gram-Negative Bacteria: Infection Prevention and Control Update 969

John P. Mills and Dror Marchaim

> Multidrug-resistant Gram-negative bacteria (MDR-GNB) pose one of the greatest challenges to health care today because of their propensity for human-to-human transmission and lack of therapeutic options. Containing the spread of MDR-GNB is challenging, and the application of multifaceted infection control bundles during an evolving outbreak makes it difficult to measure the relative impact of each measure. This article will review the utility of various infection control measures in containing the spread of various MDR-GNB and will provide the supporting evidence for these interventions.

Prevention of Infection due to *Clostridium (Clostridioides) difficile*   995

Amar Krishna and Teena Chopra

Clostridium (Clostridioides) difficile infection (CDI) causes significant morbidity and mortality in the United States every year. Prevention of CDI is difficult because of spore durability and requires implementation of multipronged strategies. Two categories of prevention strategies are infection control and prevention and risk factor reduction. Hand hygiene, contact precautions, patient isolation, and environmental decontamination are cornerstones of infection control and prevention. Risk factor reduction should focus on antibiotic stewardship to reduce unnecessary antibiotic use. If CDI incidence remains higher than the institution's goal despite these measures, then special measures should be considered.

Prevention of *Mycobacterium tuberculosis* Transmission in Health Care Settings   1013

Neeraja Swaminathan, Sarah R. Perloff, and Jerry M. Zuckerman

Patients with tuberculosis (TB) pose a risk to other patients and health care workers, and outbreaks in health care settings occur when appropriate infection control measures are not used. This article discusses strategies to prevent transmission of *Mycobacterium tuberculosis* within health care settings. All health care facilities should have an operational TB infection control plan that emphasizes the use of a hierarchy of controls (administrative, environmental, and personal respiratory protection). Resources available to clinicians who work in the prevention and investigation of nosocomial transmission of *M tuberculosis* also are discussed.

Nosocomial Fungal Infections: Epidemiology, Infection Control, and Prevention   1027

Geehan Suleyman and George J. Alangaden

Invasive fungal infections are an important cause of morbidity and mortality in hospitalized patients and in the immunocompromised population. This article reviews the current epidemiology of nosocomial fungal infections in adult patients, with an emphasis on invasive candidiasis (IC) and invasive aspergillosis (IA). Included are descriptions of nosocomial infections caused by *Candida auris,* an emerging pathogen, and IC- and IA-associated with coronavirus disease 2019. The characteristics and availability of newer nonculture-based tests for identification of nosocomial fungal pathogens are discussed. Recently published recommendations and guidelines for the control and prevention of these nosocomial fungal infections are summarized.

Health Care–Acquired Viral Respiratory Diseases   1055

Joshua G. Petrie and Thomas R. Talbot

Health care–acquired viral respiratory infections are common and cause increased patient morbidity and mortality. Although the threat of viral respiratory infection has been underscored by the coronavirus disease 2019 (COVID-19) pandemic, respiratory viruses have a significant impact in health care settings even under normal circumstances. Studies report decreased nosocomial transmission when aggressive infection control measures are implemented, with more success noted when using a multicomponent approach. Influenza vaccination of health care personnel furthers decrease rates of transmission; thus, mandatory vaccination is becoming more common. This article discusses the epidemiology, transmission, and control of health care–associated respiratory viral infections.

Pandemic Preparedness   1077

Casey E. Godshall and David B. Banach

Pandemic preparedness is a key function of any health care facility. Activities pertaining to pandemic preparedness should be developed and maintained within a broader emergency management plan. The use of a Hospital Incident Command System can centralize coordination of the response and facilitate internal and external communication. This review addresses several components of pandemic preparedness, including incident management, health care personnel safety, strategies to support ongoing clinical activities, and organizational communication during a pandemic. Preparations addressing potential ethical challenges and the psychological impact associated with pandemic response are also reviewed.

INFECTIOUS DISEASE CLINICS OF NORTH AMERICA

FORTHCOMING ISSUES

March 2022
Pediatric Infections
Jason G. Newland and Rebecca G. Same, *Editors*

June 2022
Covid-19 Infection
Rachel A. Bender Ignacio and Rajesh T. Gandhi, *Editors*

September 2022
Lyme Disease and the Expanding Spectrum of Associated Tick-Borne Illness
Robert P. Smith, *Editor*

RECENT ISSUES

September 2021
Infection Prevention and Control in Healthcare, Part I: Facility Planning
Keith S. Kaye and Sorabh Dhar, *Editors*

June 2021
Fungal Infections
Luis Ostrosky-Zeichner, *Editor*

March 2021
Skin and Soft Tissue Infections
Henry F. Chambers, *Editor*

THE CLINICS ARE AVAILABLE ONLINE!
Access your subscription at:
www.theclinics.com

Preface

Infection Prevention and Control in Health Care, Part II: Management of Infections

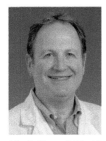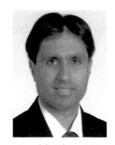

Keith S. Kaye, MD, MPH   Sorabh Dhar, MD
Editors

Infection prevention and control has grown and changed significantly since it first became nationally recognized in the early 1970s. Initially, infection control was focused on occupational health and infection surveillance in the hospital. More recently, there has been a growing emphasis on prevention and process in the hospital and other types of health care settings. Over the past several years, there has been increasing recognition of the quality and cost implications associated with health care–associated infections (HAIs) and the value of infection control. As a result of the COVID-19 pandemic, however, infection prevention has been at the forefront of global health care, thrust into the spotlight with regards to patient and health care worker safety, financial accountability, and regulatory readiness. While individual textbooks, articles, and other resources are available to address specific questions and issues pertaining to infection prevention and control, this issue (as well as the prior issue, Infection Prevention and Control in Health Care, Part I) of *Infectious Diseases Clinics of North America* serves as an inclusive, relatively concise, and focused primer on infection control.

This issue focuses on the epidemiology and prevention of different types of infections in the health care setting, which is one of the overarching and critical functions of the infection prevention department in a hospital. While the most recent 2019 Centers for Disease Control and Prevention progress report indicates reductions for several types of HAIs, recent publications indicate that there has been a relative increase in some HAIs during the COVID-19 pandemic. Multiple factors may be associated with these increases (shortages of personal protective equipment, disinfectants and medical equipment, staff, and host factors associated with increased infections), highlighting the need for continued vigilance in prevention practices. Various topics are

Infect Dis Clin N Am 35 (2021) xiii–xiv
https://doi.org/10.1016/j.idc.2021.07.010
0891-5520/21/© 2021 Published by Elsevier Inc.

id.theclinics.com

covered, including prevention of device-associated infections, surgical site infection, infections due to multidrug-resistant pathogens, and prevention of other types of HAIs.

This issue is intended to serve as a useful reference and primer for infection prevention and control, particularly with regards to key components and strategies to prevent infection acquisition in the hospital. We want to thank the authors who have contributed valuable time and effort to this issue. We hope that you will enjoy it and find it to be a wonderful resource for helping to optimize infection prevention efforts in health care settings and to improve the safety and hospital experience for patients.

Keith S. Kaye, MD, MPH
Division of Allergy, Immunology and Infectious Diseases
Robert Wood Johnson Medical School
125 Paterson Street
New Brunswick, NJ 08901, USA

Sorabh Dhar, MD
Division of Infectious Diseases
Wayne State University School of Medicine
Harper University Hospital
5 Hudson
3990 John R Street
Detroit, MI 48201, USA

E-mail addresses:
kk1116@rwjms.rutgers.edu (K.S. Kaye)
sdhar@med.wayne.edu (S. Dhar)

Prevention of Central-Line Associated Bloodstream Infections: 2021 Update

Laura M. Selby, DO, Mark E. Rupp, MD, Kelly A. Cawcutt, MD, MS*

KEYWORDS

- Bloodstream infection • Intravascular catheter • Prevention • Bacteremia

KEY POINTS

- Central line-associated bloodstream infections and catheter-related bloodstream infections are responsible for substantial morbidity, mortality, and increased health care costs.
- Many of these infections are preventable using current knowledge and prevention techniques.
- Evidence-based strategies to prevent central line-associated bloodstream infections include decision-making about appropriate catheter choice and insertion bundles.
- Techniques to increase adherence to standard of care practices such as staff training, education, appropriate staffing levels, and leadership involvement are equally important in central line-associated bloodstream infections prevention.
- Health care–associated infections rates, including central line-associated bloodstream infections, have increased during the severe acute respiratory syndrome coronavirus 2 pandemic.

INTRODUCTION AND CLINICAL SIGNIFICANCE

Vascular catheter insertion is the most common procedure in hospitalized patients.[1] Intravascular catheters are used in a wide range of clinical settings for treatment including, but not limited to, delivering medications, obtaining blood samples, hemodynamic monitoring, and facilitating life-saving procedures such as extracorporeal membrane oxygenation and renal replacement therapy. All vascular catheters carry a risk of adverse events, with infectious complications ranging from local skin and soft tissue infection to more severe bloodstream infections (BSIs).[2] Catheter-related infections increase hospital costs, extend the length of stay, and increase the risk of death. An estimated 30,000 to 40,000 episodes of CLABSI occur yearly in the United States in acute care hospitals.[3,4] Preliminary data from the coronavirus disease 2019

Division of Infectious Diseases, University of Nebraska Medical Center, 985400 Nebraska Medical Center, Omaha, NE 68198, USA
* Corresponding author.
E-mail address: Kelly.cawcutt@unmc.edu
Twitter: @KellyCawcuttMD (K.A.C.)

Infect Dis Clin N Am 35 (2021) 841–856
https://doi.org/10.1016/j.idc.2021.07.004
0891-5520/21/© 2021 Elsevier Inc. All rights reserved.

id.theclinics.com

(COVID-19) pandemic demonstrate an increase in hospital-associated infections (HAIs), including vascular catheter-related infections.[5]

DEFINITIONS AND SURVEILLANCE

Defining infections owing to vascular catheters is complicated by the variety of catheter types and imprecise terminology used. For example, CLABSI is a term defined by the Centers for Disease Control and Prevention's National Healthcare Safety Network.[3] A CLABSI is defined as a BSI in a patient with a central venous catheter (CVC), without another attributable source of infection, that occurs when the CVC has been in place for more than 2 calendar days or removed the day before the BSI.[3,6] CVCs can be inserted centrally, typically in the femoral, subclavian, or internal jugular veins, or peripherally in the cephalic or brachial veins (peripherally inserted central catheter [PICC]).[3]

CLABSI overestimates the rate of true infection and has inherent subjectivity by the requirement to assign the source of infection. Notably, midline catheters, arterial catheters, and peripheral intravascular catheters (PIVs) are excluded from the formal surveillance definition.[3] Not only are the CLABSI definition and surveillance system used to establish benchmarks, they are used for interinstitutional comparison and to drive performance improvement and third-party hospital reimbursement.

The other commonly used term is catheter-related BSI (CRBSI). CRBSI is a clinical definition that uses microbiologic data such as catheter tip cultures, differential time to positivity, or quantitative blood cultures to diagnose, and causally attribute, a BSI to a specific vascular catheter.[4] When evaluating the medical literature, it is important to not inadvertently interchange CLABSI and CRBSI.

Owing to the standardization of the CLABSI definition, it has become a common end point for both research and quality improvement studies and has been extrapolated and applied to non-CVC catheters. In the United States, efforts to decrease CLABSI rates have resulted in financial penalties for hospitals with rates of CLABSI that are higher than national targets. An increased interest in CLABSI prevention, at least partially driven by a desire to avoid financial penalties and preserve institutional reputation, has resulted in a robust literature on the topic. Unfortunately, fewer data exist regarding the prevention of BSI owing to non-CVC vascular devices.

PATHOGENESIS

Vascular catheters become inoculated through several mechanisms, and effective infection prevention techniques are needed to address each possible source. Contamination of the catheter can occur during insertion through inadequately disinfected skin of the patient, inadequate health care worker hand hygiene, or other deviations from standardized CVC insertion practices (ie, insertion bundle). Postinsertion lapses in dressing practices can result in dermal organisms gaining access to the catheter. While in place, the catheter hub and lumen may become contaminated, particularly if hub cleansing and hand hygiene are suboptimal, resulting in colonization and infection. Additionally, vascular catheters may become inoculated through hematologic spread from another site of infection, or rarely via contaminated infusates[4] (Fig. 1).

Biofilms and Their Role in Infection

The recognition of the importance of biofilms, and their impact on infection, is continually increasing. Biofilms are a distinct community of microbes that produce an extracellular polymeric substance that facilitates irreversible adherence to surfaces, such

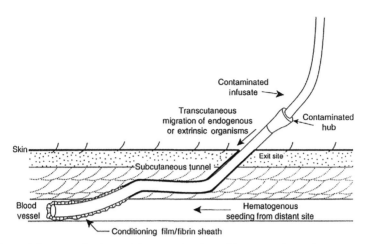

Fig. 1. Potential sources for bacterial contamination of intravascular catheters.

as the lumen of a vascular catheter. Biofilms provide opportunities for plasmid transfer between cells (bacterial conjugation) and cell-to-cell signaling (eg, quorum sensing), which can increase the fitness of the micro-organisms and result in infections that are more difficult to eradicate.[7] Bacterial colonization of vascular catheters, via mechanisms discussed elsewhere in this article, can occur in as little as 24 hours, with biofilms subsequently identified as quickly as 48 to 72 hours after catheter insertion.[8] This finding is clinically significant because biofilms also decrease the effectiveness of the immune system's phagocytes and complement system, and antibiotic susceptibility decreases around 1000-fold, causing further difficulty in eradication.[9] The recognition of the importance of biofilms has led to technological innovations, such as the development of antimicrobial-coated CVCs designed to prevent, or limit, biofilm formation.[7]

Once formed, infections with biofilms can be difficult to treat without removal of the infected catheter, so the prevention of biofilm formation is key to successful prevention of CRBSI.[9] Historically, biofilms were associated with *Staphylococcus aureus*, *Pseudomonas aeruginosa*, *Candida albicans*, *Enterococcus* species, and coagulase-negative staphylococci.[7] New pathogens are increasingly being recognized as biofilm formers, such as *Candida auris*, a known multidrug-resistant organism.[10] Given the difficulty in treating biofilm infections, strategies other than conventional antibiotics are increasingly being explored, such as antibiofilm molecules that inhibit quorum sensing, dispersion of extracellular polysaccharide substance, and molecules that disrupt biofilm adhesion mechanisms, but are not yet all available commercially.[9]

PREVENTION OF INFECTIONS
Clinical Decision-Making Regarding Catheter Type and Necessity

The first step in preventing vascular catheter infections is to optimize the choice of catheter based on the patient's clinical need. Different types of catheters have variable risks of complications, including infections; thus, the type of catheter must be considered before insertion. Vascular access algorithms may aid teams in complex device selection decisions (**Fig. 2**). Patient comfort and ease of access should also be taken into account when deciding on the optimal vascular access device.[11] Decreasing needle sticks, the possibility of complications, and the location of the vascular catheter

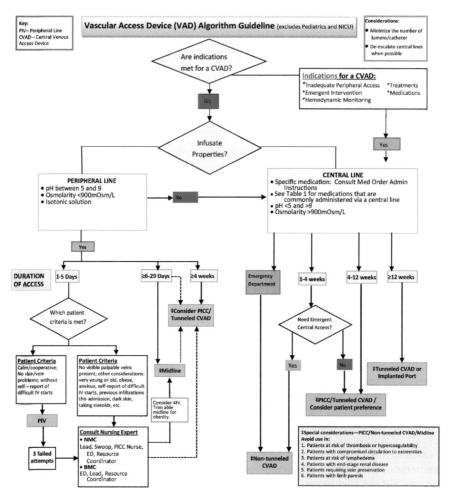

Fig. 2. Vascular access device algorithm guideline. Excludes pediatrics and the NICU. (*From* Cawcutt KA, Hankins RJ, Micheels TA, Rupp ME. Optimizing vascular-access device decision-making in the era of midline catheters. Infect Control Hosp Epidemiol. 2019;40(6):674-680; with permission.)

are factors that should be discussed with the patient before placement, if feasible, in an opportunity for shared decision-making.[11]

Length of expected need

Vascular catheters are viable for various lengths of time, from subcutaneously implanted ports that can be used for years, to PIVs that may only last a few days. CVCs can be tunneled if needed nonemergently or for more than 1 week, or nontunneled for emergent central access.[11] PIVs are ideal if the anticipated patient need for vascular access is fewer 6 days, and no other criteria for other central vascular access are met.[11] Midline catheters (midlines) can stay in place for 2 to 4 weeks, and provide an option for de-escalation from a CVC when central access is no longer required. There is mixed evidence regarding whether midlines have rates of infection similar to PIV or PICC.[12–15] Tunneled vascular catheters can remain in place for months.

Implantable devices, such as ports, provide long-term vascular access and are often used for chemotherapy regimens requiring central access over months to years.

Indications for therapeutic infusions

Certain medications such as vasopressors and vesicant chemicals, such as some chemotherapeutic agents, are recommended to be administered via a CVC rather than through a PIV. Over time, the list of medications that can be safely given through PIVs has expanded. For example, as recently as 2011, vancomycin was included in the Infusion Nursing Standards of Practice as a medication to be given through a central catheter owing to its low pH.[16] Multiple studies have now demonstrated that vancomycin can safely be given through a PIV or midline.[11] This change illustrates the importance of regular review of hospital policy around infusate requirements, and clinician familiarity with those policies, when making decisions about vascular catheter placement.

Patient monitoring

Vascular catheters are also used to monitor hemodynamic parameters such as the central venous pressure and the pulmonary artery pressure. If hemodynamic monitoring is the primary reason for placement of a CVC, consider removal of the catheter, or de-escalation to a peripheral catheter, when monitoring of those hemodynamic parameters is no longer clinically necessary or when measuring through noninvasive methods is feasible.[11]

Difficult vascular access

Patients with difficult to obtain venous access may require CVC placement. In such cases, attempts to obtain noncentral access should be considered carefully before CVC placement. For instance, ultrasound guidance can be used to maximize successful cannulation of peripheral veins in patients with difficult or tenuous vascular access.[17–19] Including the number of unsuccessful cannulation attempts before escalating to ultrasound guidance or recruitment of more experienced vascular access team personnel, and consideration for different types of vascular catheters in a hospital vascular access algorithm or policy is reasonable (see **Fig. 2** for an example of a vascular access algorithm). When placing both centrally inserted central catheters and PICCs, guidelines recommend providers use real-time ultrasound guidance to increase the rate of successful placement and minimize complications.[18]

Additional factors to consider when deciding on what type of vascular access catheter is the best option for a particular patient includes chronic kidney disease status because PICCs can affect the long-term options for dialysis by contributing to central venous stenosis, which affects hemodialysis fistula placement.[20] One study has suggested that patients with a prior history of PICC placements have an increased rate of PICC associated BSIs, so prior placement of PICCs could be considered as well.[21] Finally, the number of lumens on a catheter should be minimized to what is needed for patient care, because more lumens increase the risk of infection and thrombosis.[22]

CATHETER CHECKLIST AND BUNDLES

Using a bundle, in which a variety of interventions are combined together for placement and after care of CVCs, has been documented in many studies and quality improvement projects to decrease rates of CLABSI and CRBSI.[23–26] Bundles frequently consist of an insertion kit, hand hygiene, skin preparation, maximal barrier precautions, chlorohexidine-impregnated dressing, and checklist to ensure that all steps are performed.[27] Maximal barrier precautions include using sterile gown and gloves, a surgical mask, head covering, and a sterile drape over the patient's full body.[27] Although the relative importance of each component of a bundle is not defined clearly, the bundled approach has proven successful in preventing CLABSIs.[4] Based on this persuasive evidence, institutions should develop a bundle to decrease their rates of CLABSI and CRBSI. See **Table 1** for bundle component considerations.

Types of Catheters and Techniques and Devices to Prevent Infection

Antimicrobial-coated catheters

CVCs have been coated or impregnated with a variety of antimicrobial agents and these have been shown to decrease CRBSI in adults and pediatric population.[28,29] The most extensively studied CVC coatings are silver sulfadiazine/chlorhexidine and minocycyline/rifampin.[30] Some CVCs are coated on both the internal and external surfaces, whereas in others the material of the catheter itself is impregnated with the antimicrobial substance.[29] The latter are typically metal-based antimicrobials such as a silver or platinum product.[29] Nonantibiotic compounds are increasingly being investigated for the prevention of biofilm formation in medical devices, including vascular catheters.[29]

Using a coated CVC should be considered when the catheter is anticipated to be needed for more than 5 days. Guidelines also suggest that coated catheters can be used in hospital units when rates of CLABSI remain high despite other standard interventions or in patients who are considered high risk for CLABSI.[29,30] Although concern for the development of antimicrobial resistance when using coated CVC catheters is understandable, there is no evidence to suggest that the use of these devices is associated with increased resistance rates.[31] If an antimicrobial catheter is used, clinicians should be aware of the type of antimicrobial and what organisms are resistant to it, for example, minocycline/rifampin–coated catheters lack activity against *P aeruginosa* and *Candida* spp.[29]

Hub cleaning, connectors, and accessing catheters

Scrubbing the catheter hub before accessing the catheter is crucial in decreasing risk for infection that is, "scrub the hub."[32] The minimal needed scrub time is not well-defined. However, 1 study demonstrated that a 15-second scrub with 70% isopropyl

Table 1 Evidenced-based practices for prevention of vascular access catheter infections	
Pericatheter Insertion	Devices and Technology
Appropriate staffing	Antimicrobial catheter coatings
Education and training	Chlorhexidine impregnated dressings
Maximal sterile barriers	Passive port protectors
Insertion site selection	Silver-impregnated connectors
Cutaneous antisepsis	Sutureless catheter securement
Insertion checklist	Antimicrobial catheter locks
Bundle approach	
Postcatheter insertion	
Scrub the hub	
Chlorhexidine patient bathing	
De-escalation of unneeded catheters	
Catheter dressing maintenance	
Bundled approach	

alcohol eliminated colonization of needleless connector surfaces with a high micro-organism count and another showed no difference between 5-second and 15-second scrub times.[33,34] Lever lock systems have been shown to have higher rates of bacterial colonization than luer lock catheter connectors.[35] Some needleless connectors have been associated with an increased risk of infection, which may be related to their ease of disinfection.[32] This issue is complex and most likely relates to a variety of needleless connector characteristics, such as fluid displacement, dead space, flow dynamics, material transparency, and perhaps most important, the design of the interface be-tween the plastic components and the diaphragm contacting the catheter hub. Opti-mum design and function require an interface that can be readily disinfected in a short period of time.[36]

Needless connectors impregnated with silver have also been associated with decreased rates of CLABSI.[37,38] Standard precautions when accessing hubs and con-nectors, such as hand hygiene, should not be ignored; however, multiple studies have demonstrated, that despite education-driven initiatives, rates of nonadherence can still be high.[22]

Alcohol-containing passive hub disinfection caps have been shown to decrease CLABSI in several studies and are being used increasingly as an additional CRBSI pre-vention strategy.[22,35,39–41] Alcohol disinfection caps may also decrease blood culture contamination.[37] Although now used widely, there are limited randomized controlled trials exploring the use of passive hub disinfection, with most trials being done in a quasiexperimental manner.[22,39–41]

Closed intravenous infusions systems have been shown to have lower rates of CLABSI compared with open infusion systems. Open intravenous infusion systems use a glass bottle, burette, or semirigid plastic bottle and require external venting to allow fluid to exit the container and be infused to the patient.[42] The infusate can become contaminated during the venting processes, and open systems have been tied to numerous outbreaks of gram-negative bacteremia.[42] Closed systems include a fully collapsible bag that does not require venting, decreasing the risk of a contam-inated infusate.[42] Open systems are used more commonly in resource-limited set-tings, but if resources are available, a closed intravenous system decreased the risk of CLABSI and CRBSI.[27,42]

Dressing and dressing changes

Several types of dressings for CVCs are available. Sterile gauze dressings should be changed every 48 hours, and transparent semipermeable dressings weekly.[34,43,44] Soiled, loose, or damp dressings should be changed promptly, to prevent an increased risk of CLABSI.[34,44] Chlorhexidine-impregnated dressings can decrease micro-organisms at the insertion site of a CVC and have well-documented usefulness in the prevention of CRBSI for adults with short-term, nontunneled CVCs.[45,46] In gen-eral, administration sets should be changed no more than every 96 hours. Exceptions to the 96-hour administration set change recommendation include the following: parenteral nutrition administration sets should be changed every 24 hours, and those used to administer blood every 4 hours or at the completion of a unit.[34]

Antimicrobial locks

Antimicrobial lock is a process in which the lumen of a catheter is filled with an anti-microbial solution for a set duration. Antimicrobial lock solutions may contain antibi-otics, antiseptics, or compounds directed toward preventing bacterial adherence or biofilm formation. Primarily studied in patients requiring longer term vascular catheters or patients with prior episodes of CRBSI, and sometimes as part of an attempt to salvage an already infected catheter, there is growing evidence that lock therapy is effective in CRBSI prevention.[47] The ideal dwell time, best choice of antimicrobial solution, and potential complications remain in question. The risk of antimicrobial resistance and lumen integrity when lock therapy is used prophylactically are areas that especially need additional exploration. A study published in 2019 demonstrated that antimicrobial lock therapy to prevent CLABSI resulted in an overall cost savings when used in hemodialysis settings, oncology treatment, or home parenteral nutrition.[47] Antimicrobial lock therapy for CLABSI prevention should be considered on a case-by-case basis, and more strongly considered in long-term vascular catheter use or in patients with prior CRBSI, including pediatric patients.[48]

Chlorhexidine gluconate baths

Multiple studies have shown that chlorhexidine gluconate baths decrease the rate of CLABSI.[49,50] The majority of studies have been performed in critical care settings; however, there is reasonable evidence to suggest that daily chlorhexidine gluconate baths in patients with CVCs outside of the intensive care unit also have lower rates of CLABSI and CRBSI, and therefore should be considered in noncritical care patients.[51,52] The widespread use of chlorhexidine for bathing and methicillin-resistant S aureus decolonization has led to concern that resistance to chlorhexidine may be developed. Low-level resistance of S aureus to chlorhexidine, called tolerance, occurs by efflux pumps mediated by the qacA and qacB genes.[53] The clinical significance of tolerance remains unclear, although some evidence suggests that S aureus strains with these genes are associated with health care exposure.[54] No clinically significant resistance to chlorhexidine has been attributed to chlorhexidine gluconate bathing, but this area continues to be investigated.[53]

Implementing Standard of Care Practices to Prevent Infection

As vascular catheter infection prevention practices have become more standardized, there has been a growing body of implementation and dissemination research exploring the barriers to implementing evidence-based practices and increasing adherence to safe practices in all aspects of vascular catheter care.

Staffing

Several studies have demonstrated that the understaffing of hospital units has contributed to higher rates of CLABSI. All levels of health care professionals play a role in vascular catheter infection prevention, and when staffing is inadequate, it can lead to increased rates of infection.[55–58] Because all hospital units have unique staffing needs, from an infection prevention perspective, it is impossible to recommend exact staff to patient ratios, other than that staffing should be adequate to follow all recommended practices.[56–58] High rates of health care worker burnout have also been associated with increased risk of HAIs; thus, resiliency and wellness should be considered in the strategic planning of preventative initiatives.[59] Robust vascular access teams have also been associated with lower CLABSI rates, presumably through greater adherence to recommended practices from a dedicated team.[60]

Training and education

Adequate training and continuing education in the insertion and care of vascular catheters has been shown to decrease the rates of catheter infection.[61,62] One study showed that, after the implementation of a CLABSI prevention bundle, the rate of infection did not decrease until adherence of individual bundle elements was more than 95%, highlighting the importance of training and education in catheter-related infection prevention.[63] Quality improvement initiatives focusing on hand hygiene and catheter hub cleaning have been associated with decreased rates of CLABSI, demonstrating that effective CLABSI prevention may not require substantial upgrades to medical technology.[64] Interventions targeted directly to units with high CLABSI rates can show substantial decreases in infection rates and improvement in staff knowledge and protocol adherence when providing care.[65] Various methods of continuing education have found success at decreasing catheter infection rates, including classroom-based interventions, simulations, yearly skills checks, and the use of bedside observers and educators.[66] A robust multidisciplinary education program to optimize adherence to bundle guidelines and hospital vascular catheter policy should be a part of every hospital system infection prevention program.

Role of leadership involvement in catheter infection prevention
For successful prevention of vascular catheter infections, engagement of senior administrative leadership is necessary. A study conducted at 18 hospitals across the United States found that executive leadership engagement and manager coaching promoted prevention of HAI including CLABSI.[67] Although perhaps not feasible for all hospital systems, the involvement of executive leadership in hospital units reporting a CLABSI to provide feedback and goal setting can assist with prevention.[68]

Practices to de-escalate vascular catheters
De-escalation when a certain type of catheter is no longer indicated clinically is an important infection mitigation strategy. A multimodal strategy is needed to assist with clinically indicated de-escalation. Because vascular catheters are often hidden under clothing or blankets, clinicians can be unaware of the presence of a vascular catheter, which can be a barrier to removal.[69] Tools in electronic health records can be used to alert clinical staff to the length of time a catheter has been in place, but often need to be optimized to give accurate and easy to find information about catheters.[69]

In a critically ill patient with complex medical problems, vascular catheter de-escalation can be inadvertently deprioritized by medical providers. However, a discussion about the continued need for a CVC should occur daily among the medical team.[70,71] Checklists for use during rounds by the medical team in intensive care units are now common and should include vascular catheter considerations. It should be noted that the addition of a checklist alone has not been shown to decrease the rates of CLABSI, and checklists are but a single valuable tool in multimodal CLABSI prevention programs.[72]

For patients outside of the acute hospital setting who require vascular access for monitoring or medication administration, vascular catheters should also be removed when no longer needed. Limited data are available about rates of failure to remove ports or other long term type devices, but clinicians should monitor for continued need at regularly scheduled intervals.

EFFECTS OF THE SEVERE ACUTE RESPIRATORY SYNDROME CORONAVIRUS 2 PANDEMIC ON VASCULAR CATHETER INFECTIONS

Since the start of the severe acute respiratory syndrome coronavirus 2 pandemic, several studies have reported increased rates of CLABSI and BSI in both COVID-positive and non–COVID-infected individuals in intensive care units.[73–75] Prolonged intensive care unit admissions for patients with COVID-19, with more catheter days per patient does increase each patient's individual CLABSI risk. However, the CLABSI rate, which is expressed per 1000 CVC days, should not increase based solely on catheter dwell time. There is evidence to suggest that staffing shortages may be a strong factor, because lower nurse to patient ratios allows less time to maintain standard of care maintenance of catheters.[74,76] Health care worker burnout, which has been associated with increased risk of HAI and has been shown to have increased with the pandemic, could also be contributing.[59,77] Additionally, changes in behaviors such as moving intravenous pumps outside of rooms to minimize health care staff from entering patient rooms resulted in long tubing extensions, more tubing connectors, and an increased number of possible contamination sites.[73] The increase in prone position ventilation (patient lying face down for up to 16 hours per day, as opposed to traditional supine positioning) may make it more difficult to access vascular catheters or assess dressing integrity could also be contributing to increasing rates. Some data suggest[73] that more CVCs were placed emergently in patients with COVID-19, and higher rates of femoral catheters were used during the COVID-19 pandemic, both of which have been associated with higher rates of infection.[43,74]

Finally, the COVID-19 pandemic has resulted in a reallocation of infection prevention and antibiotic stewardship resources toward COVID-19–related issues, resulting in a neglect of other infection control efforts, which may have further exacerbated the increase in vascular catheter infections.[78]

Special Subgroups of Patients to Consider

Vascular access at home
Vascular catheter access can be required for multiple purposes outside of the acute care hospital, including home parental nutrition, outpatient antibiotic therapy, and access for administration of fluids or chemotherapy regimens.[79] The majority of research done about the prevention of CLABSI and CRBSI have been done in the acute care and critical care setting. There is a small but growing body of literature about surveillance and prevention in the home therapy setting.[80] Using data collected through home health care agencies that provide in-home care for patients with CVCs has been used to track rates of CLABSI in small studies, but there can be variability in definitions used to define CLABSI in home infusion therapy.[81] When surveyed about how CLABSI is defined, many home infusion nurses used provider documentation or a positive CVC tip culture as the sole means of defining CLABSI, although neither of these is consistent with the CLABSI definition used in the acute care setting.[81] Adherence to CLABSI/CRBSI infection prevention practices has not been well-studied in the home care setting.[82]

Patients with hematologic malignancies
Patient receiving cytotoxic chemotherapy that results in myelosuppression are at high risk of HAIs, including CLABSI.[52] Although the majority of infection prevention strategies for patients with hematologic malignancies are similar to other patients, multiple studies have examined additional prevention techniques to reduce infection in this high-risk group.[30] Chlorhexidine gluconate baths in patients outside of the intensive care unit have been shown to decrease health care–associated BSI owing to gram-positive bacteria in hematologic malignancy patients, in contrast with studies for all patients outside of the critical care setting, which has demonstrated mixed results.[52]

Arterial catheters
Arterial catheters are often placed under less stringently aseptic conditions than CVCs, and are often not tracked in CLABSI or CRBSI reporting systems.[83] However, studies have shown that arterial catheters have similar infection rates to CVCs.[84] Based on this finding, it would be reasonable to track and report BSI associated with arterial catheters and consider interventions to decrease rates.[4]

SUMMARY

Vascular catheters remain a significant source of infection despite robust research in the field of prevention. Surveillance should include all nosocomial BSIs, including PIVs, midlines, and arterial catheters, with CLABSI as a subset within the surveillance plan. Efforts to decrease BSIs from all vascular catheters portends improved outcome and costs for patients and health care organizations. Recently, the increase in CLABSIs during the COVID-19 pandemic demonstrates the continued need for research to prevent future morbidity, mortality, and cost associated with these infections, as well as research to increase adherence to proven strategies.

CLINICS CARE POINTS

- Optimal vascular access decision-making is critical and must include consideration for type of catheter needed, duration of need, and clinical indications for use.
- De-escalation of catheters is another key aspect in catheter-related risk reduction, including transitioning to a peripheral intravenous or midline as soon as central access is no longer required.
- Process improvements, including workflow, education, and the use of bundled approaches, may improve adherence to evidence-based practices across all spectrums of catheter care.
- If higher CLABSI rates persist, assess adherence to standard practices and consider implementation of coated catheters and universal chlorhexidine gluconate baths.

DISCLOSURE

The authors report no conflicts of interest related to this article. Dr M.E. Rupp reports having served as a consultant for 3M, Becton-Dickinson, Teleflex, and Citius Pharmaceuticals.

REFERENCES

1. Bodenham Chair A, Babu S, Bennett J, et al. Association of anaesthetists of Great Britain and Ireland: safe vascular access 2016. Anaesthesia 2016;71(5):573–85.
2. Zhang L, Cao S, Marsh N, et al. Infection risks associated with peripheral vascular catheters. J Infect Prev 2016;17(5):207–13.
3. 2021 NHSN patient safety component manual (n.d.). Retrieved March 22, 2021. Available at: https://www.cdc.gov/nhsn/pdfs/pscmanual/pcsmanual_current.pdf. Accesssed March 22, 2021.
4. Rupp ME, Karnatak R. Intravascular catheter-related bloodstream infections. Infect Dis Clin North Am 2018;32(4):765–87.
5. Assi M, Doll M, Pryor R, et al. Impact of coronavirus disease 2019 (COVID-19) on healthcare-associated infections: an update and perspective. Infect Control Hosp Epidemiol 2021;1–2. https://doi.org/10.1017/ice.2021.92.
6. Mayer J, Greene T, Howell J, et al. Agreement in classifying bloodstream infections among multiple reviewers conducting surveillance. Clin Infect Dis 2012; 55(3):364–70.
7. Donlan RM. Biofilms: microbial life on surfaces. Emerg Infect Dis 2002;8(9): 881–90.
8. Higgins M, Zhang L, Ford R, et al. The microbial biofilm composition on peripherally inserted central catheters: a comparison of polyurethane and hydrophobic

catheters collected from paediatric patients. J Vasc Access 2020. https://doi.org/10.1177/1129729820932423. 112972982093242.

9. Roy R, Tiwari M, Donelli G, et al. Strategies for combating bacterial biofilms: a focus on anti-biofilm agents and their mechanisms of action. Virulence 2018; 9(1):522–54.

10. Sherry L, Ramage G, Kean R, et al. Biofilm-forming capability of highly virulent, multidrug-resistant candida auris. Emerg Infect Dis 2017;23(2):328–31.

11. Cawcutt K, Hankins R, Micheels T, et al. Optimizing vascular-access device decision-making in the era of midline catheters. Infect Control Hosp Epidemiol 2019;40(6):674–80.

12. Adams D, Little A, Vinsant C, et al. The midline catheter: a clinical review. J Emerg Med 2016;51(3):252–8.

13. Xu T, Kingsley L, DiNucci S, et al. Safety and utilization of peripherally inserted central catheters versus midline catheters at a large academic medical center. Am J Infect Control 2016;44(12):1458–61.

14. Sharp R, Esterman A, McCutcheon H, et al. The safety and efficacy of midlines compared to peripherally inserted central catheters for adult cystic fibrosis patients: a retrospective, observational study. Int J Nurs Stud 2014;51(5):694–702.

15. Hogle NJ, Balzer KM, Ross BG, et al. A comparison of the incidence of midline catheter–associated bloodstream infections to that of central line–associated bloodstream infections in 5 acute care hospitals. Am J Infect Control 2020; 48(9):1108–10.

16. Infusion Nurses Society. Infusion nursing standards of practice (2011), vol. 34. Norwood, MA: Untreed Reads; 2011.

17. Egan G, Healy D, O'Neill H, et al. Ultrasound guidance for difficult peripheral venous access: systematic review and meta-analysis. Emerg Med J 2012; 30(7):521–6.

18. Franco-Sadud R, Schnobrich D, Mathews BK, et al. Recommendations on the use of ultrasound guidance for central and peripheral vascular access in adults: a position statement of the society of hospital medicine. J Hosp Med 2019;14: E1–22.

19. Xiong Z, Chen H. Interventions to reduce unnecessary central venous catheter use to prevent central-line–associated bloodstream infections in adults: a systematic review. Infect Control Hosp Epidemiol 2018;39(12):1442–8.

20. Drew D, Weiner D. Peripherally inserted central catheters (PICCs) in CKD: PICC'-ing the best access for kidney disease patients. Am J Kidney Dis 2016;67(5): 724–7.

21. Kim K, Kim Y, Peck KR. Previous peripherally inserted central catheter (PICC) placement as a risk factor for PICC-associated bloodstream infections. Am J Infect Control 2020;48(10):1166–70.

22. Barton A. The case for using a disinfecting cap for needlefree connectors. Br J Nurs 2019;28(14):S22–7.

23. Pronovost P, Needham D, Berenholtz S, et al. An intervention to decrease catheter-related bloodstream infections in the ICU. N Engl J Med 2006;355(26): 2725–32.

24. Blot K, Bergs J, Vogelaers D, et al. Prevention of central line-associated bloodstream infections through quality improvement interventions: a systematic review and meta-analysis. Clin Infect Dis 2014;59(1):96–105.

25. Lipitz-Snyderman A, Steinwachs D, Needham DM, et al. Impact of a statewide intensive care unit quality improvement initiative on hospital mortality and length of stay: retrospective comparative analysis. BMJ 2011;342(jan28 1):d219.

26. Pronovost PJ, Goeschel CA, Colantuoni E, et al. Sustaining reductions in catheter related bloodstream infections in Michigan intensive care units: observational study. BMJ 2010;340(feb04 1):c309.
27. Lutwick L, Al-Maani AS, Mehtar S, et al. Managing and preventing vascular catheter infections: a position paper of the international society for infectious diseases. Int J Infect Dis 2019;84:22–9.
28. Gilbert R, Brown M, Rainford N, et al. Antimicrobial-impregnated central venous catheters for prevention of neonatal bloodstream infection (PREVAIL): an open-label, parallel-group, pragmatic, randomized controlled trial. Lancet Child Adolesc Health 2019;3(6):381–90.
29. Francolini I, Donelli G, Crisante F, et al. Antimicrobial polymers for anti-biofilm medical devices: state-of-art and perspectives. In: Donelli G, editor. Biofilm-based Healthcare-associated Infections. Advances in experimental medicine and biology, vol. 831. Cham: Springer; 2015.
30. Malek AE, Raad II. Preventing catheter-related infections in cancer patients: a review of current strategies. Expert Rev Anti Infect Ther 2020;18(6):531–8.
31. Ramos ER, Reitzel R, Jiang Y, et al. Clinical effectiveness and risk of emerging resistance associated with prolonged use of antibiotic-impregnated catheters: more than 0.5 million catheter days and 7 years of clinical experience*. Crit Care Med 2011;39(2):245–51.
32. Rupp ME, Yu S, Huerta T, et al. Adequate disinfection of a split-septum needleless intravascular connector with a 5-second alcohol scrub. Infect Control Hosp Epidemiol 2012;33(7):661–5.
33. Devrim İ, Demiray N, Oruç Y, et al. The colonization rate of needleless connector and the impact of disinfection for 15 s on colonization: a prospective pre- and post-intervention study. J Vasc Access 2019;20(6):604–7.
34. Gorski LA, Hadaway L, Hagle ME, et al. Infusion therapy standards of practice, 8th edition. J Infus Nurs 2021;44(1S Suppl 1):S1–224.
35. Hankins R, Majorant OD, Rupp ME, et al. Microbial colonization of intravascular catheter connectors in hospitalized patients. Am J Infect Control 2019;47(12): 1489–92.
36. Jarvis WR, Murphy C, Hall KK, et al. Health care–associated bloodstream infections associated with negative- or positive-pressure or displacement mechanical valve needleless connectors. Clin Infect Dis 2009;49(12):1821–7.
37. Casey A, Karpanen T, Nightingale P, et al. Microbiological comparison of a silver-coated and a non-coated needleless intravascular connector in clinical use. J Hosp Infect 2012;80(4):299–303.
38. Jacob JT, Tejedor SC, Reyes MD, et al. Comparison of a silver-coated needleless connector and a standard needleless connector for the prevention of central line-associated bloodstream infections. Infect Control Hosp Epidemiol 2014;36(3): 294–301.
39. Wright M-O, Tropp J, Schora DM, et al. Continuous passive disinfection of catheter hubs prevents contamination and bloodstream infection. Am J Infect Control 2013;41(1):33–8.
40. Kamboj M, Blair R, Bell N, et al. Use of disinfection cap to reduce central-line–associated bloodstream infection and blood culture contamination among hematology–oncology patients. Infect Control Hosp Epidemiol 2015;36(12): 1401–8.
41. Taşdelen Öğülmen D, Ateş S. Use of alcohol containing caps for preventing bloodstream infections: A randomized controlled trial. J Vasc Access 2020. https://doi.org/10.1177/1129729820952961. 1129729820952961.

42. Maki DG, Rosenthal VD, Salomao R, et al. Impact of switching from an open to a closed infusion system on rates of central line-associated bloodstream infection: a meta-analysis of time-sequence cohort studies in 4 countries. Infect Control Hosp Epidemiol 2011;32(1):50–8.

43. O'Grady NP, Alexander M, Burns LA, et al. Guidelines for the prevention of intravascular catheter-related infections. Am J Infect Control 2011;39(4 Suppl 1): S1–34.

44. Marschall J, Mermel LA, Fakih M, et al. Strategies to prevent central line-associated bloodstream infections in acute care hospitals: 2014 update. Infect Control 2014;35(S2). https://doi.org/10.1017/s0195941700095412.

45. Timsit J-F, Mimoz O, Mourvillier B, et al. Randomized controlled trial of chlorhexidine dressing and highly adhesive dressing for preventing catheter-related infections in critically ill adults. Am J Respir Crit Care Med 2012;186(12):1272–8.

46. Timsit J-F, Bouadma L, Ruckly S, et al. Dressing disruption is a major risk factor for catheter-related infections*. Crit Care Med 2012;40(6):1707–14.

47. Pliakos EE, Andreatos N, Ziakas PD, et al. The cost-effectiveness of antimicrobial lock solutions for the prevention of central line-associated bloodstream infections. Clin Infect Dis 2019;68(3):419–25.

48. Chong CY, Ong RYL, Seah VXF, et al. Taurolidine–citrate lock solution for the prevention of central line-associated bloodstream infection in paediatric haematology–oncology and gastrointestinal failure patients with high baseline central-line associated bloodstream infection rates. J Paediatr Child Health 2019;56(1):123–9.

49. Kim HY, Lee WK, Na S, et al. The effects of chlorhexidine gluconate bathing on health care–associated infection in intensive care units: a meta-analysis. J Crit Care 2016;32:126–37.

50. Pallotto C, Fiorio M, Angelis VD, et al. Daily bathing with 4% chlorhexidine gluconate in intensive care settings: a randomized controlled trial. Clin Microbiol Infect 2019;25(6):705–10.

51. Dombecki C, Sweeney J, White J, et al. CHG skin application in non-ICU patients with central venous catheters: impact on CLABSI, MRSA bacteremia, and LabID rates. Infect Control Hosp Epidemiol 2020;41(S1). https://doi.org/10.1017/ice.2020.690.

52. Tien K, Sheng W, Shieh S, et al. Chlorhexidine bathing to prevent central line–associated bloodstream infections in hematology units: a prospective, controlled cohort study. Clin Infect Dis 2020;71(3):556–63.

53. Marolf CT, Alter R, Lyden E, et al. Susceptibility of nosocomial Staphylococcus aureus to chlorhexidine after implementation of a hospital-wide antiseptic bathing regimen. Infect Control Hosp Epidemiol 2017;38(7):873–5.

54. Addetia A, Greninger AL, Adler A, et al. A novel, widespread qacA allele results in reduced chlorhexidine susceptibility in staphylococcus epidermidis. Antimicrob Agents Chemother 2019;63(6). https://doi.org/10.1128/aac.02607-18.

55. Fridkin SK, Pear SM, Williamson TH, et al. The role of understaffing in central venous catheter-associated bloodstream infections. Infect Control Hosp Epidemiol 1996;17(3):150–8.

56. Stone PW, Pogorzelska M, Kunches L, et al. Healthcare epidemiology: hospital staffing and health care–associated infections: a systematic review of the literature. Clin Infect Dis 2008;47(7):937–44.

57. Robert J, Fridkin SK, Blumberg HM, et al. The influence of the composition of the nursing staff on primary bloodstream infection rates in a surgical intensive care unit. Infect Control Hosp Epidemiol 2000;21(1):12–7.

58. Leistner R, Thürnagel S, Schwab F, et al. The impact of staffing on central venous catheter-associated bloodstream infections in preterm neonates – results of nation-wide cohort study in Germany. Antimicrob Resist Infect Control 2013; 2(1):11.
59. Tawfik DS, Sexton JB, Kan P, et al. Burnout in the neonatal intensive care unit and its relation to healthcare-associated infections. J Perinatol 2016;37(3):315–20.
60. Holder C, Overton E, Kalaf S, et al. Impact of expansion of vascular access team on central-line–associated bloodstream infections. Infect Control Hosp Epidemiol 2020;41(S1). https://doi.org/10.1017/ice.2020.825.
61. Coopersmith CM, Rebmann TL, Zack JE, et al. Effect of an education program on decreasing catheter-related bloodstream infections in the surgical intensive care unit. Crit Care Med 2002;30(1):59–64.
62. Warren DK, Zack JE, Mayfield JL, et al. The effect of an education program on the incidence of central venous catheter-associated bloodstream infection in a medical ICU. Chest 2004;126(5):1612–8.
63. Patel PK, Olmsted RN, Hung L, et al. A tiered approach for preventing central line-associated bloodstream infection. Ann Intern Med 2019;171(7_Suppl): S16–22.
64. Kapil A, Suri A, Bhatia R, et al. Impact of continuous education and training in reduction of central line-associated bloodstream infection in neurointensive care unit. Indian J Crit Care Med 2020;24(6):414–7.
65. Evangelista T, Vosburg M, Libman R, et al. Decrease CLABSI through central line re-education on the pediatric oncology and bone marrow transplant unit. Biol Blood Marrow Transpl 2017;23(3). https://doi.org/10.1016/j.bbmt.2016.12.589.
66. Buchanan MO, Summerlin-Long S, DiBiase LM, et al. The compliance coach: a bedside observer, auditor, and educator as part of an infection prevention department's team approach for improving central line care and reducing central line-associated bloodstream infection risk. Am J Infect Control 2019;47(1): 109–11.
67. McAlearney AS, Gaughan AA, DePuccio MJ, et al. Management practices for leaders to promote infection prevention: lessons from a qualitative study. Am J Infect Control 2021;49(5):536–41.
68. Mcalearney AS, Hefner J, Robbins J, et al. The role of leadership in eliminating health care-associated infections: a qualitative study of eight hospitals. Adv Health Care Manag 2013;69–94. https://doi.org/10.1108/s1474-8231(2013) 0000014008.
69. Quinn M, Ameling JM, Forman J, et al. Persistent barriers to timely catheter removal identified from clinical observations and interviews. Jt Comm J Qual Saf 2020;46(2):99–108.
70. Exline MC, Ali NA, Zikri N, et al. Beyond the bundle–journey of a tertiary care medical intensive care unit to zero central line-associated bloodstream infections. Crit Care 2013;17(2):R41.
71. Guerin K, Wagner J, Rains K, et al. Reduction in central line-associated bloodstream infections by implementation of a postinsertion care bundle. Am J Infect Control 2010;38(6):430–3.
72. Cavalcanti AB, Bozza FA, Machado FR, et al. Effect of a quality improvement intervention with daily round checklists, goal setting, and clinician prompting on mortality of critically ill patients. JAMA 2016;315(14):1480.
73. Aldawood F, El-Saed A, Zunitan MA, et al. Central line-associated blood stream infection during COVID-19 pandemic. J Infect Public Health 2021. https://doi.org/10.1016/j.jiph.2021.01.017.

74. LeRose J, Sandhu A, Polistico J, et al. The impact of COVID-19 response on central line associated bloodstream infections and blood culture contamination rates at a tertiary care center in greater Detroit area. Infect Control Hosp Epidemiol 2020. https://doi.org/10.1017/ice.2020.1335.

75. Buetti N, Ruckly S, Montmollin ED, et al. COVID-19 increased the risk of ICU-acquired bloodstream infections: a case–cohort study from the multicentric OUT-COMEREA network. Intensive Care Med 2021;47(2):180–7.

76. Moss M, Ehni J, Herbison I, et al. 505. Use of CLABSI prevention bundle audits to decrease CLABSI rates in COVID positive ICU patients in an acute care hospital in New York City during the COVID-19 epidemic. Open Forum Infect Dis 2020; 7(Supplement_1). https://doi.org/10.1093/ofid/ofaa439.699.

77. Matsuo T, Kobayashi D, Taki F, et al. Prevalence of health care worker burnout during the coronavirus disease 2019 (COVID-19) pandemic in Japan. JAMA Netw Open 2020;3(8). https://doi.org/10.1001/jamanetworkopen.2020.17271.

78. Stevens MP, Doll M, Pryor R, et al. Impact of COVID-19 on traditional healthcare-associated infection prevention efforts. Infect Control Hosp Epidemiol 2020;41(8): 946–7.

79. Kovacevich DS, Corrigan M, Ross VM, et al. American Society for Parenteral and Enteral Nutrition Guidelines for the selection and care of central venous access devices for adult home parenteral nutrition administration. J Parenter Enter Nutr 2018;43(1):15–31.

80. Nailon RE, Rupp ME. Surveillance of home health central venous catheter care outcomes: Challenges and future directions. Am J Infect Control 2019;47(11): 1382–7.

81. Keller SC, Alexander M, Williams D, et al. Perspectives on central-line–associated bloodstream infection surveillance in home infusion therapy. Infect Control Hosp Epidemiol 2019;40(6):729–31.

82. Steffens E, Spriet I, Eldere JV, et al. Compliance with evidence-based guidelines for the prevention of central line–associated bloodstream infections in a Belgian home care setting: an observational study. Am J Infect Control 2019;47(6):723–5.

83. Cohen DM, Carino GP, Heffernan DS, et al. Arterial catheter use in the ICU. Crit Care Med 2015;43(11):2346–53.

84. Maki DG, Kluger DM, Crnich CJ. The risk of bloodstream infection in adults with different intravascular devices: a systematic review of 200 published prospective studies. Mayo Clin Proc 2006;81(9):1159–71.

Urinary Tract Infections
2021 Update

Carol E. Chenoweth, MD

KEYWORDS

- Prevention • Catheter-associated urinary tract infection
- Health care–associated infection • Urinary catheter

KEY POINTS

- Catheter-associated urinary tract infections (CAUTIs) are common and costly.
- CAUTI is often caused by hospital-based pathogens with a propensity toward antimicrobial resistance.
- Duration of urinary catheterization is the predominant risk for CAUTI; preventive measures directed at limiting placement and early removal of urinary catheters can successfully decrease catheter use and CAUTI rates.
- Intervention bundles and collaboratives are powerful tools for implementing preventive measures for health care–associated infections, including CAUTI.

INTRODUCTION

Preventive measures have improved the incidence of health care–associated urinary tract infections (UTIs) in US hospitals, but the Centers for Disease Control and Prevention (CDC) estimated that, in 2011, 93,300 catheter-associated UTIs (CAUTIs) occurred in US hospitals.[1] UTI still accounts for 12.9% of health care–associated infections (HAIs) and 23% of infections in the intensive care unit (ICU).[1–3] Most UTIs are related to indwelling urinary catheters; approximately 70% of UTIs (and 95% of UTIs occurring in ICUs) develop in patients with urinary catheters.[4]

CAUTI has significant impact on clinical outcomes, including mortality, length of hospital stay, and cost.[5,6] It is estimated that 65% to 70% of these infections are preventable,[7,8] thus the Centers for Medicare and Medicaid Services (CMS) has not reimbursed hospitals for the extra costs of managing patients with hospital-acquired CAUTI for more than a decade.[9] As a result, prevention of CAUTI has become a priority for most hospitals. This article reviews the epidemiology and pathogenesis, with a focus on preventing CAUTI.

Division of Infectious Diseases, Department of Internal Medicine, University of Michigan Medical School, F4141 South University Hospital, 1500 E. Medical Center Drive, Ann Arbor, MI 48109-5226, USA

E-mail address: cchenow@umich.edu

Infect Dis Clin N Am 35 (2021) 857–870
https://doi.org/10.1016/j.idc.2021.08.003   id.theclinics.com

PATHOGENESIS

Humans have innate defense mechanisms, such as length of urethra and micturition, that prevent attachment and migration of pathogens into the bladder; urinary catheters interfere with these natural defenses.[2,10] Biofilms, composed of clusters of microorganisms and extracellular matrix, deposit on all surfaces of urinary catheters and allow bacterial attachment.[11,12] Biofilms also provide a protective environment from immune cells and antimicrobials. In addition, microorganisms grow more slowly in biofilms, decreasing the effects of many antimicrobials.[11,12] Despite slow growth, microorganisms within the biofilm may ascend the catheter to the bladder in 1 to 3 days. Typically, the biofilm is composed of 1 type of microorganism, although polymicrobial biofilms are possible.[11,12]

Most microorganisms causing CAUTI are endogenous organisms colonizing the patient's intestinal tract and perineum, entering the bladder by ascending the urethra from the perineum.[13] Approximately 66% of the time, organisms migrate in the biofilm on the external surface of the catheter. A smaller proportion of infections (~34%) are acquired from intraluminal contamination of the collection system from exogenous sources resulting from cross-transmission of organisms from the hands of health care personnel.[12,13] Rarely, organisms such as Staphylococcus aureus spread from a hematogenous source and cause upper UTI.

Most CAUTIs are caused by microorganisms from the patient's own gastrointestinal tract; however, approximately 15% of episodes of health care–associated bacteriuria occur in clusters from intrahospital transmission from one patient to another.[2,12] Most of these hospital-based outbreaks have been associated with improper hand hygiene by health care personnel.

EPIDEMIOLOGY OF CATHETER-ASSOCIATED URINARY TRACT INFECTION

Rates of CAUTI in US hospitals have declined significantly since 1990, because of increased emphasis on prevention.[14] Rates of CAUTI in ICUs, reported through the National Healthcare Safety Network (NHSN) in 2013, ranged from to 1.3 UTIs/1000 catheter-days in small medical/surgical ICUs to 5.3 UTIs/1000 catheter-days in neurosurgical ICUs. General care wards had rates of CAUTI similar to the ICU setting, ranging from 0.2 to 3.2/1000 catheter-days; the highest rates occurred in hematology and rehabilitation wards.[15] CAUTIs in pediatric ICUs occur at a rate of 0 to 3.4 UTIs/1000 catheter-days; CAUTI rates in pediatric ICUs in the United States may not be decreasing as in other ICUs.[15,16] In a community hospital consortium, rates of CAUTI were found to be similar in ICU and non-ICU care units, but 72% of CAUTIs occurred in non-ICU patients, suggesting targeted prevention efforts for non-ICU patients may have a significant impact.[17] In non-US settings, rates of CAUTI reported through the International Nosocomial Infection Control Consortium 2010 to 2015, were generally higher than those reported through NHSN, with a range of 1.66 CAUTIs/1000 catheter-days in surgical cardiothoracic ICUs to 17.17 CAUTIs/1000 catheter-days in neurologic ICUs.[18] In addition, NHSN has recently reported CAUTI surveillance data collected between 2013 and 2016, in long-term care facilities in the United States; rates of CAUTI (0.49 CAUTI/1000 catheter-days) were lower than previously reported rates from hospitals discussed earlier.[19]

Microbial Cause of Catheter-associated Urinary Tract Infection

Enterobacteriaceae are the most common pathogens associated with CAUTI,[20] but, in the ICU setting, Pseudomonas sp, Candida sp, and Enterococcus sp become more prevalent.[20,21] Antimicrobial resistance in CAUTI isolates from ICU patients has increased in recent decades; in summary reports from the NHSN 2015 to 2017, 31.1% of *Escherichia coli* isolates from patients with CAUTIs were nonsusceptible to fluoroquinolones.[20] In addition, 16.6% of *Klebsiella* sp and 16% of *E coli* isolates from patients with CAUTIs produced extended-spectrum beta-lactamases (ESBLs).[20] Resistance to antibiotics in CAUTI isolates was even greater in long-term acute care hospitals, where 48.2% of *Klebsiella* sp showed ESBL-mediated (48%) or carbapenem resistance (23.1%).[20]

Risk Factors for Catheter-associated Urinary Tract Infection

Up to 95% of UTIs in the ICU are associated with an indwelling urinary catheter; duration of catheterization is the most important risk factor for CAUTI.[17,22] The precursor of CAUTI is bacteriuria, which develops at an average rate of 3% to 10% per day of catheterization. Virtually all patients catheterized for a month develop bacteriuria, so catheterization for longer than 1 month is generally defined as long-term catheterization.[22]

Table 1 outlines major risk factors for CAUTI. Women have a higher risk of bacteriuria than men, and heavy bacterial colonization of the perineum increases that risk. Other patient factors identified in 1 or more studies include rapidly fatal underlying illness, age greater than 50 years, nonsurgical disease, hospitalization on an orthopedic or urologic service, catheter insertion after the sixth day of hospitalization, catheter inserted outside the operating room, diabetes mellitus, and serum creatinine level greater than 2 mg/dL at the time of catheterization. Nonadherence to aseptic catheter care recommendations has been associated with increased risk of bacteriuria, whereas systemic antimicrobial agents have a protective effect on bacteriuria (relative risk = 2.0–3.9).[22] Additional risk factors for hospitalized children include prematurity, underlying urogenital abnormalities, neurologic disorders, and immune compromised state.[23,24]

Catheter-associated bacteremia occurs in fewer than 4% of CAUTIs[25,26]; therefore, risk factors for UTI-associated bacteremia are incompletely understood. Risk factors for bloodstream infections from a urinary source from early studies included infections caused by *Serratia marcescens*, male sex, immunosuppressant therapy, history of malignancy, cigarette use in the past 5 years, and number of hospital days before bacteriuria.[26,27] In more recent studies, independent predictors of bloodstream infection included neutropenia, diabetes mellitus, malignancy, renal disease, and male sex[26,28]; prevention strategies for those patients at highest risk of bacteremia should be considered in an overall CAUTI prevention program.

Table 1	
Risk factors for catheter-associated urinary tract infection	
Modifiable Risk Factors	**Nonmodifiable Risk Factors**
Duration of catheterization	Female sex
Nonadherence to aseptic catheter care (ie, opening closed system)	Severe underlying illness
Lower professional training of inserter	Nonsurgical disease
Catheter insertion outside operating room	Age>50 y
Catheter insertion after sixth day of hospitalization	Diabetes mellitus
—	Serum creatinine >2 mg/dL

SURVEILLANCE FOR CATHETER-ASSOCIATED URINARY TRACT INFECTIONS

An essential element of any improvement initiative is to measure the prevalence of the condition or surrogate marker, with feedback of the results of interventions to clinical care providers. The NHSN surveillance definition for health care–associated UTI has been the standard for interhospital comparison of CAUTI rates.[29]

Clinical diagnosis of CAUTI remains challenging, because bacteriuria is not a reliable indicator of symptomatic UTI in the setting of catheterization.[30,31] However, results of cultures may be affected by collection technique; improperly handled cultures may grow significant numbers of bacteria.[32,33]

Urine cultures are often collected for inappropriate reasons or as part of a generic fever evaluation, without symptoms referable to the urinary tract.[34,35] In such cases, asymptomatic bacteriuria may result in designation of CAUTI in surveillance data, even when another source of fever has been identified.[2] Interventions promoting the stewardship of cultures, as part of a multifaceted approach, have resulted in improvement in CAUTI rates in ICUs.[36] In addition to lack of specificity, the culture-based definitions of CAUTI may lack sensitivity.[37]

Positive urine cultures often lead to inappropriate treatment of asymptomatic UTI.[38–40] However, the distinction of asymptomatic versus symptomatic UTI is clinically important, because asymptomatic catheter-associated bacteriuria rarely results in adverse outcomes[30,41] and treatment is not recommended.[41]

The NHSN symptomatic CAUTI rate (UTIs per 1000 urinary catheter-days) is the most widely accepted measure for infection surveillance, and is endorsed by the CDC and Society for Healthcare Epidemiology of America/Infectious Diseases Society of America practice recommendation. However, as hospitals decrease their catheterization use, a paradoxic increase in rate of UTI per 1000 catheter-days may be observed.[42] This increase has led some experts to recommend the rate of UTIs per patient-days or device use as a more appropriate outcome measure for CAUTI prevention initiatives.[43–45] A recent study suggests that health care–associated CAUTI may be common within 30 days after hospital discharge, suggesting that surveillance efforts may need to be expanded[46]; more studies will be necessary to confirm the significance of this finding.

Because CMS has included CAUTI as one of the hospital-acquired complications that will not be reimbursed, hospitals have had increased attention on CAUTI rates.[9,47,48] In addition, beginning in 2012, CMS has required, as a condition of participation, that hospitals submit ICU-level CAUTI rates to NHSN. To date, the CMS hospital-acquired conditions policy does seem to have resulted in immediate reductions, followed by possible leveling off, in billing rates for CAUTI from US hospitals.[47,48]

PREVENTING CATHETER-ASSOCIATED URINARY TRACT INFECTION

Several guidelines have been developed for prevention of CAUTI.[49–51] It has been estimated that an intervention resulting in a feasible reduction in urinary catheter use could lead to a ~50% reduction in CAUTI-related costs.[52] General strategies have been formulated for prevention of all HAIs, whereas specific strategies have been targeted at risk factors for CAUTI (**Box 1**).

General Strategies for Prevention

Most outbreaks of urinary pathogens have been linked to inadequate employee hand hygiene; strict adherence to hand hygiene is essential for prevention of all HAIs, including UTI.[53] The urinary tract of hospitalized patients, especially those in an ICU setting, represents a significant reservoir for multidrug-resistant organisms

Box 1
Key strategies for prevention of catheter-associated urinary tract infection

Avoid insertion of indwelling urinary catheters
- Placement only for appropriate indications (see **Box 2**)
- Institutional protocols for placement, including perioperative setting

Early removal of indwelling catheters
- Checklist or daily reminder
- Nurse-based or physician-based interventions
- Electronic reminders
- Automatic stop orders

Consider alternatives to indwelling catheterization
- Intermittent catheterization
- Condom catheter
- Portable bladder ultrasonography scanner

Proper techniques for insertion and maintenance of catheters
- Sterile insertion
- Secure catheter to prevent movement
- Maintain closed drainage system
- Maintain unobstructed urine flow
- Avoid routine bladder irrigation

Institutional support for CAUTI prevention program
- Policy development and implementation
- Education
- Surveillance for catheter use, CAUTI

Data from Refs.[49-51]

(MDROs).[20] Indwelling devices, including urinary catheters, increase the risk of colonization with MDROs, and therefore limiting their use is an important strategy for prevention of MDRO transmission in health care settings.[54]

Judicious use of antibiotics, as part of an overall antimicrobial stewardship program, is an important strategy to prevent development of antimicrobial resistance related to urinary catheters.[54,55] Inappropriate antimicrobial treatment of bacteriuria in hospitalized patients, especially those with indwelling catheterization, is a significant risk for colonization with MDROs.[35,39,40,55] Educational sessions and audit and feedback to care providers have been used successfully to decrease overdiagnosis of CAUTI and associated inappropriate antibiotic use.[56,57]

Systemic antimicrobial therapy reduces the risk of CAUTI.[22] However, because of issues of cost, potential adverse effects, and selection for multidrug-resistant organisms, systemic antimicrobial therapy for the purpose of preventing CAUTI is not currently recommended.[50] A recent meta-analysis suggests that antimicrobial treatment at the time of removal of a short-term (<14 days) urinary catheter, reduces the risk of UTI.[58] Studies are needed to further define those patients in whom the benefit of reducing UTI outweigh these risks of antimicrobial therapy at the time of urinary catheter removal.[58]

Specific Strategies for Prevention

Limitation of use of urinary catheters
The dominant risk factor for health care–associated UTI is the presence of an indwelling urinary catheter; therefore, the most important strategy for CAUTI prevention is avoiding or limiting urinary catheterization.[49,50] Regional geographic variations

in urinary catheter use have been identified, suggesting there is room for improvement of catheter usage.[59]

Decreasing catheter usage requires interventions at several stages of the life cycle of a urinary catheter.[60] A critical first step is avoiding placement of indwelling urinary catheters; catheters should be inserted only for appropriate indications (**Box 2**).[50] Despite these recommendations, urinary catheters are placed for inappropriate indications in 21% to 50% of catheterized patients.[59,62,63] Many institutions, believing they followed national guidelines, allowed indications for urinary catheter use that were not currently recommended in guidelines.[62] In addition, multiple perceptions of risk, some non–evidence based, were used by health care providers to determine whether urinary catheter use was necessary; CAUTI prevention initiatives should be formulated with the awareness of these other perceived risks with strategies to address those that are not evidence based.[64]

In a statewide CAUTI prevention initiative, barriers to reducing catheterization included catheter insertion practices in the emergency department.[65] Therefore, successful interventions may be targeted at hospital locations where initial urinary catheter placement usually occurs, such as emergency departments and operating rooms.[45]

Once placed, strategies for early removal of urinary catheters become essential. Urinary catheter management based on physicians' orders alone may be inadequate because physicians are frequently unaware that a patient has a urinary catheter. In 1 study, 28% of physicians were unaware that their patients had catheters, with lack of awareness increasing with level of training.[63] In addition, surveys of house staff reported that although house staff were aware of CAUTI prevention guidelines,

---

Box 2
Indications for indwelling urinary catheters

Urinary retention
- Acute urinary retention without bladder outlet obstruction
- Acute urinary obstruction with bladder outlet obstruction caused by noninfectious, nontraumatic diagnosis
- Chronic urinary retention with bladder outlet obstruction

Stage III, IV, or unstageable pressure ulcer or other severe wounds that cannot be kept clean despite other strategies

Urinary incontinence that cannot be addressed by noncatheter methods

Accurate monitoring of urine output or urine collection
- Hourly measurement of urine volume required for treatment
- Daily measurement of urine volume that is required and cannot be assessed by other urine collection strategies
- Single 24-hour urine sample collection for a diagnostic test that cannot be collected through other means

Management of gross hematuria with blood clots in urine

Improvement of patient comfort
- Address patient and family goals for dying patients
- Reduce acute, severe pain with movement when other urine management strategies are difficult
- Clinical condition for which intermittent catheterization or external catheter placement was difficult or bladder emptying was inadequate

Data from Refs.[49,50,61]

application of catheter prevention practices generally fell short of national goals.[66,67] Nurse- or computer-generated reminders or automatic stop orders are important tools for early removal of urinary catheters; a systematic review and meta-analysis reported that urinary catheter reminder systems and stop orders seemed to reduce mean duration of catheterization by 37% and CAUTI by 52%.[68]

Nurse-driven interventions have shown effectiveness in reducing duration of catheterization.[69,70] Such interventions are easy to implement and may consist of either a written notice or a verbal contact with the physician regarding the presence of a urinary catheter and alternative options. A statewide CAUTI initiative, using this strategy, resulted in a significant decrease in catheter use and increase in appropriate indications of catheters.[69] Physician-initiated reminders may be more effective than nurse-initiated reminders for decreasing duration of urinary catheterization.[71] Barriers to implementation of nurse-driven intervention included difficulty with physician and nurse engagement[45]; strategies for health care worker engagement are discussed later.

Computerized physician order entry systems may offer a more cost-effective and efficient system to reduce both placement of catheters and duration of catheterization.[68,72,73] Cornia and colleagues[73] found that a computerized reminder reduced the duration of catheterization by 3 days. A more recent study of a computerized clinical decision support system decreased urinary catheter use from 0.22 to 0.19 (P<.001) and CAUTI from 0.84 CAUTI/1000 patient-days to 0.51 CAUTI/1000 patient-days (P<.001).[72]

Perioperative management of urinary catheters

Most patients undergoing major surgical procedures have a perioperative indwelling urinary catheter.[74,75] Those catheterized longer than 2 days are much more likely to develop UTIs and are less likely to be discharged to home. Older surgical patients are at highest risk for prolonged catheterization; 23% of surgical patients older than 65 years of age were discharged to skilled nursing facilities with an indwelling catheter in place and had more rehospitalization or death within 30 days.[2]

Postoperative urinary retention developed in 2.1% of patients undergoing one of the Surgical Care Improvement Project (SCIP) surgeries.[75] Patients who developed postoperative retention were more likely to be older men undergoing knee, hip, or colon surgery. This group has significance because they are at risk of requiring recatheterization. Combining the use of a portable bladder ultrasonography scanner with intermittent catheterization may reduce the need for indwelling catheterization in postsurgical patients with urinary retention.[50]

Alternatives to indwelling urinary catheters

Avoiding urinary catheter placement with use of alternative urinary drainage systems has been used successfully in some situations. Patients with neurogenic bladder and long-term urinary catheters, in particular, may benefit from intermittent catheterization instead of indwelling urinary catheterization.[49,50] Combining the use of a portable bladder ultrasonography scanner with intermittent catheterization has been recommended to reduce the need for indwelling urinary catheterization.[50]

Condom catheters may also be considered in place of indwelling catheters in male patients without urinary retention or bladder outlet obstruction. A randomized trial showed a decrease in bacteriuria, symptomatic UTI, or death in patients with condom catheters, compared with those with indwelling catheters; the benefit was primarily seen in men without dementia.[76] In addition, condom catheters may cause less discomfort than indwelling catheters in some men.[76]

Aseptic techniques for insertion and maintenance of urinary catheters

If indwelling urinary catheterization is deemed necessary, proper aseptic technique during catheter insertion and catheter care is essential for prevention of CAUTI. During 81 catheter insertions observed in a busy emergency department, 59% of the insertions were associated with major breeches of aseptic technique.[77] It is also important that urinary catheters be inserted by a trained health care professional using aseptic technique.[49,50] Cleaning the urethral meatus at the time of catheter insertion is recommended, but daily meatal cleaning thereafter with an antiseptic may increase rates of bacteriuria compared with routine care with soap and water.[49,50]

Closed urinary catheter collection systems reduce the risk of CAUTI; sampling urine may be performed aseptically from a port or from the drainage bag when large, non-sterile samples are required.[49,50] Prophylactic instillation of antiseptic agents or irrigation of the bladder with antimicrobial or antiseptic agents leads to increased infections and is not recommended.[49,50]

Bacteriuria may be reduced with exchange of catheters, but this reduction is transient. Therefore, routine exchange of urinary catheters is not recommended, except for mechanical reasons.[49,50] However, exchange of long-term catheters with treatment of symptomatic UTI is likely beneficial.[78]

Use of anti-infective catheters

Antimicrobial-impregnated catheters, typically coated with nitrofurazone, minocycline, or rifampin, and antiseptic catheters have been studied extensively as an adjunctive measure for CAUTI prevention, with variable results.[79,80] A multicenter, randomized controlled trial that used symptomatic CAUTI as the end point reported no significant clinical benefit with use of silver alloy–coated or nitrofural-impregnated catheters during short-term (<14 days) catheterization.[80] A Cochrane Review similarly found that silver alloy catheters did not significantly reduce the incidence of symptomatic UTI in adult patients.[79] Therefore, current guidelines do not recommend routine use of anti-infective urinary catheters to prevent CAUTI.[50]

Other preventive measures

Body surface decolonization with a short course of intranasal mupirocin and chlorhexidine bathing was found to decrease candiduria and bacteriuria in men, but not in women.[81] Another study of chlorhexidine bathing in ICUs found no benefit in the prevention of CAUTI. More studies are needed to describe whether targeted chlorhexidine bathing could benefit high-risk patients.[82]

Implementation: the role of bundles and collaboratives

Despite CAUTI prevention guidelines having been published for several decades, prevention measures have been inconsistently applied in US hospitals. A national survey of US hospitals from 2005 to 2013 showed that use of catheter reminder systems increased from 9% in 2005 to 53.3% in 2013. Surveillance for CAUTI increased from 46.9% of hospitals to 85.1% during the same time period.[83] There still remains much room for improvement in implementation of CAUTI prevention measures.

Recently, bundles of interventions, often in association with hospital collaborations, have been used with success for prevention of HAIs, including CAUTI.[84,85] A multifaceted approach was used successfully in 2 Veterans' Affairs hospitals with good success.[86,87] Similar improvement projects have been implemented effectively in pediatric hospitals[23,88] and community long-term care facilities.[89] A national collaborative program to prevent CAUTI in Veterans Health Administration nursing homes was less effective, presumably because of a low baseline rate of infection.[90]

Box 3
The bladder bundle for preventing catheter-associated urinary tract infection

- Adherence to general infection control principles (eg, hand hygiene, surveillance and feedback, aseptic insertion, proper maintenance, education) is important

- Bladder ultrasonography may avoid indwelling catheterization

- Condom catheters or other alternatives to an indwelling catheter, such as intermittent catheterization, should be considered in appropriate patients

- Do not use the indwelling catheter unless you must!

- Early removal of the catheter using a reminder or nurse-initiated removal protocol seems warranted

From Saint S, Olmsted RN, Fakih MG, et al. Translating health care-associated urinary tract infection prevention research into practice via the bladder bundle. Jt Comm J Qual Patient Saf. 2009;35:449-455; with permission

---

A bladder bundle, outlined in **Box 3**, was successfully adopted by the Michigan Hospital Association Keystone initiative[61,69] and resulted in more Michigan hospitals using key prevention practices and a lower rate of CAUTI compared with hospitals in the rest of the country. This type of collaborative program has been expanded to national initiatives for hospitals[84,85] and nursing homes.[89]

SUMMARY

CAUTIs are common, costly, and cause significant patient morbidity. Despite studies showing benefit of interventions for prevention of CAUTI, adoption of these practices has not occurred consistently in many health care facilities in the United States. Duration of urinary catheterization is the predominant risk for CAUTI; preventive measures directed at limiting placement and early removal of urinary catheters have a significant impact on decreasing CAUTIs. Intervention bundles, collaboratives, and hospital leadership are powerful tools for implementing preventive measures for HAIs, including CAUTIs.

CLINICS CARE POINTS

- The need for indwelling urinary catheters should be assessed daily, with removal of catheters as soon as possible.

- Alternatives to indwelling urinary catheters, such as external catheters and intermittent straight catheterization can decrease risk of CAUTI.

- Institutional initiatives focused on limiting use of indwelling urinary catheters have been successful in decreasing CAUTI in multiple settings.

DISCLOSURE

None.

REFERENCES

1. Magill S, Edward J, Bamberg W, et al. Multistate point-prevalence survey of health care-associated infections. N Engl J Med 2014;370(13):1198–208.

2. Chenoweth CE, Saint SS. Urinary tract infections. Infec Dis Clinic N Amer 2016; 30:869–85.

3. Zingg W, Metsini A, Balmelli C, et al. National point prevalence survey on healthcare-associated infections in acute care hospitals, Switzerland, 2017. Euro Surveill 2019;24(32):1–11.

4. Burton D, Edwards J, Srinivasan A, et al. Trends in catheter-associated urinary tract infection in adult intensive care units-United States, 1990–2007. Infect Control Hosp Epidemiol 2011;32:748–56.

5. Mitchell B, Ferguson J, Anderson M, et al. Length of stay and mortality associated with healthcare-associated urinary tract infections: a multistate model. J Hosp Infect 2016;93(1):92–9.

6. Zimlichman E, Henderson D, Tamir O, et al. Health care-associated infections: a meta-analysis of costs and financial impact on the US care system. JAMA Intern Med 2013;173(22):2039–46.

7. Schreiber PW, Sax H, Wolfensberger A, et al. The preventable proportion of healthcare-associated infections 2005-2016: systematic review and meta-analysis. Infect Control Hosp Epidemiol 2018;39:1277–95.

8. Umsheid C, Mitchell M, Doshi J, et al. Estimating the proportion of healthcare-associated infections that are reasonably preventable and the related mortality and costs. Infect Control Hosp Epidemiol 2011;32:101–14.

9. Saint S, Meddings J, Calfee D, et al. Catheter-associated urinary tract infection and the Medicare rule changes. Ann Intern Med 2009;150:877–84.

10. Nicolle LE. Catheter-related urinary tract infection. Drugs Aging 2005;22:627–39.

11. Donlan RM, Costertan JW. Biofilms: survival mechanisms of clinically relevant microorganisms. Clin Microbiol Rev 2002;15:167–93.

12. Saint SS, Chenoweth C. Biofilms and catheter-associated urinary tract infections. Infect Dis Clin N Am 2003;17:411–32.

13. Tambyah PA, Halvorson KT, Maki DG. A prospective study of pathogenesis of catheter-associated urinary tract infections. Mayo Clin Proc 1999;74:131–6.

14. Magill SS, O'Leary E, Janelle SJ, et al. Changes in prevalence of health care-associated infections in U.S. hospitals. N Engl J Med 2018;379(18):1732–44.

15. Dudeck M, Edwards J, Allen-Bridson K, et al. National Healthcare Safety Network report, data summary for 2013, device associated module. Am J Infect Control 2015;43(3):206–21.

16. Patrick S, Kawai A, Kleinman K, et al. Health care-associated infection among critically ill children in the US, 2007-2012. Pediatrics 2014;134(4):705–7012.

17. Weber D, Sickbert-Bennett E, Gould C, et al. Incidence of catheter-associated and non-catheter-associated urinary tract infections in a healthcare system. Infect Control Hosp Epidemiol 2011;32:822–3.

18. Rosenthal V, Al-Aabdeli H, El-Kholy A, et al. International nosocomial infection control consortium report, data summary of 50 countries for 2010-2015; device-associated module. Am J Infect Control 2016;44:1495–504.

19. Palms DL, Mungai E, Eure T, et al. The National Healthcare Safety Network long-term care facility component early reporting experience: Jan 2013-December 2015. Am J Infect Control 2018;46:637–42.

20. Weiner-Lastinger LM, Abner S, Edwards JR, et al. Antimicrobial-resistant pathogens associated with adult healthcare-associated infections: Summary of data reported to the National Healthcare Safety Network, 2015-2017. Infect Control Hosp Epidemiol 2020;41(1):1–18.

21. Chitnis A, Edwards J, Ricks P, et al. Device-associated infection rates, device utilization, and antimicrobial resistance in long-term acute care hospitals reporting

to the National Healthcare Safety Network, 2010. Infect Control Hosp Epidemiol 2012;33:933–1000.

22. Shuman EK, Chenoweth C. Urinary catheter-associated infections. Infec Dis Clinic N Amer 2018;32:886–97.

23. Davis KF, Colebaugh AM, Eithun BL, et al. Reducing catheter-associated urinary tract infections: a quality-improvement initiative. Pediatrics 2014;134:e8557–864.

24. Langley JM, Hanakowski M, LeBlanc JC. Unique epidemiology of nosocomial urinary tract infection in children. Am J Infect Control 2001;29:94–8.

25. Chang R, Greene MT, Chenoweth CE, et al. Epidemiology of hospital-acquired urinary tract-related bloodstream infection at a university hospital. Infect Control Hosp Epidemiol 2011;32:1127–9.

26. Greene MT, Chang R, Kuhn L, et al. Predictors of hospital-acquired urinary tract-related bloodstream infection. Infect Control Hosp Epidemiol 2012;33:1001–7.

27. Krieger JN, Kaiser DL, Wenzel RP. Urinary tract etiology of bloodstream infections in hospitalized patients. J Infect Dis 1983;148:57–62.

28. Patel P, Greene MT, Rogers MAM, et al. The epidemiology of hospital-acquired urinary tract-related bloodstream infection in veterans. Am J Infect Control 2018;46(7):747–50.

29. CDC. Urinary tract infection (Catheter-associated urinary tract infection {CAUTI} and non-catheter-associated urinary tract infection [UTI] Events. 2021. Available at: https://wwwcdcgov/nhsn/pdfs/validation/2020/pcsmanual_2020-508pdf. Accessed June 11, 2021.

30. Tambyah PA, Maki D. Catheter-associated urinary tract infection is rarely symptomatic: a prospective study of 1,497 catheterized patients. Arch Intern Med 2000;160:678–82.

31. Tambyah PA, Maki D. The relationship between pyuria and infection in patients with indwelling urinary catheters: a prospective study of 761 patients. Arch Intern Med 2000;160:673–7.

32. Jones K, Sibaie J, Battjes R, et al. How and why nurses collect urine cultures on catheterized patients: a survey of 5 hospitals. Am J Infect Control 2016;44:173–6.

33. LaRocco M, Franek J, Leibach E, et al. Effectiveness of preanalytic practices on contamination and diagnostic accuracy of urine cultures: a laboratory medicine best practices systematic review and meta-analysis. Clin Micro Rev 2016;29(1):105–46.

34. Advani SD, Gao CA, Sann L, et al. Knowledge and practices of physicians and nurses related to urine cultures in catheterized patients: an assessment of adherence to IDSA guidelines. Open Forum Infect Dis 2019;6(8):ofz305.

35. Hartley S, Valley S, Kuhn L, et al. Inappropriate testing for urinary tract infection in hospitalized patients: an opportunity for improvement. Infect Control Hosp Epidemiol 2013;34(11):1204–7.

36. Mullin KM, Kovacs CS, Fatica C, et al. A multifaceted approach to reduction of catheter-associated urinary tract infections in the intensive care unit with an emphasis on "stewardship of culturing. Infect Control Hosp Epidemiol 2017;38(2):186–8.

37. Greene MT, Ratz D, Meddings J, et al. Potential misclassification of urinary tract-related bacteremia upon applying the 2015 NHSN catheter-associated urinary tract infection surveillance definition. Infect Control Hosp Epidemiol 2016;37(4):469–71.

38. Grein J, Kahn K, Eells S, et al. Treatment of positive urine cultures in hospitalized adults: a survey of prevalence and risk factors. Infect Control Hosp Epidemiol 2016;37(3):319–26.

39. Hartley S, Valley S, Kuhn L, et al. Overtreatment of asymptomatic bacteriuria: Identifying targets for intervention. Infect Control Hosp Epidemiol 2015;36(4): 470–3.

40. Trautner B, Petersen N, Hysong S, et al. Overtreatment of asymptomatic bacteriuria: identifying barriers to evidence-based care. Am J Infect Control 2014;42: 653–8.

41. Nicolle LE, Gupta K, Bradley SF, et al. Clinical practice guideline for the management of asymptomatic bacteriuria: 2019 update by the Infectious Disease Society of America. Clin Infect Dis 2019;68(10):e83–110.

42. Wright M-O, Kharasch M, Beaumont J, et al. Reporting catheter-associated urinary tract infections: denominator matters. Infect Control Hosp Epidemiol 2011; 32:635–40.

43. Advani SD, Fakih M. The evolution of catheter-associated urinary tract infection (CAUTI): is it time for more inclusive metrics? Infect Control Hosp Epidemiol 2019;40:681–5.

44. Fakih M, Gould C, Trautner B, et al. Beyond infection: device utilization ratio as a performance measure for urinary catheter harm. Infect Control Hosp Epidemiol 2016;37(3):327–33.

45. Fakih M, Pena M, Shemes S, et al. Effect of establishing guidelines on appropriate urinary catheter placement. Acad Emerg Med 2010;17:337–40.

46. Elman MR, Williams CD, Bearden DT, et al. Health-care associated urinary tract infections with onset post hospital discharge. Infect Control Hosp Epidemiol 2019;40:863–71.

47. Kawai A, Calderwood M, Jin R, et al. Impact of the Centers for Medicare and Medicaid Services hospital acquired conditions policy on billing rates of 2 targeted healthcare-associated infections. Infect Control Hosp Epidemiol 2015; 36(2):871–7.

48. Waters T, Daniels M, Bazzoli G, et al. Effect of Medicare's nonpayment for hospital-acquired conditions: lessons for future policy. JAMA Intern Med 2015; 175(3):347–54.

49. Gould C, Umscheid C, Agarwal R, et al. CDC Guideline for prevention of catheter-associated infections 2009. Infect Control Hosp Epidemiol 2010;31:319–26.

50. Lo E, Nicolle L, Coffin S, et al. Strategies to prevent catheter-associated urinary tract infections in acute care hospitals: 2014 update. Infect Control Hosp Epidemiol 2014;35(S2):S32–47.

51. Rebmann T, Greene L. Preventing catheter-associated urinary tract infections: an executive summary of the Association for Professionals in Infection Control and Epidemiology. Am J Infect Control 2010;38:644–6.

52. Kennedy E, Greene M, Saint S. Estimating hospital costs of catheter-associated urinary tract infection. J Hosp Med 2013;2013(8):644–6.

53. Boyce J, Pittet D. Guideline for hand hygiene in health-care settings. Recommendations of the Healthcare Infection Control Practices Advisory Committee and the HICPAC/SHEA/APIC/IDSA Hand Hygiene Task Force. MMWR Recomm Rep 2002;51:1–45.

54. Dellit T, Owens R, McGowan J Jr, et al. Infectious Diseases Society of America and the Society for Healthcare Epidemiology of America guidelines for developing an institutional program to enhance antimicrobial stewardship. Clin Infect Dis 2007;44:159–77.

55. Gandhi T, Flanders S, Markovitz E, et al. Importance of urinary tract infection to antibiotic use among hospitalized patients. Infect Control Hosp Epidemiol 2009;30:193–5.

56. Trautner B, Grigoryan L, Petersen N, et al. Effectiveness of an antimicrobial stewardship approach for urinary catheter-associated asymptomatic bacteriuria. JAMA Intern Med 2015;175(7):1120–7.

57. Trautner B, Kelly P, Petersen N, et al. A hospital-site controlled intervention using audit and feedback to implement guidelines concerning inappropriate treatment of catheter-associated asymptomatic bacteriuria. Implement Sci 2011;6:41.

58. Marshall J, Carpenter C, Fowler S, et al. Antibiotic prophylaxis for urinary tract infections after removal of urinary catheter: metanalysis. BMJ 2013;2013(356): f3147.

59. Greene M, Fakih M, Fowler K, et al. Regional variation in urinary catheter-associated urinary tract infections in acute care hospitals. Infect Control Hosp Epidemiol 2014;35(S3):S99–106.

60. Meddings J, Saint S. Disrupting the life cycle of the urinary catheter. Clin Infect Dis 2011;52:1291–3.

61. Saint S, Olmsted RN, Fakih MG, et al. Translating health care-associated urinary tract infection prevention research into practice via the bladder bundle. Jt Comm J Qual Patient Saf 2009;35:449–55.

62. Greene MT, Kiyoshi-Teo H, Reichert H, et al. Urinary catheter indications in the United States: results from a national survey of acute care hospitals. Infect Control Hosp Epidemiol 2014;35(S3):S96–8.

63. Saint S, Weise J, Amory JK, et al. Are physicians aware of which of their patients have indwelling catheters? Am J Med 2000;109:476–80.

64. Harrod M, Kowalski C, Saint S, et al. Variation in risk perceptions: a qualitative study of why unnecessary urinary catheter use continues to be problematic. BMC Health Serv Res 2013;13:151.

65. Krein S, Kowalski C, Harrod M, et al. Barriers to reducing urinary catheter use: a qualitative assessment of a statewide initiative. JAMA Intern Med 2013;173(10): 881–6.

66. Apisarnthanarak A, Damronglerd P, Meesing A, et al. Impact on physicians' mindfulness attitudes toward prevention of catheter-associated urinary tract infections. Infect Control Hosp Epidemiol 2014;35(9):1198–9.

67. Paras M, Shenoy E, Hsu H, et al. Housestaff knowledge related to urinary catheter use and catheter-associated urinary tract infections. Infect Control Hosp Epidemiol 2015;36(11):1355–7.

68. Meddings J, Rogers MA, Macy M, et al. Systematic review and meta-analysis: reminder systems to reduce catheter-associated urinary tract infections and urinary catheter use in hospitalized patients. Clin Infect Dis 2010;51:550–60.

69. Fakih M, Watson S, Greene MT, et al. Reducing inappropriate urinary catheter use: a statewide effort. Arch Intern Med 2012;172:255–60.

70. Huang WC, Wann S, Lin SL, et al. Catheter-associated urinary tract infections in intensive care units can be reduced by prompting physicians to remove unnecessary catheters. Infect Control Hosp Epidemiol 2004;25:974–8.

71. Felix L, Smith B, Santos E, et al. Physician-initiated daily verbal reminders decrease the duration of indwelling urinary catheter use compared to nurse-initiated reminders. Am J Infect Control 2016;44:346–8.

72. Baillie C, Epps M, Hanish A, et al. Usability and impact of a computerized clinical decision support intervention designed to reduce urinary catheter utilization and catheter-associated urinary tract infections. Infect Control Hosp Epidemiol 2014; 35(1):1147–55.

73. Cornia PB, Amory JK, Fraser S, et al. Computer-based order entry decreases duration of indwelling urinary catheterization in hospitalized patients. Am J Med 2003;114:404–7.

74. Stephan F, Sax H, Wachsmuth M, et al. Reduction of urinary tract infection and antibiotic use after surgery: a controlled, prospective, before-after intervention study. Clin Infect Dis 2006;42:1544–51.

75. Wu A, Aurback A, Aaronson D. National incidence and outcomes of postoperative urinary retention in the Surgical Care Improvement Project. Am J Surg 2012;204:167–71.

76. Saint S, Kaufman SR, Rogers MA, et al. Condom versus indwelling urinary catheters: a randomized trial. J Am Geriatr Soc 2006;54:1055–61.

77. Manojlovich M, Saint S, Meddings J, et al. Indwelling urinary catheterization insertion practices in the emergency department: an observational study. Infect Control Hosp Epidemiol 2016;37(1):117–9.

78. Raz R, Schiller D, Nicolle LE. Chronic indwelling catheter replacement before antimicrobial therapy for symptomatic urinary tract infection. J Urol 2000;164:1254–8.

79. Lam T, Omar M, Fisher E, et al. Types of indwelling urethral catheters for short-term catheterisation in hospitalized patients. Cochrane Database Syst Rev 2014;9:CD004013.

80. Pickard R, Lam T, MacLennon G, et al. Antimicrobial catheters for reduction of symptomatic urinary tract infection in adults requiring short-term catheterisation in hospital: a multicentre randomised controlled trial. Lancet 2012;380:1927–35.

81. Noto M, Domenico H, Byrne D, et al. Chlorhexidine bathing and healthcare-associated infections: a randomized clinical trial. JAMA 2015;313(4):369–78.

82. Huang S, Hayden M, Kleinman K, et al. Effect of body surface decolonisation on bacteriuria and candiduria in intensive care units: an analysis of a cluster-controlled trial. Lancet Infect Dis 2016;15:70–9.

83. Krein S, Fowler K, Ratz D, et al. Preventing device-associated infection in US hospitals from 2005-2013. BMJ Qual Saf 2015;24:385–92.

84. Fakih M, George C, Edson B, et al. Implementing a national program to reduce catheter-associated urinary tract infection: a quality improvement collaboration of state hospital associations, academic medical centers, professional societies, and government agencies. Infect Control Hosp Epidemiol 2013;34(10):1048–54.

85. Saint S, Greene MT, Krein S, et al. A program to prevent catheter-associated urinary tract infection in acute care. N Engl J Med 2016;374(22):2111–9.

86. Knoll B, Wright D, Ellingson L, et al. Reduction of inappropriate urinary catheter use at a Veterans Affairs hospital through a multifaceted quality improvement project. Clin Infect Dis 2011;52:1283–90.

87. Miller B, Krein S, Fowler K, et al. A multimodal intervention to reduce urinary catheter use and associated infection at a Veterans Affairs Medical Center. Infect Control Hosp Epidemiol 2013;34(6):631–3.

88. Foster CB, Ackerman K, Hupertz V, et al. Catheter-associated urinary tract infection reduction in pediatric safety engagement network. Pediatrics 2020;146(4):e20192057.

89. Mody L, Greene M, Meddings J. A national implementation project to prevent catheter-associated urinary tract infection in nursing home residents. JAMA Intern Med 2017;177(8):1154–62.

90. Krein S, Greene MT, King B, et al. Assessing a national collaborative program to prevent catheter-associated urinary tract infection in Veterans Health Administration nursing home cohort. Infect Control Hosp Epidemiol 2018;39:820–5.

Ventilator-Associated Events

Epidemiology, Risk Factors, and Prevention

Jeremy Weinberger, MD[a,b,c], Noelle Cocoros, DSc, MPH[a],
Michael Klompas, MD, MPH[a,b,]*

KEYWORDS

- Ventilator-associated events • Ventilator-associated pneumonia
- Mechanical ventilation • Quality improvement • Infection control and prevention

KEY POINTS

- Ventilator-associated events definitions were designed to improve the objectivity, breadth, and seriousness of adverse event surveillance in mechanically ventilated populations
- The most common conditions that trigger ventilator-associated events are pneumonia, fluid overload, acute respiratory distress syndrome, and atelectasis
- Promising strategies to prevent ventilator-associated events include minimizing sedation, enhancing paired daily spontaneous awakening and breathing trials, promoting early mobility, setting low tidal volume ventilation, using intravenous fluids conservatively after resuscitation, and implementing restrictive transfusion thresholds.
- An increasing number of reports document that multifaceted quality improvement initiatives are associated with lower ventilator-associated event rates

INTRODUCTION

Up to 800,000 patients per year receive mechanical ventilation in the United States and the incidence is increasing over time.[1–3] This procedure can be lifesaving for patients with acute respiratory failure, but being on a ventilator also increases the risk of an array of complications that can prolong ventilator dependence and sometimes hasten death. Some of these complications are caused directly by mechanical ventilation, others only indirectly. The objective of this article is to provide an up-to-date review on the epidemiology, outcomes, risk factors, and prevention strategies for ventilator-associated

Conflicts of Interest: None.
[a] Department of Population Medicine, Harvard Medical School, Harvard Pilgrim Health Care Institute, 401 Park Street, Suite 401, Boston, MA 02215, USA; [b] Department of Medicine, Brigham and Women's Hospital, Boston, MA, USA; [c] Division of Pulmonary, Critical Care, and Sleep Medicine, Tufts Medical Center, 200 Washington Street, Boston, MA 02111, USA
* Corresponding author. Department of Population Medicine, 401 Park Street, Suite 401, Boston, MA 02215.
E-mail address: mklompas@partners.org

Infect Dis Clin N Am 35 (2021) 871–899
https://doi.org/10.1016/j.idc.2021.07.005
0891-5520/21/© 2021 Elsevier Inc. All rights reserved.

id.theclinics.com

events (VAEs), including pneumonia. We focus on the adult patient population, but also briefly describe relevant work in pediatric and neonatal populations.

VENTILATOR-ASSOCIATED EVENTS VERSUS VENTILATOR-ASSOCIATED PNEUMONIA

Before January 2013, the Centers for Disease Controls and Prevention's (CDC) National Healthcare Safety Network (NHSN) only provided surveillance definitions for ventilator-associated pneumonia (VAP). The NHSN switched the focus of surveillance from VAP to VAE in early 2013, however, in response to increasing concerns about the suitability of traditional VAP definitions to support quality improvement and benchmarking initiatives.[4]

The VAE framework includes a nested set of definitions designed to detect both infectious and noninfectious complications in mechanically ventilated patients.[5] Some of these complications may be direct adverse consequences of mechanical ventilation (such as pneumonia), whereas others are indirect events that can complicate the course of mechanical ventilation (such as pulmonary edema). **Fig. 1** provides a summary of adult VAE surveillance definitions. The core definition in the VAE set is called a ventilator-associated condition (VAC). A VAC is designed to detect respiratory deterioration after a period of stability or improvement. To be eligible for a VAC, a patient must first demonstrate at least 2 days of stable or improving ventilator settings, namely, the daily minimum fraction of inspired oxygen (Fio_2) or positive end-expiratory pressure (PEEP). If a patient subsequently requires an increase in the daily minimum Fio_2 by 0.20 or more or an increase in the daily minimum PEEP by 3 or more cm H_2O, and the increase is sustained for at least 2 calendar days relative to both baseline days, then the patient meets VAC criteria and has a VAE. The increase in ventilator settings is presumed to indicate that the patient may have suffered a complication or deleterious change in their clinical status, but does not in and of itself indicate what might have gone wrong. There are consequently additional VAE criteria to identify the subset of VACs that may be attributable to infection and the subset of those that might be due to pneumonia. An infection-related ventilator-associated complication (IVAC) occurs in a patient with VAC who has concurrent inflammatory changes (abnormal white blood cell count or temperature) and in whom clinicians begin and continue a new course of antibiotics ($\geq$4 days of new antimicrobials starting within 2 days of the VAC). Both VAC and IVAC intentionally capture both pulmonary and nonpulmonary complications.[6] The last surveillance tier of the VAE definition set identifies the subset of IVACs that are possible VAPs (PVAP). This final tier is flagged by a case of IVAC with concurrent inflammatory pulmonary secretions and/or positive respiratory cultures. IVAC-plus refers to IVACs that include PVAPs (whereas IVAC-alone is IVAC excluding PVAPs).

Why the Shift to Ventilator-associated Events?

Numerous concerns catalyzed the shift from VAP to VAE. From a technical and practical perspective, the old NHSN VAP criteria were challenging.[7] The definitions included multiple pathways for different patient populations and many of the surveillance criteria were subjective, insensitive, and nonspecific (eg, "new or progressive infiltrates," "change in the character of sputum," or "worsening cough").[8] The definition correlated poorly with histologic pneumonia and the clinical information needed to apply traditional VAP definitions was hard to collect, making surveillance difficult to implement.[9,10] The subjective components of the VAP definition led to high rates of interobserver variability.[11–14] Finally, VAP criteria did not consistently identify patients at increased risk for poor outcomes, and interventions that decreased VAP rates often had no effect on more patient-centered outcomes, such as the duration of mechanical

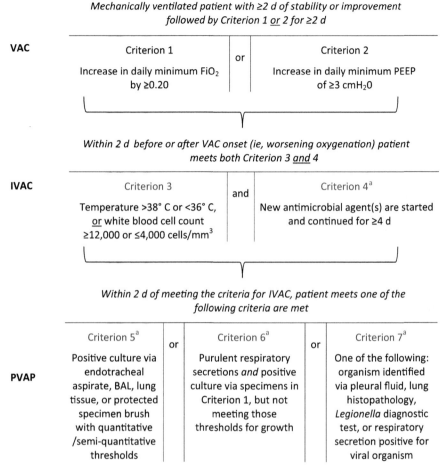

VAC

Mechanically ventilated patient with ≥2 d of stability or improvement followed by Criterion 1 or 2 for ≥2 d

Criterion 1	or	Criterion 2
Increase in daily minimum FiO₂ by ≥0.20		Increase in daily minimum PEEP of ≥3 cmH₂0

Within 2 d before or after VAC onset (ie, worsening oxygenation) patient meets both Criterion 3 and 4

IVAC

Criterion 3	and	Criterion 4[a]
Temperature >38° C or <36° C, or white blood cell count ≥12,000 or ≤4,000 cells/mm³		New antimicrobial agent(s) are started and continued for ≥4 d

Within 2 d of meeting the criteria for IVAC, patient meets one of the following criteria are met

PVAP

Criterion 5[a]	or	Criterion 6[a]	or	Criterion 7[a]
Positive culture via endotracheal aspirate, BAL, lung tissue, or protected specimen brush with quantitative /semi-quantitative thresholds		Purulent respiratory secretions *and* positive culture via specimens in Criterion 1, but not meeting those thresholds for growth		One of the following: organism identified via pleural fluid, lung histopathology, *Legionella* diagnostic test, or respiratory secretion positive for viral organism

Fig. 1. National surveillance definitions for VAEs in adults. [a]See the full CDC NHSN protocol for details related to each criterion (CDC 2020). BAL, bronchoalveolar lavage. Surveillance "day 1" is the day of intubation and initiation of mechanical ventilation; the earliest day VAE criteria can be fulfilled is day 4 and the earliest event date for VAE is day 3 of mechanical ventilation.

ventilation or hospital mortality.[15–19] Indeed, recent estimates suggest that the attributable mortality of VAP is only about 10%.[20,21]

The failure of most VAP prevention strategies to yield better outcomes for ventilated populations begs the question of whether VAP is the best target to drive surveillance and prevention programs. Quality improvement initiatives should ideally focus on identifying and preventing objective, morbid complications that are unambiguously associated with poor outcomes. By broadening the scope of surveillance from VAP to VAE, CDC acknowledged that both infectious and noninfectious complications can arise in ventilated patients and all should be considered when designing prevention programs.

VAE surveillance is based on quantitative clinical criteria that can be collected, detected, and reported electronically.[22–27] Although some of the VAE criteria reflect underlying clinical judgment—such as adjusting ventilator settings, starting and continuing antimicrobial treatment, and obtaining respiratory cultures—the definition components themselves are clear and reproducible, the key characteristics of good case definitions for public health surveillance.[28] The objective criteria associated with VAEs have comparable meanings and can be collected in comparable ways across institutions.

EPIDEMIOLOGY AND OUTCOMES
Descriptive Epidemiology of Ventilator-associated Events

The proportion of mechanically ventilated patients who develop a VAE has generally been reported as 5% to 10%, although studies that restricted eligibility to patients on mechanical ventilation for longer periods of time have reported rates of more than 20%.[15,19,25,27,29–36] Incidence rates reported to the CDC for the first full year of VAE surveillance (2014) varied from 2.59 to 11.79 per 1000 ventilator-days, with higher rates found in larger teaching hospitals.[37] VAE incidence varies by intensive care unit (ICU) type, a finding common to VAP as well. One large academic medical center, for example, observed VAE rates per 1000 ventilator days of 16.0, 15.7, 12.9, and 12.1 in the general surgery, medical, thoracic surgery, and cardiac medicine units, respectively, compared with rates of 9.8 and 5.8 in the neuroscience and cardiac surgery units, respectively.[30] The rates of probable or possible pneumonia, based on older versions of the PVAP surveillance definition, also varied by ICU type ranging from 1.7 to 4.5 events per 1000 ventilator days. Likewise, the fraction of VACs that qualify as IVACs vary by ICU type and ranges from about one-third to one-half, with higher fractions in trauma, burn, and surgical ICUs compared with medical ICUs.[29,30,37]

An increasing number of large case series are being published from around the world describing VAE epidemiology. VAE rates in recent series largely mirror earlier reports.[27,33,34,36] A study of more than 6000 ventilated patients in 5 ICUs across medical and surgical specialties at an academic medical center in China, for example, reported VAC, IVAC, and PVAP rates of 13.7, 6.3, and 2.2 per 1000 ventilator days, respectively.[36] However, lower rates were reported in a study of 7 urban hospitals in Japan (6.4 VAEs per 1000 ventilator days) and higher rates within a multinational cohort in Europe (40.8 VAEs per 1000 ventilator days).[38,39] Interestingly, the European cohort reported that 96% of VAEs qualified as IVACs or PVAPs (vs one-third to one-half in most US studies), a finding that may represent differences in patient populations and/or local practices in antimicrobial prescribing. **Table 1** summarizes these and other key findings related to the epidemiology of VAEs.

Stevens and colleagues[25] found that patients with a VAE were more likely to be male and younger (unadjusted analyses) compared with mechanically ventilated patients without a VAE. Some investigators have found that patients who develop VAEs have more severe illness at baseline compared with those who do not.[19,40] Most studies, however, have not found significant demographic differences between patients with and without VAEs.[15,24,27,31,32,34–36,38,39,41]

Like VAP, most VAEs occur early in the course of mechanical ventilation. One study found a mean daily rate of 2.9 per 100 patients on day 3 and 2.0 per 100 patients on day 7, with a steady decrease to between 1.0 and 1.5 per 100 patients from day 14 onwards.[30] Another found that 68% of VAEs occurred before day 7, 86% before day 14, and that the rate decreased to less than 1 VAE per 1000 ventilator days after day 21.[27] The median time to VAE onset is typically 5 to 6 days after the initiation of mechanical ventilation.[29,30,35,37,38,42]

Adverse Outcomes Among Patients with a Ventilator-associated Event

Most studies report that patients with VAEs are approximately 1.5 to 2.0 times more likely to die in the hospital compared with similar patients without

Table 1
The epidemiology of VAE in adults

	Incidence	Hospital Mortality	Ventilation Duration	ICU and Hospital Length of Stay
Klompas et al,[15] 2011 (VAC) N = 597 patients, half ventilated 2–7 d and half ventilated >7 d	21/1000 vent days	OR 2.0 (1.3–3.2)	14.2 (12.5–16.0) vs 9.1 (8.2–10.0) days of ventilation	25.4 (224–29.0) vs 23.7 (21.6–25.9) days, hospital LOS 17.4 (15.4–19.7) vs 13.1 (11.9–14.4) days, ICU LOS
Klompas et al,[10] 2012 (VAC) N = 8735 ventilation episodes (no restrictions)	12.0/1000 vent days	OR 2.4 (1.6–3.6)	1.9 (1.7–2.1), ratio of ventilator days from VAC to extubation in cases vs controls	1.4 (1.2–1.5), ratio of hospital days from VAC to hospital discharge in cases vs controls
Muscedere et al,[31] 2013 N = 1320 patients ventilated >48 h		VAC: 49.6% vs 31.7% IVAC: 44.6% vs 33.0%	VAC: Median 15.4 vs 6.2 d of ventilation IVAC: Median 16.9 vs 6.4 d of ventilation	VAC: Median 31.7 vs 21.8 d, hospital LOS VAC: Median 18.9 vs 9.0 d, ICU LOS IVAC: Median 34.6 vs 22.5 d, hospital LOS IVAC: Median 22.0 vs 9.3 d, ICU LOS
Hayashi et al,[32] 2013 (VAC) N = 543 patients ventilated ≥48 h		HR 0.9 (0.6–1.4) for days to ICU death	HR 0.7 (0.6–0.8) for days of ventilation	HR 0.8 (0.5–1.1) for days to hospital discharge HR 0.5 (0.4–0.6) for days to ICU discharge
Klein Klouwenberg et al,[24] 2014 N = 2080 patients ventilated ≥2 d	VAC: 10/1000 vent days IVAC: 4.2/1000 vent days Possible or probable VAP: 3.2/1000 vent days	VAC: HR 3.9 (2.9–5.3) IVAC: HR 2.5 (1.5–4.1) Possible or probable VAP: 2.0 (1.1–3.6)		VAC: HR for ICU discharge 0.38 (0.3–0.6) IVAC: HR for ICU discharge 0.47 (0.3–0.7) Possible or probable VAP HR for ICU discharge: 0.6 (0.3–1.1)

(continued on next page)

Table 1
(continued)

	Incidence	Hospital Mortality	Ventilation Duration	ICU and Hospital Length of Stay
Klompas et al,[30] 2014 N = 20,356 ventilation episodes (no restrictions)	VAC: 6–16/1000 vent days, variable by ICU type IVAC: 3–7/1000 vent days, variable by ICU type PVAP: 0.8–2/1000 vent days, variable by ICU type	VAC: OR 2.4 (1.9–2.9) IVAC: OR 1.9 (1.4–2.4) PVAP: OR 2.2 (1.4–3.2)	VAC: OR for days to extubation 3.1 (2.9–3.3) IVAC: OR for days to extubation 3.5 (3.2–3.7) Possible VAC: OR for days to extubation 3.2 (2.8–3.5)	VAC: OR for days to hospital discharge 1.5 (1.4–1.6) IVAC: OR for days to hospital discharge 1.5 (1.4–1.6) Possible VAC: OR for hospital discharge 1.4 (1.2–1.6)
Stevens et al,[25] 2014 (VAE) N = 10,998 patients ventilated ≥4 d		38% vs 24% OR 1.9 (1.5–2.4)		Mean 24 vs 18 d, hospital LOS Mean 18 vs 11 d, ICU
Boyer et al,[29] 2015 N = 1209 patients ventilated ≥2 d	VAC: 7.0/1000 vent days IVAC: 3.6/1000 vent days	66% vs 14%	14.7 vs 6.3 d of ventilation	
Lilly et al,[132] 2014 N = 8408 episodes of mechanical ventilation	VAC: 13.8/1000 vent days IVAC: 8.8/1000 vent days	VAC: 42% vs 24% OR 1.84 (0.95, 3.6) IVAC: 43% vs 24% OR 1.32 (0.66, 2.6)	14.8 (VAC) and 14.5 (IVAC) vs 4.8 d of ventilation	25.3 (VAC) and 25.1 (IVAC) vs 15.1 d, hospital LOS
Fan et al,[44] 2016 N = Meta-analysis of 18 studies, 61,489 patients receiving mechanical ventilation	VAC: 13.8% (9%–18.6%) IVAC: 6.4% (4.8%–8.1%) PVAP: Possible, Probable 1.1% (0.5%–1.7%), 0.9% (0.6%–1.2%)			
Magill et al,[37] 2016 N = 1824 health care facilities representing 32,772 mo of VAE data	VAE (any): 2.59–11.79/1000 vent days, variable by ICU type IVAC plus: 0.4–5.46/1000 vent days, variable by ICU type	VAC: 33.65% I VAC plus: 27.43%		

Study				
Kobayashi et al,[34] 2017 N = 407 patients ventilated ≥4 d	VAC: 13.4% IVAC plus: 5.7%	VAC: 57.4%, HR 1.45 (0.97–2.18) IVAC plus: 65.2%, HR 2.42 (1.39–4.2) Without VAE and VAP: 34.9%	VAC: 15 d IVAC plus: 13 d Without VAE and VAP: 6 d	17 (VAC) and 15 (IVAC) days for median ICU LOS 47 (VAC) and 47 (IVAC) days for median hospital LOS
Rawat et al,[121] 2017 N = 120,519 ventilator days (no restrictions)	VAE rate from first study quarter to after 2 y of study intervention: VAE 7.34–4.58/1000 vent days IVAC: 3.15–1.56/1000 vent days PVAP: 1.41–0.31/1000 vent days			
Chao et al,[33] 2018 N = 1158 patients ventilated (no restrictions)	VAE: 7.7/1000 vent days, 7.3% VAC: 2.9/1000 vent days IVAC: 2.6/1000 vent days PVAP: 2.1/1000 vent days	Non-PVAP (VAC + IVAC): 66.1% PVAP: 60.9%	Non-PVAP 17 d (11–29.3) vs PVAP 22 d (12–38) PVAP: 22 d (12–38)	ICU LOS: Non-PVAP 18.5 d (13–26.3) vs PVAP 20 d (12–33) Hospital LOS: Non-PVAP 30 d (18.3–48) vs PVAP 41 d (26–53)
Meagher et al,[19] 2018 N = 1533 trauma patients ventilated ≥3 d	VAE: 8.1% VAP: 7.4% Both: 4.1%	VAE vs VAP: HR 2.86 (1.44–5.68) VAE vs no-VAP: HR 2.83 (1.83–4.38)	Ventilator-free days, mean (SD): VAE: 8.9 (8.8), VAP 10.9 (7.9), both 7.6 (6.9)	ICU LOS, mean (SD): VAE 19.2 (±13.3), VAP 18.8 (±11.2), both 26.3 (±16.2) Hospital LOS, mean (SD): VAE 31.9 (28.6), VAP 31.4 (22.4), both 36.7 (19.9)
Nakahashi et al,[39] 2018 N = 785 patients ventilated ≥2 d	VAE: 5.7% of patients ventilated ≥2 6.4/1000 vent days. VAC: 2.20/1000 vent days IVAC: 1.90/1000 vent days PVAP: 2.29/1000 vent days	ICU mortality rate: VAE: 42.9% No VAE: 15.4% Unadjusted OR: 4.13	VAE: 22.4 d No VAE: 8.7 d	ICU LOS: VAE: 25.2 d No VAE: 13.6 d

(continued on next page)

Table 1
(continued)

	Incidence	Hospital Mortality	Ventilation Duration	ICU and Hospital Length of Stay
Ramirez-Estrada et al,[38] 2018 N = 244 patients ventilated ≥2 d	VAC: 1.2/1000 vent days IVAC plus: 39.6/1000 vent days PVAP: 22.3/1000 vent days	30-d mortality rate: VAE: 43% No VAE: 29%	VAE: 31 d (17–54) No VAE: 12 d (7–20)	ICU LOS: VAE: 23 d (10–36) No VAE: 12 d (7–20) Hospital LOS: VAE: 31 d (17–54) No VAE: 19 d (10–38)
Liu et al,[35] 2019 N = 428 patients ventilated ≥4 d	VAC: 7.53/1000 vent days IVAC: 3.52/1000 vent days PVAP: 2.26/1000 vent days	VAE: 56.7% No VAE: 11.8% Relative risk, 9.77 (4.66–21.38)	VAE: 11 d (7–15), P < .001 No VAE: 7 d (5–10)	ICU LOS: VAE: 13 d (8–19), P = .01 No VAE: 9.5 d (7–150 Hospital LOS: VAE: 20 d (11.5–33.25), P = .77 No VAE: 21 d (10–33)
He et al,[27] 2021 N = 6252 patients ventilated ≥4 d	VAC plus: 7.29–23.72/1000 vent days, variable by ICU type IVAC plus: 3.59–9.44/1000 vent days, variable by ICU type PVAP: 0.62–2.18/1000 vent days, variable by ICU type	Non-VAE: 13.7% VAC plus: 20.7% IVAC plus: 19.9% PVAP: 22.3%	Non-VAE: 8 d (5–13) VAC plus: 14 d (8–22) IVAC plus: 15 d (10–25) PVAP: 20 d (11–31)	ICU LOS: Non-VAE: 13 (8–21) VAC plus: 20 (12–33) IVAC plus: 21 (14–33) PVAP: 23 (15–35) Hospital LOS: Non-VAE: 22 (15–34) VAC plus: 28 (17–43) IVAC plus: 30 (19–44) PVAP: 30 (21–46)
Zhu et al,[36] 2021 N = 6426 patients ventilated ≥4 d	VAE: 22.2/1000 vent days VAC: 13.7/1000 vent days IVAC: 6.3/1000 vent days PVAP: 2.2/1000 vent days	ICU Mortality VAE: 18.8% No VAE: 12.3%	VAE: 13 (8–22) No VAE: 7 (5–13)	ICU LOS: VAE: 19 (11–30) No VAE: 12 (8–20) Hospital LOS: VAE: 27 (17–42) No VAE: 22 (15–34)

Caution should be used directly comparing rates and outcomes between the listed studies given varying inclusion criteria for ventilated patients in the VAE denominator. Note that some of the studies reported here did not apply the current specific VAE definitions (CDC 2020).

Abbreviations: HR, hazard ratio; IVAC, infection-related VAC; LOS, length of stay; OR, odds ratio; vent, ventilator.

VAEs.[10,15,19,24,25,27,30,31,36,39,43] VAEs are also associated with more time on mechanical ventilation, longer ICU stays, and longer hospital stays, as summarized in **Table 1**. These findings have been observed across a variety of ICU types with heterogeneous patient populations. Studies that have compared VAE mortality with VAP mortality generally report that patients with VAEs are about 50% more likely to die compared with patients with VAP.[44] Patients with IVAC and PVAP have longer attributable ventilator and hospital days relative to patients with VAC alone. Patients with PVAP have outcomes similar to those with IVAC alone.[27,30,33,36,38]

Higher rates of antimicrobial use have been reported for patients with VAEs compared with matched controls.[45] Some investigators have suggested that the strong association between antimicrobial consumption and VAEs allows for the possibility that VAE surveillance in general and the ratio of IVACs to VACs in particular may be useful metrics for antimicrobial stewardship programs.[8]

CLINICAL TRIGGERS AND RISK FACTORS FOR VENTILATOR-ASSOCIATED EVENTS
Clinical Triggers Identified in Case Series

Table 2 summarizes findings from studies that assessed the clinical etiologies of consecutive VAEs within defined populations. These studies used medical chart reviews to identify the clinical conditions that necessitated the acute and sustained increase in ventilator settings that triggered VAE criteria. Respiratory infections, fluid overload, acute respiratory distress syndrome (ARDS), and atelectasis were the most common conditions that triggered VAEs.[15,24,29,32,33,38,40,46] Pneumonia and respiratory infections accounted for approximately 25% to 40% of cases, pulmonary edema and/or fluid overload accounted for 20% to 40% of cases, atelectasis for 10% to 15%, and ARDS for 10% to 20%. The proportion of cases with no identified trigger ranged from 6% to 41%, depending on the series.[15,24,32,38] Prospective studies were more apt to identify causes for VAEs compared with retrospective studies. Hayashi and colleagues[32] found that although more than 30% of VAC patients did not have a particular diagnosis documented in the chart at the time of VAE, many of these were functionally treated for presumed respiratory infections and/or pulmonary edema with antibiotics and/or furosemide.

Potential Risk Factors for ventilator-associated Events

Fluid overload
Excess fluid balance has been identified across multiple studies as a risk factor for VAE. Lewis and colleagues[47] identified positive fluid balance as a risk factor (odds ratio [OR]. 1.2 per liter; 95% confidence interval [CI], 1.0–1.4) and congestive heart failure (CHF) as protective, presumably because patients with a history of CHF were given about one-third less fluid compared with patients without CHF. An analysis of VAEs among 1608 patients admitted to the medical ICU of a tertiary care center in Taiwan identified renal replacement therapy (OR, 8.9; 95% CI, 1.5–54.6), and a positive cumulative 2-day fluid balance (OR, 1.5 per liter increase; 95% CI, 1.2–2.0) as independently associated with VAEs owing to pulmonary edema.[33] A 2018 case-control study including 186 VAEs from an academic medical center in Ohio identified total parenteral nutrition as a risk factor for VAC, whereas CHF was protective.[48] A study of 2 ICUs in Eastern China including 5532 patients also found a strong association between positive fluid balance and VAEs (relative risk, 8.4; 95% CI, 3.0–23.5).[35] Blood transfusions are associated with volume overload and may increase risk for ARDS, and in multiple logistic regression analysis have been associated with the development of VAE after cardiac surgery (OR, 19.7; 95% CI, 7.3–41.4).[49]

Table 2
Clinical triggers identified among adult patients with VAE

	Klompas et al,[15] 2011	Hayashi et al,[32] 2013	Klein Klouwenberg et al,[24] 2014		Boyer et al,[29] 2015		Whiting et al,[46] 2015	Nakahashi et al,[40] 2016	Chao et al,[33] 2018	Ramirez-Estrada et al,[38] 2018
	n = 44 VAE	n = 153 VAE	n = 81 VAE	n = 31 IVAC	n = 67 VAE	n = 34 IVAC	n = 19 VAE	n = 37 VAE	n = 85 VAE	n = 49 IVAC
Pneumonia and/or aspiration	10 (23%)	66 (43%)	28 (35%)	15 (48%)	22 (33%)	21 (62%)	4 (21%)	14 (38%)	22 (26%)	-
Pulmonary edema, pleural effusion, and/or fluid overload	8 (18%)	40 (26%)	23 (28%)	12 (39%)	10 (15%)	-	5 (26%)	15 (41%)	19 (22%)	2 (4%)
ARDS	7 (16%)	10 (7%)	-	-	14 (21%)	3 (9%)	2 (11%)	5 (14%)	7 (8%)	6 (13%)
Atelectasis/mucous plugging	6 (13%)	25 (16%)	12 (15%)	5 (19%)	6 (9%)	-	4 (21%)	8 (22%)	20 (24%)	26 (55%)
Extrapulmonary infection/sepsis syndrome	1 (2%)	-	9 (11%)	5 (16%)	3 (5%)	-	-	-	12 (14%)	-
Pulmonary embolism	2% (1)	3 (2%)	0 (0%)	0 (0%)	-	-	-	-	-	-
Pneumothorax	-	-	2 (2%)	-	2 (3.0%)	-	-	-	4 (5%)	-
TRALI/TACO	-	-	-	-	2 (3.0%)	-	-	-	-	-
Abdominal compartment syndrome/distention	1 (2%)	2 (1%)	9 (11%)	4 (13%)	-	-	-	-	1 (1%)	-
Radiation pneumonitis	1 (2%)	-	-	-	-	-	-	-	-	-
Acute neurologic event	-	-	10 (12%)	3 (10%)	-	-	4 (21%)	-	-	-
Other	-	-	10 (12%)	-	7 (13%)	4 (12%)	-	-	-	-
No trigger identified	41% (18)	11 (17%)	10 (12%)	2 (6%)	6 (9%)	6 (18%)	-	-	-	13 (28%)

Abbreviations: ARDS, acute respiratory distress syndrome; TRALI, transfusion-related acute lung injury; TACO, transfusion-associated circulatory overload; Totals per study do not equal 100% because multiple triggers could be identified and reported per VAC event.

Sedation
Deep sedation and paralysis are also associated with increased risk of VAE. The afore-mentioned study out of Eastern China found sedative administration between the first and fourth days of mechanical ventilation to be associated with VAE development (relative risk, 15.7; 95% CI, 1.6–152.1).[35] Klompas and colleagues[50] analyzed 9603 consecutive episodes of mechanical ventilation in a large academic hospital to mea-sure associations between different kinds of sedatives and VAEs. The analysis took into account the day-to-day patterns of sedative exposures for each patient. The au-thors found that benzodiazepines and propofol were associated with an increased risk for VAEs, whereas dexmedetomidine was not. They also found that propofol and dex-medetomidine were associated with less time to extubation compared with benzodi-azepines, and that dexmedetomidine was associated with less time to extubation compared with propofol. In a matched case-control study, Lewis and colleagues[47] identified exposures to paralytics (OR, 2.3; 95% CI, 0.79–80), sedation with benzodi-azepines (OR, 5.0; 95% CI, 1.3–29), and total opioid exposure (OR, 2.3; 95% CI, 0.9–16) as risk factors for VAEs. They found liver disease to be protective against VAE, and that physicians used opioids and sedatives more sparingly among this population; pa-tients with liver disease were given about one-quarter fewer opioids compared with patients without liver disease.[47]

Mandatory ventilation and driving pressure
Mandatory modes of mechanical ventilation as well as high tidal volumes or driving pressures have also been associated with increased risk of VAE. Mandatory modes of ventilation, defined as all mechanical ventilation modes other than pressure sup-port, were associated with an OR of 3.4 (95% CI, 1.6–8.0) for VAEs.[47] Higher driving pressures were also risk factors for VAEs on multivariate analysis of 303 ventilated pa-tients at an academic center in Japan (HR 1.12; 95% CI, 1.04–1.22). Ogbu and col-leagues[42] found an association between tidal volumes and VAE risk. They matched 167 patients with VAEs with 668 controls. On multivariable conditional logistic regres-sion, the odds of VAE increased by 1.21 for each milligram per kilogram of tidal volume greater than 6 mL/kg of predicted body weight ($P = .03$).

As pointed out by Lewis and associates,[47] mandatory modes of ventilation may or may not be independent predictors of VAEs. On the one hand, mandatory modes may cause more volume and pressure trauma to patients' alveoli than spontaneous modes. This could trigger or worsen ARDS and thus cause VAEs. On the other hand, the as-sociation between mandatory modes of mechanical ventilation and VAE may be confounded by severity of illness. Patients with severe, progressive pulmonary dis-ease are more likely to require mandatory modes of mechanical ventilation and pro-gressively higher ventilator settings that might trigger VAE criteria. Similarly, a high driving pressure is associated with poorly compliant lungs that may be at greater risk for volume and pressure trauma. There may also be an interplay between manda-tory modes of mechanical ventilation and other risk factors for VAEs: patients who require mandatory modes of ventilation are also more likely to require heavy sedation and/or neuromuscular blockade, which in turn could also increase their risk for VAEs.

Aspiration
Aspiration has been identified as a potential trigger for VAE. Not surprisingly then, many risk factors for aspiration have also been identified as risk factors for VAEs.[13,29,32,33,40,46] These include gastric residuals or more than 200 mL (relative risk, 9.3; 95% CI, 1.9–45.5),[35] oral care with chlorhexidine where aspiration may cause

a chemical pneumonitis and ARDS (OR, 1.42; $P = .03$),[51] and tube feeds (which can inhibit upper and lower esophageal sphincter function).[48]

Risk factors for infection-related ventilator-associated complications

Risk factors for IVAC have been evaluated by fewer studies. Lewis and colleagues[47] identified benzodiazepines started between admission and intubation (OR, 5.0; 95% CI, 1.3–29), prescriptions for opioids (OR, 3.3 per 100 µg fentanyl equivalents per kg; 95% CI, 0.9–16), and the use of paralytics while intubated (OR, 2.3; 95% CI, 0.8–8.0). There were also trends toward more IVACs with higher minimum tidal volumes (OR, 1.5 per mL/kg; 95% CI, 0.91–2.9) and positive daily fluid balances (OR, 1.1 per liter positive; 95% CI, 0.90–1.5). Kubbara and colleagues[48] identified COPD, tube feeds, and total parenteral nutrition as risk factors for IVAC plus, whereas morphine and prednisone use were protective. Morphine use may have been in place of longer acting sedatives, leading to shorter and lighter sedation. The mechanisms by which prednisone may decrease the rate of IVAC plus are numerous, with blunting of the fever response as one plausible explanation.

Care-related risk factors

Bouadma and colleagues[45] noted that patient transport was associated with 17% of VAEs in their multicenter retrospective dataset of 2331 cases. Nakahashi and colleagues[40] identified 4 care-related variables (as opposed to host-related variables) associated with VAEs among 3122 patients admitted to a Japanese ICU: absence of intensivist participation in managing ventilated patients, the use of higher ventilator driving pressures, development of edema, and greater body weight increases.

PREVENTION INTERVENTIONS

Because only a small proportion of VAEs are attributable to pneumonia, standard VAP prevention bundles may only partially lower VAE rates. A logical framework for preventing VAEs is to select interventions that decrease the duration of mechanical ventilation (and hence the time at risk for VAEs) and/or prevent one or more of the major conditions associated with VAEs (pneumonia, fluid overload, atelectasis, and ARDS).[52] Using this framework, 6 interventions have been proposed to prevent VAEs: minimize sedation, speed extubation by optimizing the performance of daily paired spontaneous awakening and breathing trials, mobilize patients, use conservative fluid management, ventilate patients with low tidal volumes, and set restrictive thresholds for transfusions (**Fig. 2**).[53] There are likely additional institution-specific strategies to improve care for ventilated patients that could be identified by conducting root-cause analyses of individual VAEs.[29,45] **Table 3** provides an overview of studies to date assessing interventions to prevent VAEs.

Minimize Sedation

Deep and sustained sedation is associated with numerous adverse events, including increased mortality, prolonged mechanical ventilation, and a higher risk for VAEs.[54–57] Deep and/or sustained sedation may trigger VAEs by prolonging time on mechanical ventilation, increasing the need for mandatory modes of mechanical ventilation (which in turn may increase the risk of lung injury), decreasing clearance of respiratory secretions, and increasing the risk of atelectasis and aspiration.[58] Collectively, these effects predispose patients to pneumonia, atelectasis, and/or ARDS, 3 of the 4 clinical conditions most commonly associated with VAEs.

Because sedation is associated with ICU-acquired infection—via a number of potential mechanisms—minimizing sedatives and opioids is recommended to decrease

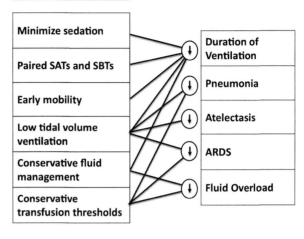

VAE Risk Factors   VAE Prevention Elements

Fig. 2. Potential strategies to prevent VAEs. Interventions that decrease duration of mechanical ventilation and target 1 or more of the conditions that most commonly trigger VAEs are highlighted. SATs, spontaneous awakening trials; SBTs, spontaneous breathing trials.

time on the ventilator and time in the ICU.[59,60] The short-acting sedatives propofol and dexmedetomidine have been associated with less time to extubation compared with benzodiazepines, and dexmedetomidine has been associated with a lower risk for VAEs. Conversely benzodiazepines, opioids, and paralytics have been associated with an increased risk for IVACs.[47,50,61]

Daily Coordinated Spontaneous Awakening Trials and Spontaneous Breathing Trials

Spontaneous awakening trials and spontaneous breathing trials are 2 of the best-studied interventions to decrease VAEs. Spontaneous awakening and spontaneous breathing trials are designed to decrease sedation and the duration of mechanical ventilation by identifying the lowest level of sedation a patient needs to be comfortably ventilated and the earliest time at which they can safely be extubated. Both interventions reduce time at risk for VAEs.[56,62–64] Coordinating spontaneous awakening trials and spontaneous breathing trials to perform spontaneous breathing trials during sedative interruptions (so that patients are more awake and hence more likely to pass their spontaneous breathing trials) further decreased the time to extubation compared with spontaneous breathing trials alone.[56,65]

Multiple studies have documented inverse associations between spontaneous awakening trials and/or spontaneous breathing trials and VAEs. Muscedere and colleagues[31] found that the percentage of ventilator days with spontaneous awakening trials and spontaneous breathing trials was associated with lower VAC and IVAC rates. Other investigators reported decreased rates of VAEs and IVAC in hospitals compliant with spontaneous breathing trial guidelines.[66] A prospective quality improvement collaborative among 12 ICUs subsequently confirmed that increasing the performance rate of paired daily spontaneous awakening trials/spontaneous breathing trials can lower VAE rates.[56] Over a 19-month period, the collaborative noted 37% fewer VAEs

Table 3
Interventions to prevent VAE in adults

Study	Intervention	Impact
Muscedere et al,[31] 2013	Retrospective analysis after implementation of VAP clinical practice guidelines sequentially introduced over 24 mo	Overall VAE rate decreased by 29% over the study period. Rates of VAC decreased, although the IVAC rates remained steady. Those who developed VAC were more likely to be orally intubated and had less frequent humidifier and suction system exchanges. The percentage of ventilator days with SATs and SBTs was associated with a trend toward lower VAC and IVAC rates.
Mekontso Dessap et al,[85] 2014	Retrospective analysis of a randomized controlled trial targeting depletive fluid management using BNP in ventilated patients	In the BNP guided group, patients received more diuretics, had a more-negative daily fluid balance (mean −640 mL vs −37 mL), and shorter time to extubation (42.4 h vs 58.6 h). There was a 50% lower incidence of VAE in the fluid depletive group vs usual care (8.6% vs 17.8%)
Klompas et al,[56] 2015	Prospective study of a protocol for increasing paired daily SAT and SBT (collaborative group) over a 19-month period	Among intervention ICUs, SAT performance rate increased from 14% to 77% of days where indicated. SBT performance rates increased from 49% to 75% of days where indicated. Mean duration of mechanical ventilation decreased by 2.4 d, but there was no change in ICU mortality. The VAE rate went from 9.7 events per 100 episodes of mechanical ventilation to 5.2 events per 100 episodes of mechanical ventilation. IVAC rates went from 3.5 to 0.52 events per 100 episodes of mechanical ventilation. PVAP rates did not significantly change. There was no change in VAE rate in the surveillance group ICUs.

(continued on next page)

Table 3 (continued)		
Study	**Intervention**	**Impact**
Rawat et al,[121] 2017	Multifaceted collaborative including unit teamwork, safety culture and adherence to 6 evidence-based interventions (head of bed elevation, subglottic suctioning, oral care, chlorhexidine mouth care, SAT, and SBT)	Over a 24-month period, there was a 37% decrease in VAE (7.34–4.58 VAE per 1000 ventilator days). IVAC (3.16–1.56) and PVAP (1.41–0.31) cases per 1000 ventilator days also decreased. Compositive compliance in the 6 interventions increased from 14% to 20% over the study. Regression analysis suggested that a 10% increase in composite compliance was associated with a 12% VAE decrease.
Anand et al,[122] 2018	Quality improvement intervention to improve VAP bundle (head of bed elevation, oral care, peptic ulcer prophylaxis, daily SAT/SBT) adherence among trauma patients	Compliance with the VAP bundle increased from 65% at baseline to more than 90% within 1 year of the quality initiatives. Mean ventilator days did not change over the course of the study, but PVAP rates fell from 12% at baseline to 3% at 1 y, 2% at 2 y, and then 0%.
Chumpia et al,[67] 2019	Multifaceted intervention including education around electronic order sets and nurse and respiratory driven protocols to improve SAT/SBT adherence	SAT and SBT order rates increased and duration of mechanical ventilation decreased (mean 7.2 d at baseline to 4.7 d after the intervention) This was associated with a drop in VAEs from 5.2 per 100 episodes at baseline to 0.7 per 100 episodes after intervention.
Seaver et al,[79] 2020	Multidisciplinary team collaboration on VAE prevention including electronic health record optimization and protocol driven ventilator liberation	The rate of VAE decreased from 12.8 VAE per 1000 ventilator days at baseline to 2.8 VAE per 1000 ventilator days after intervention. As part of the intervention, PEEP was initiated at 6 cm H_2O instead of historically used 5 cm H_2O such that VAE would not be triggered by an increase of PEEP to 8 cm H_2O.

Abbreviation: BNP, B-type natriuretic peptide.

(OR, 0.63; 95% CI, 0.42–0.97) and 65% fewer IVACs (OR, 0.35; 95% CI, 0.17–0.71) per episode of mechanical ventilation. These improvements were also associated with a 2.4-day decrease in the mean duration of mechanical ventilation, a 3.0-day decrease in ICU length of stay, and a 6.3-day decrease in hospital length of stay. A 2019 study at a Los Angeles Veterans Affairs Hospital aimed to decrease VAE rates by decreasing duration of mechanical ventilation via improved spontaneous awakening/spontaneous breathing trial protocols and adherence. Spontaneous awakening and spontaneous breathing trial order rates increased and duration of mechanical ventilation decreased (mean of 7.2 days at baseline to 4.7 days after the intervention; $P = .049$). This strategy was associated with a decrease in VAEs from 5.2 per 100 episodes at baseline to 0.7 per 100 episodes after the intervention; $P = .06$).[67]

Importantly, spontaneous awakening trials and spontaneous breathing trials are means, not ends. The intent of these 2 interventions is to decrease the overall level of sedation and to lessen the period from readiness for extubation to actual extubation. Merely checking the box on spontaneous awakening trial or spontaneous breathing trial performance is not sufficient to decrease VAE rates if not paired with active attempts to decrease sedative use and speed extubation. A well-rounded quality improvement initiative will thus include not only mechanisms to increase spontaneous awakening trial and spontaneous breathing trial rates, but also education around best practices for sedation and protocols to move patients from successful spontaneous breathing trials to extubation. This need was evident in a clinical trial that found that adding daily sedation interruptions to a sedation protocol did not decrease the duration of mechanical ventilation or hospital stay compared with a sedation protocol alone.[68] The patients randomized to sedative interruptions in this trial paradoxically received more boluses and higher daily doses of midazolam and fentanyl compared with patients being managed by protocol alone. Presumably this outcome reflected a persistent culture of sedation, wherein patients who became agitated during sedative interruptions were reflexively managed with more sedation rather than trying to manage their agitation using nonsedating strategies.

Programs for Early Exercise and Mobility

Immobility is associated with atelectasis and pneumonia—common triggers for VAEs—as well as a longer duration of hospital stay and time on the ventilator. To date, no studies that have examined the independent impact of early mobility on VAE risk; however, multiple studies have reported better patient outcomes after the introduction of early exercise and mobility programs.[69–72] Early physical and/or occupational therapy can decrease time on the ventilator, and has been associated with lower rates of complications and VAP in some studies.[73,74] Although there are challenges with mobilizing someone on a ventilator and surveys of practice suggest that early mobility is not yet commonly used, adverse outcomes have not been observed when such programs are instituted.[75–78] A small prospective study of quality improvement programs around ventilator liberation, including daily exercise and ambulation, observed a decrease in the VAE rate after the intervention, although the data for adherence to the exercise component were not provided.[79]

Low Tidal Volume Ventilation

Low tidal volume ventilation has been associated with improved outcomes in ventilated patients with and without ARDS and it may prevent several triggers of VAEs, namely ARDS, atelectasis, and lung infections.[80–84] Neto and colleagues[82,83] performed 2 meta-analyses of the impact of low tidal volume ventilation on patients without lung injury at the start of ventilation. Lower tidal volumes were associated with a lower risk for ARDS, fewer pulmonary infections, and less atelectasis when compared with higher tidal volumes. A shorter hospital length of stay and decreased mortality were also observed. Ogbu and colleagues[42] affirmed the potential value of lower tidal volumes to prevent VAEs in a case-control study that documented an increased odds of VAE with each milligram er kilogram of tidal volume that is greater than 6 mL/kg.

Conservative Fluid Management

A positive fluid balance has consistently been associated with VAEs.[15,29,32,40,47,85] Excess fluids increase the risk of pulmonary edema, ARDS, and pneumonia, 3 of the 4 most common conditions that trigger VAEs.[86] Conversely, conservative fluid management is associated less time to extubation, shorter ICU stays, and lower hospital mortality rates, particularly among patients with ARDS.[87,88]

One randomized controlled trial thus far has affirmed that conservative fluid management can prevent VAEs. Mekonsto Dessap and colleagues[85] retrospectively applied VAE definitions to data from a randomized controlled trial of conservative fluid management versus usual practice during the weaning phase of mechanical ventilation. Conservative fluid management in this trial was driven by daily measurements of B-type natriuretic peptide (BNP). Patients randomized to daily measurement of BNP levels were administered less fluids and more diuretics, and had greater negative fluid balances compared with patients in the usual practice arm. Conservative fluid management was associated with more ventilator-free days and substantially lower VAE rates. There were 52% fewer VAEs in the intervention group compared with usual care group.

What remains to be seen is how conservative fluid management is best operationalized. Wiedemann and colleagues used a complex protocol that included invasive monitoring devices and a complicated management algorithm, whereas Mekontso Dessap and colleagues used daily BNP levels.[85,87] Neither of these approaches is optimal: invasive monitoring devices can be harmful, overly complex protocols are difficult to generalize and error prone, and daily BNP levels can be expensive and challenging to interpret in patients with renal impairment. Additional approaches are required. Possibilities include daily weight monitoring, noninvasive ultrasound measurements, or simplified protocols for interpreting common physiological data.[89] Work in this area is ongoing.

Conservative Blood Transfusion Thresholds

Restrictive red blood cell transfusion strategies have been associated with decreased risk for hospital-acquired infections, including pneumonia.[90] In addition, blood transfusions may increase the risk of ARDS and pulmonary edema.[80,86,91] Two recent studies, one among adult patients in the cardiac ICU and another in 6 pediatric hospitals, found associations between blood transfusions and VAE risk.[49,92] No studies to date, however, have directly evaluated whether restrictive transfusion thresholds can decrease VAE rates.

Ventilator-associated Pneumonia Prevention

The VAE prevention bundle proposed in this article is designed to include and supersede VAP prevention bundles. VAP accounts for about one-third of VAEs and thus VAE prevention bundles must by right include VAP prevention strategies. The proposed VAE prevention bundle includes most of the VAP prevention practices associated with shorter durations of mechanical ventilation and/or lower mortality rates as recommended in the Society for Healthcare Epidemiology of America's Compendium of Strategies to Prevent VAP.[93] Some of the additional strategies classically used to prevent VAP such as elevating the head of the bed, oral care with chlorhexidine, and subglottic secretion drainage are discussed elsewhere in this article. There are still grounds to include some of these interventions in comprehensive prevention bundles for ventilated patients, particularly head of bed elevation.

Elevating the head of the bed to prevent VAP is common practice in almost all US hospitals.[94] Although there are compelling physiologic arguments to support this practice, there are very few data describing its impact on patients' outcomes. In a Cochrane review encompassing 10 randomized controlled trials and 878 participants, the semirecumbent position ($\geq30°$) significantly decreased the risk of clinically suspected VAP, but had no impact on objective outcomes such as duration of ventilation, ICU length of stay, or mortality.[95] There are very few data, however, suggesting any risk of harm associated with elevating the head of the bed, the practice is free of charge, and it is possible that larger studies in the future may yet document clear benefits. As such, elevating the head of the bed still seems to be a reasonable practice to include in prevention bundles for ventilated patients.

Routine oral care with chlorhexidine, by contrast, may be a source of harm for some fraction of patients. Recent meta-analyses question the association between oral care with chlorhexidine and lower VAP rates in non–cardiac surgery patients and note that there may be a signal toward higher mortality rates in patients randomized to chlorhexidine.[96–98] The mechanism of increased mortality risk is unknown, but a possible explanation may be occasional episodes of aspiration of antiseptic precipitating ARDS.[99–102] Note that the concern with oral care with chlorhexidine is specifically with the chlorhexidine component of the regimen. Oral care alone still seems very reasonable for patient hygiene and comfort. Few studies have rigorously assessed the impact of oral care alone without an antiseptic on VAP and other outcomes, but in contrast with chlorhexidine there is no suggestion of a safety signal.[103–106]

One area of ongoing controversy is whether selective digestive decontamination with a combination of oral and parenteral antibiotics can be helpful for patients. A series of large randomized controlled trials have suggested that this strategy may not only prevent VAP but also decrease mortality rates.[107–109] The practice is controversial, however, owing to fear that prescribing antibiotics for all ICU patients or all ventilated patients may cultivate and promote multidrug-resistant organisms that might ultimately compromise the care of future ICU patients.[110] A 2018 multicenter cluster randomized controlled trial of selective digestive decontamination specifically conducted in ICUs with higher rates of antibiotic use and higher baseline prevalences of antibiotic resistant organisms, however, reported no impact on mortality rates (or the frequency of multidrug resistant infections).[106] The decontamination regimen in this study did not include a course of parenteral third-generation cephalosporin antibiotics, in contrast with prior studies of digestive decontamination that reported mortality benefits. It is unknown, whether this factor accounts for the lack of a mortality signal in this study or if other factors were at play. The literature on the long-term impact of selective digestive decontamination on ICU resistance rates and patient outcomes is still relatively sparse, but studies thus far have not clearly confirmed enhanced risk.[111–113] Indeed, some studies suggest that digestive decontamination may paradoxically lower overall antibiotic use, presumably by averting some infections. Many hospitals in Europe routinely practice selective digestive decontamination, but it is almost never practiced in North America.

An additional practice commonly adopted to prevent VAP is endotracheal tubes with subglottic secretion drainage. These devices are designed to minimize the pooling of secretions above the endotracheal tube cuff and hence to diminish the volume of microbe-laden secretions seeping around the cuff and into the lungs. Early meta-analyses of this strategy suggested that these devices can both decrease VAP rates and shorten the duration of mechanical ventilation, leading to a recommendation in favor of subglottic secretion drainage in VAP prevention guidelines.[93,114–117] These analyses were based on a possible misinterpretation of 1 key trial, however, that was responsible for much of the signal toward shorter ventilator episodes.[118] A 2016 meta-analysis that excluded this trial failed to find any improvements in the duration of mechanical ventilation, ICU length of stay, or mortality.[119] A more recent systemic review and meta-analysis did report a mortality improvement, but double-abstracted 1 article and used per-protocol rather than intention-to-treat results for another.[120]

Ventilator Bundle Compliance and Ventilator-associated Pneumonia

An increasing number of centers and quality improvement collaboratives have published data showing that bundling together multiple measures to prevent VAEs is effective at decreasing VAE rates. A 2017 study including 56 ICUs from 2 states tested a bundle of 6 interventions traditionally used for VAP prevention: head of bed elevation, subglottic suctioning, oral care, chlorhexidine mouth care, spontaneous awakening trials, and spontaneous breathing trials.[121] The study was collaborative by nature, encouraged peer learning, and used a structured change management process. Rates of VAC, IVAC, and PVAP per 1000 ventilator days all significantly decreased over the course of the study. The incidence of VAC in particular decreased by 37.6%. Each 10% increase in composite compliance was estimated to decrease the VAE rate by 12% (incident rate ratio, 0.88; 95% CI, 0.78–0.99; $P = .032$). The authors noted that head of bed elevation and subglottic suctioning compliance did not change over the course of the study, and thus it seemed that oral care, chlorhexidine mouth rinse, and/or increased compliance with spontaneous awakening trials and spontaneous breathing trials were responsible for the decrease in VAE rates. Alternatively, given only modest increases in these measures and the potential for chlorhexidine to be associated with harm, the drop in VAE may have been due to other unmeasured factors, such as improvements in safety culture.

A 2018 study at a large academic medical center further investigated the association between ventilator bundle compliance and the incidence of VAE.[51] Among 273 VAEs and 984 controls, there was no association between overall bundle scores in the 3 days before VAE, and a risk of VAE trigger (OR, 1.15, $P = .34$). During this time period, the same bundle implementation was associated with decreased rates of VAP, highlighting the limited overlap between VAE and VAP. Compliance with oral chlorhexidine was associated with a higher risk of VAE (OR, 1.45; $P = .007$) as well as IVAC plus (OR, 1.73; $P = .0006$), a finding that persisted on multivariate analysis. In a retrospective single center trauma surgical ICU population, improved compliance with a VAP prevention bundle after a multifaceted educational intervention was associated with decreased PVAP rates (12% from 2009 to 2010, 0% in from 2013 to 2016) and a near 50% decrease in mortality, although ventilator days remained similar.[122]

All told, the data on ventilator bundles are promising but more work is needed to identify the ideal components to include in ventilator bundles and to better determine their impact on VAE and other outcomes.

Pediatric Ventilator-Associated Conditions

Investigators continue to explore the application of VAE surveillance to children and neonates. Cocoros and colleagues[123] examined whether adult VAC criteria should be revised for a pediatric VAC definition given the inherent differences between adults, children, and neonates. They evaluated a range of potential alternative approaches to identify pediatric VAC and ultimately recommended identifying worsening oxygenation by increases in daily minimum Fio_2 or mean airway pressure (MAP) after a period of ventilator improvement or stability. The authors opted for MAP instead of PEEP because MAP more accurately reflects lung compliance, whereas PEEP is set by clinicians. They reported incidence rates of approximately 3 per 1000 ventilator days in the pediatric ICU (PICU), neonatal ICU, and cardiac ICU. They also reported a substantially increased risk of hospital mortality, increased hospital and ICU lengths of stay, and a longer ventilation duration among children with a VAC compared with matched patients without a VAC across all ICU types.

The need for a VAC definition tailored to children and neonates led to CDC developing a Pediatric VAE (PedVAE) definition (**Fig. 3**). PedVAEs, like adult VAEs, are identified by a deterioration in respiratory status after a period of stability or improvement on the ventilator.[124] There are important differences, however, including the use of MAP in lieu of PEEP and the exclusion of nested VAE subtypes, namely, IVAC and

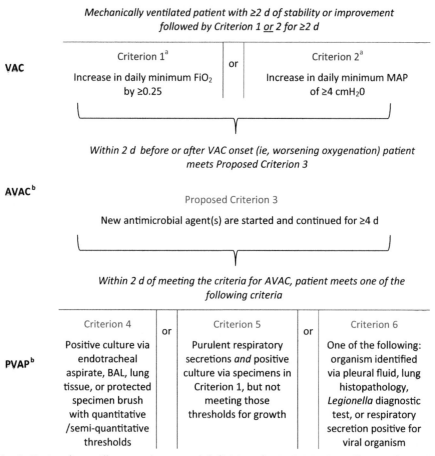

Fig. 3. National surveillance and proposed definitions for PedVAEs. Surveillance "day 1" is the day of intubation and initiation of mechanical ventilation; the earliest day PedVAE criteria can be fulfilled is day 4 and the earliest event date for PedVAE is day 3 of mechanical ventilation. [a]See the full CDC NHSN protocol for details related to each criterion (CDC 2021). For patients <30 days old, daily minimum MAP values of 0 to 8 cm H_2O are considered equal to 8 cm H_2O for the purposes of surveillance and for patients ≥30 days old, 0 to 10 cm H_2O are considered equal to 10 cm H_2O for the purposes of surveillance. [b]AVAC and Pediatric PVAP are proposed definitions and not currently included in CDC guidelines. AVAC, pediatric VAC with antimicrobial use; MAP, mean airway pressure; PVAP, pediatric possible VAP.

PVAP. However, a simplified algorithm encompassing pediatric VAC with antimicrobial use has been proposed as an alternative to IVAC.[125] This pediatric VAC with antimicrobial use definition differs from IVAC insofar as the only additional criterion beyond VAC is the initiation of new antimicrobials within 2 days of the PedVAE; abnormal temperature and white blood cell counts are not required, a reflection of the fact that most ventilated patients have abnormal white blood cell counts and/or temperatures, and these criteria have minimal impact on case counts and add little specificity.

Several studies have now applied adult and PedVAE definitions to real-world pediatric populations. Phongjitsiri and colleagues[126] applied the adult VAE definitions to patients in a PICU and found that approximately 15% of patients met the adult VAC definition (21/1000 ventilator days) and about half had an IVAC (13/1000 ventilator days). Those with a VAC had increased hospital mortality and longer ventilator, hospital, and ICU stays compared with those without. These findings of worse outcomes among those with VAC were affirmed in a 2018 study from a tertiary care PICU.[127] Beardsley and colleagues[128] assessed 300 episodes of mechanical ventilation in the PICU and identified 30 episodes of IVAC (2.16 events per 1000 ventilator days). There was little overlap in the diagnosis of IVAC, traditional VAP, and tracheobronchitis with only 9 episodes meeting more than 1 definition.

A 2018 study compared clinical outcomes between patients who met criteria for VAP, traditional VAE, and a modified PedVAE algorithm based on a more liberal definition for PEEP or Fio_2 increases.[129,130] Among 656 children, there were 7 VAEs (2.74 per 1000 ventilator days), 29 PedVAEs (11.34 per 1000 ventilator days), and 11 VAPs or VATs (4.3 per 1000 ventilator days). VAEs were associated with significant increases in ventilator duration and mortality, PedVAE was only associated with increased duration of ventilation, and VAP was not associated with worse outcomes. The authors expressed concern that the adult VAE definition is too restrictive in identifying only the most severely ill patients. They noted that VAE rates in children tend to be lower than adults, and associated mortality higher, and that the less restrictive PedVAE definition may, therefore, be more suitable for pediatric populations. This concern was shared by Cirulis and colleagues,[129] who noted in a single-center study that 80% of VAP cases did not meet VAC criteria, but were associated with similarly poor outcomes.

Risk factors for VAEs in pediatric and adult populations may differ, requiring new analyses and perhaps different approaches for prevention in neonates and children. Recent studies, however, have identified overlap of VAE risk factors between adult and pediatric patients. A case-control study of 192 pediatric VAC cases and controls across 6 hospitals in the United Stated identified neuromuscular blockade (OR, 2.3; 95% CI, 1.1–4.9), positive fluid balance (OR, 7.8; 95% CI, 2.1–28.6), and blood product use (OR, 1.52; 95% CI, 0.7–3.3) as potential risk factors for VAC.[92] These risk factors were shared between PICU, cardiac ICU, and neonatal ICU patients, and a recent surgical procedure was also associated with increased risk in neonatal ICU patients. Weaning from sedation or sedation interruption was protective against VAC across ICU types. A 2018 case control study of 70 VAE and 140 controls using adult VAE definitions identified a higher mean peak inspiratory pressure (OR, 1.1; 95% CI, 1.0–1.2) and acute kidney injury (OR, 2.9; 95% CI, 1.4–5.7) as risk factors for VAC.[127] These risk factors were also observed in a case-control study conducted in a tertiary care PICU, which identified a composite score for fluid overload and kidney injury (FOKIS score) to be associated with VAC.[131] The degree of fluid overload, kidney injury severity, and high peak inspiratory pressure were independently associated risk factors for both VAC and IVAC.

SUMMARY

The introduction of VAE definitions transformed national surveillance for complications in adults receiving mechanical ventilation. VAE definitions expanded the purview of surveillance to include both infectious and noninfectious conditions and transitioned hospitals toward using objective data to measure events. VAEs are associated with higher mortality rates, prolonged mechanical ventilation, and longer lengths of stay. Excess fluid balance, blood transfusions, deeper levels of sedation, prolonged sedation, high tidal volumes, high inspiratory driving pressures, oral care with chlorhexidine, and stress ulcer prophylaxis are risk factors for VAEs. The most common and consistent complications that trigger VAE criteria are pneumonia, pulmonary edema, ARDS, and atelectasis. Conservative fluid management, enhancing the performance of spontaneous awakening trials and spontaneous breathing trials, and minimizing sedation can prevent VAEs and combining these measures into VAE prevention bundles in multidiscipline collaboratives can facilitate implementation and maximize their impact.

REFERENCES

1. Behrendt CE. Acute respiratory failure in the United States: incidence and 31-day survival. Chest 2000;118(4):1100–5.
2. Wunsch H, Linde-Zwirble WT, Angus DC, et al. The epidemiology of mechanical ventilation use in the United States. Crit Care Med 2010;38(10):1947–53.
3. Mehta AB, Syeda SN, Wiener RS, et al. Epidemiological trends in invasive mechanical ventilation in the United States: a population-based study. J Crit Care 2015;30(6):1217–21.
4. Magill SS, Fridkin SK. Improving surveillance definitions for ventilator-associated pneumonia in an era of public reporting and performance measurement. Clin Infect Dis 2012;54(3):378–80.
5. Centers for Disease Control and Prevention. Ventilator-associated event protocol. 2021. Available at: https://www.cdc.gov/nhsn/pdfs/pscmanual/10-vae_final.pdf. Accessed February 27, 2021.
6. Magill SS, Klompas M, Balk R, et al. Developing a new, national approach to surveillance for ventilator-associated events. Crit Care Med 2013;41(11):2467–75.
7. Horan TC, Andrus M, Dudeck MA. CDC/NHSN surveillance definition of health care-associated infection and criteria for specific types of infections in the acute care setting. Am J Infect Control 2008;36(5):309–32.
8. Klompas M. Complications of mechanical ventilation–the CDC's new surveillance paradigm. N Engl J Med 2013;368(16):1472–5.
9. Klompas M, Kleinman K, Khan Y, et al. Rapid and reproducible surveillance for ventilator-associated pneumonia. Clin Infect Dis 2012;54:370–7.
10. Klompas M, Magill S, Robicsek A, et al. Objective surveillance definitions for ventilator-associated pneumonia. Crit Care Med 2012;40(12):3154–61.
11. Klompas M. Interobserver variability in ventilator-associated pneumonia surveillance. Am J Infect Control 2010;38(3):237–9.
12. Stevens JP, Kachniarz B, Wright SB, et al. When policy gets it right: variability in U.S. hospitals' diagnosis of ventilator-associated pneumonia. Crit Care Med 2014;42(3):497–503.
13. Klein Klouwenberg PM, Ong DS, Bos LD, et al. Interobserver agreement of centers for disease control and prevention criteria for classifying infections in critically Ill patients. Crit Care Med 2013;41(10):2373–8.

14. Kerlin M, Trick W, Anderson D, et al. Interrater reliability of surveillance for ventilator-associated events and pneumonia. Infect Control Hosp Epidemiol 2016;38:1–7.

15. Klompas M, Khan Y, Kleinman K, et al. Multicenter evaluation of a novel surveillance paradigm for complications of mechanical ventilation. PLoS One 2011; 6(3):e18062.

16. Klompas M. The paradox of ventilator-associated pneumonia prevention measures. Crit Care 2009;13(5):315.

17. Bonten MJ. Healthcare epidemiology: ventilator-associated pneumonia: preventing the inevitable. Clin Infect Dis 2011;52(1):115–21.

18. Khan R, Al-Dorzi HM, Al-Attas K, et al. The impact of implementing multifaceted interventions on the prevention of ventilator-associated pneumonia. Am J Infect Control 2016;44(3):320–6.

19. Meagher AD, Lind M, Senekjian L, et al. Ventilator-associated events, not ventilator-associated pneumonia, is associated with higher mortality in trauma patients. J Trauma Acute Care Surg 2019;87(2):307–14.

20. Nguile-Makao M, Zahar JR, Francais A, et al. Attributable mortality of ventilator-associated pneumonia: respective impact of main characteristics at ICU admission and VAP onset using conditional logistic regression and multi-state models. Intensive Care Med 2010;36(5):781–9.

21. Melsen WG, Rovers MM, Groenwold RH, et al. Attributable mortality of ventilator-associated pneumonia: a meta-analysis of individual patient data from randomised prevention studies. Lancet Infect Dis 2013;13(8):665–71.

22. Nuckchady D, Heckman MG, Diehl NN, et al. Assessment of an automated surveillance system for detection of initial ventilator-associated events. Am J Infect Control 2015;43(10):1119–21.

23. Mann T, Ellsworth J, Huda N, et al. Building and validating a computerized algorithm for surveillance of ventilator-associated events. Infect Control Hosp Epidemiol 2015;36(9):999–1003.

24. Klein Klouwenberg PM, van Mourik MS, Ong DS, et al. Electronic implementation of a novel surveillance paradigm for ventilator-associated events: feasibility and validation. Am J Respir Crit Care Med 2014;189(8):947–55.

25. Stevens JP, Silva G, Gillis J, et al. Automated surveillance for ventilator-associated events. Chest 2014;146(6):1612–8.

26. Resetar E, McMullen KM, Russo AJ, et al. Development, implementation and use of electronic surveillance for ventilator-associated events (VAE) in adults. AMIA Annu Symp Proc 2014;2014:1010–7.

27. He Q, Wang W, Zhu S, et al. The epidemiology and clinical outcomes of ventilator-associated events among 20,769 mechanically ventilated patients at intensive care units: an observational study. Crit Care 2021;25(1):44.

28. Smith PF, Hadler JL, Stanbury M, et al. "Blueprint version 2.0": updating public health surveillance for the 21st century. J Public Health Manag Pract 2013;19(3): 231–9.

29. Boyer AF, Schoenberg N, Babcock H, et al. A prospective evaluation of ventilator-associated conditions and infection-related ventilator-associated conditions. Chest 2015;147:68–81.

30. Klompas M, Kleinman K, Murphy MV. Descriptive epidemiology and attributable morbidity of ventilator-associated events. Infect Control Hosp Epidemiol 2014; 35(5):502–10.

31. Muscedere J, Sinuff T, Heyland D, et al. The clinical impact and preventability of ventilator-associated conditions in critically ill mechanically ventilated patients. Chest 2013;144(5):1453–60.

32. Hayashi Y, Morisawa K, Klompas M, et al. Toward improved surveillance: the impact of ventilator-associated complications on length of stay and antibiotic use in patients in intensive care units. Clin Infect Dis 2013;56(4):471–7.

33. Chao WC, Chang WL, Wu CL, et al. Using objective fluid balance data to identify pulmonary edema in subjects with ventilator-associated events. Respir Care 2018;63(11):1413–20.

34. Kobayashi H, Uchino S, Takinami M, et al. The impact of ventilator-associated events in critically Ill subjects with prolonged mechanical ventilation. Respir Care 2017;62(11):1379–86.

35. Liu J, Zhang S, Chen J, et al. Risk factors for ventilator-associated events: a prospective cohort study. Am J Infect Control 2019;47(7):744–9.

36. Zhu S, Wang W, Kang Y, et al. Clinical outcomes and risk factors for mortality from ventilator-associated events: a registry-based cohort study among 30,830 intensive care unit patients. Infect Control Hosp Epidemiol 2021;1–8.

37. Magill SS, Li Q, Gross C, et al. Incidence and characteristics of ventilator-associated events reported to the National Healthcare Safety Network in 2014. Crit Care Med 2016;44(12):2154–62.

38. Ramírez-Estrada S, Lagunes L, Peña-López Y, et al. Assessing predictive accuracy for outcomes of ventilator-associated events in an international cohort: the EUVAE study. Intensive Care Med 2018;44(8):1212–20.

39. Nakahashi S, Imai H, Imanaka H, et al. Ventilator-associated events: prevalence and mortality in Japan. J Thorac Dis 2018;10(12):6942–9.

40. Nakahashi S, Yamada T, Ogura T, et al. Association of patient care with ventilator-associated conditions in critically Ill patients: risk factor analysis. PLoS One 2016;11(4):e0153060.

41. Rello J, Ramírez-Estrada S, Romero A, et al. Factors associated with ventilator-associated events: an international multicenter prospective cohort study. Eur J Clin Microbiol Infect Dis 2019;38(9):1693–9.

42. Ogbu OC, Martin GS, Sevransky JE, et al. High tidal volumes are independently associated with development of a ventilator-associated condition in the ICU. Am J Respir Crit Care Med 2015;191:A3117.

43. Khan RM, Al-Juaid M, Al-Mutairi H, et al. Implementing the comprehensive unit-based safety program model to improve the management of mechanically ventilated patients in Saudi Arabia. Am J Infect Control 2019;47(1):51–8.

44. Fan Y, Gao F, Wu Y, et al. Does ventilator-associated event surveillance detect ventilator-associated pneumonia in intensive care units? A systematic review and meta-analysis. Crit Care 2016;20(1):338.

45. Bouadma L, Sonneville R, Garrouste-Orgeas M, et al. Ventilator-associated events: prevalence, outcome, and relationship with ventilator-associated pneumonia. Crit Care Med 2015;43(9):1798–806.

46. Whiting J, Edriss H, Nugent K. Frequency and etiology of ventilator-associated events in the medical intensive care unit. Am J Med Sci 2015;350(6):453–7.

47. Lewis SC, Li L, Murphy MV, et al. Risk factors for ventilator-associated events: a case-control multivariable analysis. Crit Care Med 2014;42(8):1839–48.

48. Kubbara A, Barnett WR, Safi F, et al. Case-control study investigating parameters affecting ventilator-associated events in mechanically ventilated patients. Am J Infect Control 2019;47(4):462–4.

49. He S, Wu F, Wu X, et al. Ventilator-associated events after cardiac surgery: evidence from 1,709 patients. J Thorac Dis 2018;10(2):776–83.
50. Klompas M, Li L, Szumita P, et al. Associations between different sedatives and ventilator-associated events, length-of-stay, and mortality in mechanically ventilated patients. Chest 2016;149:1373–9.
51. Harris BD, Thomas GA, Greene MH, et al. Ventilator bundle compliance and risk of ventilator-associated events. Infect Control Hosp Epidemiol 2018;39(6):637–43.
52. Klompas M. Ventilator-associated events surveillance: a patient safety opportunity. Curr Opin Crit Care 2013;19(5):424–31.
53. Klompas M. Potential strategies to prevent ventilator-associated events. Am J Respir Crit Care Med 2015;192(12):1420–30.
54. Shehabi Y, Bellomo R, Reade MC, et al. Early intensive care sedation predicts long-term mortality in ventilated critically ill patients. Am J Respir Crit Care Med 2012;186(8):724–31.
55. Shehabi Y, Chan L, Kadiman S, et al. Sedation depth and long-term mortality in mechanically ventilated critically ill adults: a prospective longitudinal multicentre cohort study. Intensive Care Med 2013;39(5):910–8.
56. Klompas M, Anderson D, Trick W, et al. The preventability of ventilator-associated events. The CDC prevention epicenters wake up and breathe collaborative. Am J Respir Crit Care Med 2015;191(3):292–301.
57. Aragón RE, Proaño A, Mongilardi N, et al. Sedation practices and clinical outcomes in mechanically ventilated patients in a prospective multicenter cohort. Crit Care 2019;23(1):130.
58. Metheny NA, Clouse RE, Chang YH, et al. Tracheobronchial aspiration of gastric contents in critically ill tube-fed patients: frequency, outcomes, and risk factors. Crit Care Med 2006;34(4):1007–15.
59. Nseir S, Makris D, Mathieu D, et al. Intensive care unit-acquired infection as a side effect of sedation. Crit Care 2010;14(2):R30.
60. Barr J, Fraser GL, Puntillo K, et al. Clinical practice guidelines for the management of pain, agitation, and delirium in adult patients in the intensive care unit. Crit Care Med 2013;41(1):263–306.
61. Zhang Z, Chen K, Ni H, et al. Sedation of mechanically ventilated adults in intensive care unit: a network meta-analysis. Sci Rep 2017;7(1):44979.
62. Esteban A, Frutos F, Tobin MJ, et al. A comparison of four methods of weaning patients from mechanical ventilation. Spanish Lung Failure Collaborative Group. N Engl J Med 1995;332(6):345–50.
63. Ely EW, Baker AM, Dunagan DP, et al. Effect on the duration of mechanical ventilation of identifying patients capable of breathing spontaneously. N Engl J Med 1996;335(25):1864–9.
64. Kress JP, Pohlman AS, O'Connor MF, et al. Daily interruption of sedative infusions in critically ill patients undergoing mechanical ventilation. N Engl J Med 2000;342(20):1471–7.
65. Girard TD, Kress JP, Fuchs BD, et al. Efficacy and safety of a paired sedation and ventilator weaning protocol for mechanically ventilated patients in intensive care (Awakening and Breathing Controlled trial): a randomised controlled trial. Lancet 2008;371(9607):126–34.
66. Posa P, Barnes D, Bogan B, et al. Compliance with spontaneous breathing trial protocol associated with lower VAE rates. Crit Care Med 2014;42(Suppl 1):A1547.

67. Chumpia MM, Ganz DA, Chang ET, et al. Reducing the rare event: lessons from the implementation of a ventilator bundle. BMJ Open Qual 2019;8(2):e000426.

68. Mehta S, Burry L, Cook D, et al. Daily sedation interruption in mechanically ventilated critically ill patients cared for with a sedation protocol: a randomized controlled trial. JAMA 2012;308(19):1985–92.

69. Needham DM, Korupolu R, Zanni JM, et al. Early physical medicine and rehabilitation for patients with acute respiratory failure: a quality improvement project. Arch Phys Med Rehabil 2010;91(4):536–42.

70. Engel HJ, Tatebe S, Alonzo PB, et al. Physical therapist-established intensive care unit early mobilization program: quality improvement project for critical care at the University of California San Francisco Medical Center. Phys Ther 2013;93(7):975–85.

71. Fraser D, Spiva L, Forman W, et al. Original research: implementation of an early mobility program in an ICU. Am J Nurs 2015;115(12):49–58.

72. Klein K, Mulkey M, Bena JF, et al. Clinical and psychological effects of early mobilization in patients treated in a neurologic ICU: a comparative study. Crit Care Med 2015;43(4):865–73.

73. Schweickert WD, Pohlman MC, Pohlman AS, et al. Early physical and occupational therapy in mechanically ventilated, critically ill patients: a randomised controlled trial. Lancet 2009;373(9678):1874–82.

74. Titsworth WL, Hester J, Correia T, et al. The effect of increased mobility on morbidity in the neurointensive care unit. J Neurosurg 2012;116(6):1379–88.

75. Nydahl P, Ruhl AP, Bartoszek G, et al. Early mobilization of mechanically ventilated patients: a 1-day point-prevalence study in Germany*. Crit Care Med 2014;42(5):1178–86.

76. The Team Study Investigators. Early mobilization and recovery in mechanically ventilated patients in the ICU: a bi-national, multi-centre, prospective cohort study. Crit Care 2015;19:81.

77. Morris PE, Goad A, Thompson C, et al. Early intensive care unit mobility therapy in the treatment of acute respiratory failure. Crit Care Med 2008;36(8):2238–43.

78. Bailey P, Thomsen GE, Spuhler VJ, et al. Early activity is feasible and safe in respiratory failure patients. Crit Care Med 2007;35(1):139–45.

79. Seaver J, Grant K, Lunn J, et al. A multidisciplinary approach to reducing ventilator-associated events in a busy urban hospital. Am J Infect Control 2020;48(7):828–30.

80. Determann RM, Royakkers A, Wolthuis EK, et al. Ventilation with lower tidal volumes as compared with conventional tidal volumes for patients without acute lung injury: a preventive randomized controlled trial. Crit Care 2010;14(1):R1.

81. Li G, Malinchoc M, Cartin-Ceba R, et al. Eight-year trend of acute respiratory distress syndrome: a population-based study in Olmsted County, Minnesota. Am J Respir Crit Care Med 2011;183(1):59–66.

82. Serpa Neto A, Cardoso SO, Manetta JA, et al. Association between use of lung-protective ventilation with lower tidal volumes and clinical outcomes among patients without acute respiratory distress syndrome: a meta-analysis. JAMA 2012; 308(16):1651–9.

83. Serpa Neto A, Simonis FD, Barbas CS, et al. Lung-protective ventilation with low tidal volumes and the occurrence of pulmonary complications in patients without acute respiratory distress syndrome: a systematic review and individual patient data analysis. Crit Care Med 2015;43:2155–63.

84. Gajic O, Frutos-Vivar F, Esteban A, et al. Ventilator settings as a risk factor for acute respiratory distress syndrome in mechanically ventilated patients. Intensive Care Med 2005;31(7):922–6.

85. Mekontso Dessap A, Katsahian S, Roche-Campo F, et al. Ventilator-associated pneumonia during weaning from mechanical ventilation: role of fluid management. Chest 2014;146:58–65.

86. Jia X, Malhotra A, Saeed M, et al. Risk factors for ARDS in patients receiving mechanical ventilation for > 48 h. Chest 2008;133(4):853–61.

87. Wiedemann HP, Wheeler AP, Bernard GR, et al. Comparison of two fluid-management strategies in acute lung injury. N Engl J Med 2006;354(24): 2564–75.

88. Rosenberg AL, Dechert RE, Park PK, et al. Review of a large clinical series: association of cumulative fluid balance on outcome in acute lung injury: a retrospective review of the ARDSnet tidal volume study cohort. J Intensive Care Med 2009;24(1):35–46.

89. Grissom CK, Hirshberg EL, Dickerson JB, et al. Fluid management with a simplified conservative protocol for the acute respiratory distress syndrome. Crit Care Med 2015;43(2):288–95.

90. Rohde JM, Dimcheff DE, Blumberg N, et al. Health care-associated infection after red blood cell transfusion: a systematic review and meta-analysis. JAMA 2014;311(13):1317–26.

91. Mitchell KH, Carlbom D, Caldwell E, et al. Volume overload: prevalence, risk factors, and functional outcome in survivors of septic shock. Ann Am Thorac Soc 2015;12(12):1837–44.

92. Cocoros N, Priebe G, Gray J, et al. Factors associated with pediatric ventilator-associated conditions in six U.S. hospitals: a nested case-control study. Pediatr Crit Care Med 2017;18:1.

93. Klompas M, Branson R, Eichenwald EC, et al. Strategies to prevent ventilator-associated pneumonia in acute care hospitals: 2014 update. Infect Control Hosp Epidemiol 2014;35(8):915–36.

94. Krein SL, Fowler KE, Ratz D, et al. Preventing device-associated infections in US hospitals: national surveys from 2005 to 2013. BMJ Qual Saf 2015;24:385–92.

95. Wang L, Li X, Yang Z, et al. Semi-recumbent position versus supine position for the prevention of ventilator-associated pneumonia in adults requiring mechanical ventilation. Cochrane Database Syst Rev 2016;2016(1):CD009946.

96. Klompas M, Speck K, Howell MD, et al. Reappraisal of routine oral care with chlorhexidine gluconate for patients receiving mechanical ventilation: systematic review and meta-analysis. JAMA Intern Med 2014;174(5):751–61.

97. Price R, MacLennan G, Glen J. Selective digestive or oropharyngeal decontamination and topical oropharyngeal chlorhexidine for prevention of death in general intensive care: systematic review and network meta-analysis. BMJ 2014; 348:g2197.

98. Deschepper M, Waegeman W, Eeckloo K, et al. Effects of chlorhexidine gluconate oral care on hospital mortality: a hospital-wide, observational cohort study. Intensive Care Med 2018;44(7):1017–26.

99. Hirata K, Kurokawa A. Chlorhexidine gluconate ingestion resulting in fatal respiratory distress syndrome. Vet Hum Toxicol 2002;44(2):89–91.

100. Orito K, Hashida M, Hirata K, et al. Effects of single intratracheal exposure to chlorhexidine gluconate on the rat lung. Drug Chem Toxicol 2006;29(1):1–9.

101. Xue Y, Zhang S, Yang Y, et al. Acute pulmonary toxic effects of chlorhexidine (CHX) following an intratracheal instillation in rats. Hum Exp Toxicol 2011; 30(11):1795–803.

102. Seguin P, Laviolle B, Dahyot-Fizelier C, et al. Effect of oropharyngeal povidone-iodine preventive oral care on ventilator-associated pneumonia in severely brain-injured or cerebral hemorrhage patients: a multicenter, randomized controlled trial. Crit Care Med 2014;42:1–8.

103. Panchabhai TS, Dangayach NS, Krishnan A, et al. Oropharyngeal cleansing with 0.2% chlorhexidine for prevention of nosocomial pneumonia in critically ill patients: an open-label randomized trial with 0.01% potassium permanganate as control. Chest 2009;135(5):1150–6.

104. Mori H, Hirasawa H, Oda S, et al. Oral care reduces incidence of ventilator-associated pneumonia in ICU populations. Intensive Care Med 2006;32(2):230–6.

105. Alhazzani W, Smith O, Muscedere J, et al. Toothbrushing for critically ill mechanically ventilated patients: a systematic review and meta-analysis of randomized trials evaluating ventilator-associated pneumonia. Crit Care Med 2013;41(2):646–55.

106. Wittekamp BH, Plantinga NL, Cooper BS, et al. Decontamination strategies and bloodstream infections with antibiotic-resistant microorganisms in ventilated patients: a randomized clinical trial. JAMA 2018;320(20):2087–98.

107. de Smet AM, Kluytmans JA, Cooper BS, et al. Decontamination of the digestive tract and oropharynx in ICU patients. N Engl J Med 2009;360(1):20–31.

108. de Smet AM, Kluytmans JA, Blok HE, et al. Selective digestive tract decontamination and selective oropharyngeal decontamination and antibiotic resistance in patients in intensive-care units: an open-label, clustered group-randomised, crossover study. Lancet Infect Dis 2011;11:372–80.

109. Silvestri L, van Saene HK, Milanese M, et al. Selective decontamination of the digestive tract reduces bacterial bloodstream infection and mortality in critically ill patients. Systematic review of randomized, controlled trials. J Hosp Infect 2007;65(3):187–203.

110. Buelow E, Gonzalez TB, Versluis D, et al. Effects of selective digestive decontamination (SDD) on the gut resistome. J Antimicrob Chemother 2014;69(8): 2215–23.

111. Daneman N, Sarwar S, Fowler RA, et al. Effect of selective decontamination on antimicrobial resistance in intensive care units: a systematic review and meta-analysis. Lancet Infect Dis 2013;13(4):328–41.

112. Noteboom Y, Ong DS, Oostdijk EA, et al. Antibiotic-induced within-host resistance development of gram-negative bacteria in patients receiving selective decontamination or standard care. Crit Care Med 2015;43(12):2582–8.

113. Houben AJ, Oostdijk EA, van der Voort PH, et al. Selective decontamination of the oropharynx and the digestive tract, and antimicrobial resistance: a 4 year ecological study in 38 intensive care units in the Netherlands. J Antimicrob Chemother 2014;69(3):797–804.

114. Muscedere J, Rewa O, McKechnie K, et al. Subglottic secretion drainage for the prevention of ventilator-associated pneumonia: a systematic review and meta-analysis. Crit Care Med 2011;39(8):1985–91.

115. Dezfulian C, Shojania K, Collard HR, et al. Subglottic secretion drainage for preventing ventilator-associated pneumonia: a meta-analysis. Am J Med 2005; 118(1):11–8.

116. Wang F, Bo L, Tang L, et al. Subglottic secretion drainage for preventing ventilator-associated pneumonia: an updated meta-analysis of randomized controlled trials. J Trauma Acute Care Surg 2012;72(5):1276–85.

117. Frost SA, Azeem A, Alexandrou E, et al. Subglottic secretion drainage for preventing ventilator associated pneumonia: a meta-analysis. Aust Crit Care 2013;26:180–8.
118. Valles J, Artigas A, Rello J, et al. Continuous aspiration of subglottic secretions in preventing ventilator-associated pneumonia. Ann Intern Med 1995;122(3): 179–86.
119. Caroff DA, Li L, Muscedere J, et al. Subglottic secretion drainage and objective outcomes: a systematic review and meta-analysis. Crit Care Med 2016;44(4): 830–40.
120. Pozuelo-Carrascosa DP, Herráiz-Adillo Á, Alvarez-Bueno C, et al. Subglottic secretion drainage for preventing ventilator-associated pneumonia: an overview of systematic reviews and an updated meta-analysis. Eur Respir Rev 2020; 29(155):190107.
121. Rawat N, Yang T, Ali KJ, et al. Two-state collaborative study of a multifaceted intervention to decrease ventilator-associated events. Crit Care Med 2017; 45(7):1208–15.
122. Anand T, Ponce S, Pakula A, et al. Results from a quality improvement project to decrease infection-related ventilator events in trauma patients at a community teaching hospital. Am Surg 2018;84(10):1701–4.
123. Cocoros NM, Kleinman K, Priebe GP, et al. Ventilator-associated events in neonates and children-a new paradigm. Crit Care Med 2016;44(1):14–22.
124. Centers for Disease Control and Prevention. Pediatric Ventilator-Associated Event (PedVAE) protocol. 2021. Available at: https://www.cdc.gov/nhsn/pdfs/pscmanual/pedvae-current-508.pdf. Accessed February 27, 2021.
125. Cocoros NM, Priebe GP, Logan LK, et al. A pediatric approach to ventilator-associated events surveillance. Infect Control Hosp Epidemiol 2017;38(3): 327–33.
126. Phongjitsiri S, Coss-Bu J, Kennedy C, et al. The centers for disease control and prevention's new definitions for complications of mechanical ventilation shift the focus of quality surveillance and predict clinical outcomes in a PICU. Crit Care Med 2015;43(11):2446–51.
127. Guess R, Vaewpanich J, Coss-Bu JA, et al. Risk factors for ventilator-associated events in a PICU. Pediatr Crit Care Med 2018;19(1):e7–13.
128. Beardsley AL, Nitu ME, Cox EG, et al. An evaluation of various ventilator-associated infection criteria in a PICU. Pediatr Crit Care 2016;17:73–80.
129. Cirulis MM, Hamele MT, Stockmann CR, et al. Comparison of the new adult ventilator-associated event criteria to the centers for disease control and prevention pediatric ventilator-associated pneumonia definition (PNU2) in a population of pediatric traumatic brain injury patients. Pediatr Crit Care Med 2016; 17(2):157–64.
130. Peña-López Y, Pujol M, Campins M, et al. Assessing prediction accuracy for outcomes of ventilator-associated events and infections in critically ill children: a prospective cohort study. Clin Microbiol Infect 2018;24(7):732–7.
131. Vaewpanich J, Akcan-Arikan A, Coss-Bu JA, et al. Fluid overload and kidney injury score as a predictor for ventilator-associated events. Front Pediatr 2019;7:204.
132. Lilly CM, Landry KE, Sood RN, et al. Prevalence and test characteristics of national health safety network ventilator-associated events. Crit Care Med 2014;42: 2019–28.

Surgical Site Infections

Jessica Seidelman, MD, MPH[a,b,*], Deverick J. Anderson, MD, MPH[a,b]

KEYWORDS

- Surgical site infection • Health care–associated infection • Risk • Prevention
- Outcome

KEY POINTS

- Surgical site infections (SSIs) are associated with prolonged hospitalizations, death, and overall poor patient outcomes.
- SSIs are typically caused by pathogens inoculated at the time of surgery from the patient's own flora.
- SSI acquisition depends on exposure to bacteria and the host's ability to control the inevitable bacterial contamination of the surgical wound.
- The 9 core best practices to reduce SSIs address preoperative bathing, antimicrobial prophylaxis, preoperative surgical site preparation, surgical hand preparation, normothermia, hyperoxygenation, wound protectors, glucose control, and perioperative checklist.
- SSI surveillance and feedback decrease SSI rates and are recommended by Centers for Disease Control and Prevention.

INTRODUCTION

Surgical site infections (SSIs) are a leading cause of health care–associated infections (HAIs). These infections can range in severity from nuisance to life threatening; overall, they contribute to substantial patient suffering. A large portion of SSIs are preventable, and SSI prevention is a key patient safety matter that requires teamwork among multiple health care personnel, including surgeons, nurses, anesthetists, and infection preventionists. This article provides updates to the epidemiology and diagnosis of SSIs with particular emphasis on risk factors, evidence-based prevention strategies, and surveillance.

[a] Division of Infectious Diseases and International Health, Department of Medicine, Duke University School of Medicine, Duke University, Durham, NC, USA; [b] Duke Center for Antimicrobial Stewardship and Infection Prevention, Duke University Medical Center, Durham, NC, USA
* Corresponding author. 315 Trent Dr Hanes House, Room 145, Durham, NC 27710.
E-mail address: jessica.seidelman@duke.edu

Infect Dis Clin N Am 35 (2021) 901–929
https://doi.org/10.1016/j.idc.2021.07.006
0891-5520/21/© 2021 Elsevier Inc. All rights reserved.

EPIDEMIOLOGY

SSIs are the most common and most costly HAI in the United States, accounting for almost a quarter of all HAIs.[1,2] Although the risk of SSI is generally low, SSIs are common because of the volume of surgical procedures performed across the United States. In the United States in 2014, 17.2 million hospital visits (ambulatory or inpatient) included invasive, therapeutic surgeries.[3] SSIs occur in 1% to 5% of patients undergoing inpatient surgery.[4,5] Rates are generally lower among procedures performed in outpatient settings. Overall, approximately 300,000 SSIs occur each year, although this estimate likely underrepresents the true SSI burden because of limitations in surveillance and diagnosis.[4,5] SSIs are even more common in low-income and middle-income countries, occurring in 1% to 24% of procedures performed.[6]

Overall, rates of SSI are decreasing in the United States. Among 148 hospitals participating in serial point prevalence surveys performed by the Centers for Disease Control and Prevention (CDC), the rate of SSI decreased from 0.97 per 100 procedures in 2011 (n = 11,282 patients reviewed) to 0.56 per 100 procedures in 2015 (n = 12,299 patients reviewed; P = .001).[7] Similarly, the publicly reported rates of SSI following abdominal hysterectomy and colon surgery decreased approximately 10% in 2017 compared with the national baseline reported in 2016, although the decreases were not statistically significant.[8] However, decreases in SSI have been modest compared with decreases observed in several other HAIs, including central line–associated bloodstream infection, catheter-associated urinary tract infection, methicillin-resistant *Staphylococcus aureus* (MRSA) bacteremia, and *Clostridioides difficile* infection.

Rates of SSI vary by type of procedure and by setting. The CDC's National Healthcare Safety Network (NHSN) no longer routinely reports national rates of SSI following commonly performed procedures; therefore, most nationwide estimates currently used are from data reported almost 10 years ago. Clean-contaminated and dirty procedures, including procedures that enter a nonsterile viscera, have higher rates of SSI than clean procedures. For example, rates of SSI following colon, rectal, or other gastrointestinal (GI) procedures range from 4% to 25%, whereas the rate of SSI following coronary artery bypass grafting is approximately 3% and following hip or knee arthroplasty is 1% or lower.[9] In most cases, rates of SSI at surgical centers are inversely associated with surgical volume. That is, the more procedures performed, the lower the rate of SSI.[8] Although referral centers typically care for more complex patients and perform higher-risk procedures, these risks are often offset by high surgical volume and experience. Small community hospitals with low volume have higher rates of SSI than higher-volume community hospitals.[10]

CLINICAL OUTCOMES

SSIs lead to significant patient morbidity and mortality. Each SSI is associated with approximately 7 to 11 additional postoperative hospital days.[2,11] In total, patients with SSIs have 3.7 million excess hospital days each year.[12] Surgical patients who develop an SSI have a risk of death that is, between 2-fold and 11-fold higher than patients without an SSI[13]; 77% of deaths in patients with SSI are directly attributable to SSI.[14] Investigators from the Agency for Healthcare Research and Quality (AHRQ) estimated excess mortality related to SSI was 0.026 (95% confidence interval [CI], 0.009–0.059, meaning 26 deaths occur for every 1000 SSIs).[15] Each SSI leads to approximately $25,000 of additional costs, although attributable costs of SSI vary depending on the type of operative procedure and the type of infecting pathogen.[11,13,15] Overall,

SSIs are estimated to account for $3.5 billion to $10 billion annually in United States health care expenditures using the CPI (consumer price index for inpatient hospital services with all cost estimates adjusted for 2007 dollars).[5]

EVALUATION

Clinically, a surgical wound is considered infected when purulent drainage is present at the incision site or there is evidence of abscess involving the surgical bed. However, other presentations of surgical wound infections also occur, including wound dehiscence, nonpurulent drainage, local erythema, induration, pain, or systemic signs of infection. Because of the varied presentation of SSIs, many of which overlap with noninfectious causes, no single clinical definition of SSI exists. Instead, the diagnosis of SSI is typically made based on a constellation of clinical and examination features, laboratory and microbiologic data, and radiography results.

Despite the variability in clinical presentations of SSIs, specific definitions of SSI are used for epidemiologic and surveillance purposes. The NHSN provides the most commonly used SSI definitions. These definitions were designed to be objective and easy to apply but also flexible enough to identify clinically relevant SSIs with varied presentations.[16] NHSN categorizes SSIs into 3 groups: superficial incisional (involving the skin or subcutaneous tissue layers of the incision), deep incisional (involving muscle or connective tissue layers of the incision), and organ/space (involving structures, organs, or spaces deep to the incision) (**Fig. 1, Table 1**). Examples of organ/space infection include intra-abdominal abscess following colon surgery, periprosthetic joint infection following joint arthroplasty, and mediastinitis following cardiac surgery. Per NHSN definitions, surveillance for superficial-incisional infections is conducted for 30 days, whereas surveillance for deep-incisional and organ/space infections is conducted for 30 or 90 days, depending on the index surgical procedure.

Note that surveillance definitions have changed over time and that various epidemiologic surveys and studies of SSI prevention have used variable case-finding methods (eg, active vs passive surveillance), criteria for inclusion (eg, index procedure vs all procedures), depth of infection (eg, superficial-incisional, deep-incisional, or organ/space infection), and surveillance periods (eg, 30 vs 90 days). For example, 10% fewer SSIs were identified when, compared with previously used NHSN definitions, updated 2013 NHSN definitions that shortened surveillance periods were applied retrospectively to SSI surveillance data from a network of 35 hospitals and 2 ambulatory surgery centers.[17] Therefore, it is important to understand the surveillance criteria used when interpreting SSI data from different surveys or time periods, and how different criteria can affect reported rates.

CURRENT EVIDENCE

SSIs are typically caused by pathogens inoculated at the time of surgery. Most SSIs are caused by the patients' endogenous flora. However, exogenous sources of wound contamination are possible.[14,18] Most SSIs are caused by skin pathogens, although enteric pathogens are frequently seen in SSIs following GI procedures (**Table 2**).[19] Overall, S aureus is the most common cause of SSI. Although MRSA was previously a more frequent cause of SSI than methicillin-sensitive S aureus (MSSA), rates of MRSA SSI have declined; MSSA is now a more common cause of SSI than MRSA.[9] This trend is important because SSIs caused by resistant pathogens such as MRSA lead to worse clinical outcomes than SSIs caused by susceptible pathogens.[11] Outbreaks involving atypical organisms such as *Mycoplasma, Ureaplasma, Candida*

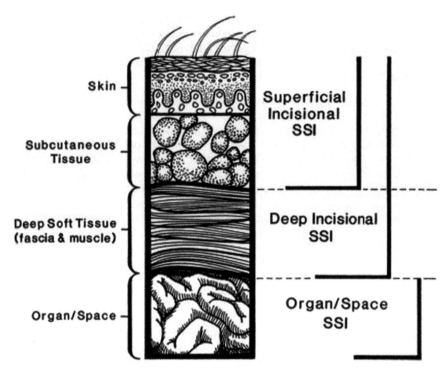

Fig. 1. NHSN categorization of SSIs. (*From* Horan TC, Gaynes RP, Martone WJ, Jarvis WR, Emori TG. CDC definitions of nosocomial surgical site infections, 1992: a modification of CDC definitions of surgical wound infections. Infect Control Hosp Epidemiol. 1992;13(10):606-608; with permission)

and other fungi, *Nocardia*, *Rhodococcus*, and nontuberculous mycobacteria (including rapidly growing mycobacteria) are uncommon, but have been described.[20–22]

Endogenous Contamination

Most SSIs are caused by the patients' endogenous flora contaminating the surgical site.[18] Even an inoculum as low as 100 colony-forming units into the wound can lead to an SSI.[23] Several factors may modify the risk of surgical wound contamination by endogenous flora.

Perioperative antibiotics

The absence of antibiotic prophylaxis also significantly increases the risk of SSI.[24] Contamination of operative sites, even clean ones, is unavoidable despite the best preparation and operative technique. The goal of antimicrobial prophylaxis is to reduce the risk of SSI by reducing the burden of microorganisms at the surgical site during the operative procedure.

Skin antisepsis

In addition, lack or inappropriate application of preoperative skin antiseptics increases the risk of SSI by failing to remove transient organisms from the skin where a surgical incision will be made. Effectiveness of incisional site preparation depends on correct application. Although skin disinfection before surgery drastically reduces the number

Table 1
Summary of National Healthcare Safety Network surveillance criteria for surgical site infection based on 2021 definitions

Superficial Incisional	Deep Incisional	Organ/Space
Any of the following: • Purulent drainage • Organism identified from aseptically obtained specimen or superficial incision deliberately opened by surgeon, attending physician, or designee • Diagnosis of superficial incisional SSI by surgeon, attending physician, or other designee culture not obtained	Any of the following: • Purulent drainage from the deep incision • A deep incision that spontaneously dehisces or is deliberately opened or aspirated by a surgeon, attending physician, or designee, and organism identified from deep soft tissues of the incision and 1 or more of the following symptoms: fever >38°C, localized pain or tenderness • Abscess or other evidence of infection involving the deep incision that is detected on gross anatomic or histopathologic examination, or imaging test	Any of the following: • Purulent drainage from a drain that is placed into the organ/space • Organism identified from fluid or tissue in the organ/space • Abscess or other evidence of infection involving the organ/space that is detected on gross anatomic or histopathologic examination, or imaging test evidence suggestive of infection

Deep incisional involves part of the incision deeper than the fascial layer. Organ/space involves any part of the body that is deeper than the muscle/fascial layers and was manipulated or entered during the operative procedure.

Modified from Centers for Disease Control and Prevention. Surgical Site Infection (SSI) Event Web site. https://www.cdc.gove/nhsn/pdfs/pscmanual/9pscssicurrent.pdf. Accessed 11/20/20.

of bacteria on the skin's surface, recolonization of the skin with bacteria from deeper skin layers and hair follicles may occur during the operation.[25]

Preoperative hair removal

Preoperative shaving of the surgical site is associated with a significantly higher SSI risk than either the use of depilatory agents or no hair removal.[14] One study found that SSI rates for patients who shaved before surgery was 5.6% compared with an SSI rate of 0.6% in patients who removed hair via depilatory agent or did not remove hair at all. The increased risk of SSI with shaving is attributed to microscopic cuts in the skin that later serve as niduses for bacteria to multiply. In addition, timing of hair removal is a key factor for development of SSI. One study found that patients who shaved immediately before the operation compared with patients who shaved within 24 hours preoperatively had lower rates of SSI (3.1% vs 7.1%).[26] Furthermore, if patients shaved more than 24 hours before operation, their SSI rates exceeded 20%.[26] Similarly, clipping hair immediately before an operation is associated with a lower risk of SSI than shaving or clipping the night before surgery (1.8% vs 4.0%).[27] Depilatory agents are associated with lower SSI risk compared with shaving or clipping[26]; however, these products can produce hypersensitivity reactions, which can compromise the integrity of the skin.[26]

	Clean Cardiac Bypass and Joint Arthoplasties[81,a] N = 6263 n (%); Rank	Community Hospitals[9,b] N = 3988 SSIs n (%); Rank
Table 2 Common causes of surgical site infections		
Organism		
S aureus	2704 (41); 1	1357 (34); 1
MSSA	1520 (23)	683 (17)
MRSA	1184 (18)	674 (17)
Coagulase-negative staphylococci	1085 (17); 2	340 (9); 4
Enterococcus species	433 (7); 3	467 (12); 3
Pseudomonas aeruginosa	339 (5); 4	168 (4); 7
Escherichia coli	314 (5); 5	482 (12); 2
Streptococcus species	278 (4); 6	242 (6); 5

Abbreviation: MSSA, methicillin-sensitive S aureus.
 [a] 6263 complex SSIs identified after 680,489 procedures performed in 880 hospitals over a 4-year period.
 [b] 3,988 complex SSIs identified after 532,694 procedures performed in 29 community hospitals over a 5-year period.

Exogenous Contamination

Length of operation
Prolonged operative time may increase the risk of SSI. The increased risk may be related to increased wound contamination, increased tissue damage (eg, bleeding, cautery, suture), or some combination of these factors.[28]

Surgical technique
Poor surgical technique is widely thought to increase SSI risk.[14] Examples of poor surgical technique that may increase subsequent SSI risk include failure to maintain adequate blood supply, rough manipulation of tissues, accidental entry into a hollow viscus, leaving behind devitalized tissue, and inappropriate use of drains and sutures. In general, the impact of poor surgical technique is difficult to quantify or study.

Foreign material
Any foreign material, such as sutures or drains, promotes inflammation at the surgical site and increases the risk of SSI.[29] Furthermore, the presence of foreign material decreases the inoculum required to cause an SSI from 10^6 to 10^2 organisms.[30]

Wound contamination from operating room personnel
Health care personnel's hands and fingernails harbor bacteria that may be introduced into the surgical site.[31] Application of surgical gloves substantially reduces but does not prevent the potential passage of microorganisms to the patient. Gloves can become perforated during surgery and bacteria on gloved hands can multiply rapidly. Therefore, absence of appropriate hand antisepsis can expose patients to potential pathogens harbored on operating room personnel's hands. Furthermore, watches, long finger nails, artificial nails, and finger rings can increase bacterial counts on the hands of operating room personnel.[32,33] The number of SSIs caused by exogenous flora is unknown, although several outbreaks of SSI have been attributed to operating room personnel.

Airborne contamination

Transmission of bacteria from operating room personnel to patients can occur through several other routes, including shedding of bacteria from the personnel's hair, skin, and clothing. Actions that increase bacterial air counts are strongly associated with SSI risk.[34] Most of the airborne contamination comes from persons present in the operating room and their movements.[35] Several studies investigated the impact of operating room door openings on air quality, and the results were mixed.[36] However, some data suggest a positive correlation between high door opening rates and numbers of microorganisms in air samples.[37]

Wound care

Postoperative wound care practices are thought to modify risk of SSI.[38] Wounds that remain uncovered after surgery may be subject to environmental contamination or ongoing drainage that decreases the integrity of the surrounding skin.[39]

Intra-articular steroid injections

The relationship between intra-articular steroid injections and incidence of SSIs is under ongoing investigation. Infection may be introduced at the time of injection, especially if rigorous antisepsis is not applied.[40] In addition, the intra-articular steroid may decrease the host immune response to the introduction of such bacteria. Although some studies have shown an increase in SSI incidence in patients who receive intra-articular steroid injections,[41] other trials show no difference in SSI risk between patients who receive intra-articular steroid injections and those who do not.[42] Current clinical guidelines from the American Academy of Orthopedic Surgeons (AAOS) do not outline specific recommendations for intra-articular injection administration and SSI prevention.[43]

Periarticular injections

Recently, surgeons have incorporated local analgesia into pain management regimens for patients undergoing joint replacement surgery in order to improve postoperative pain control and promote early activity.[44] Physicians inject a wide variety of medications and often prepare them without the use of a sterile hood. Infection can be introduced when these injections are compounded or at the time of injection. Although no definitive evidence shows an increased risk of SSI associated with use of periarticular injections, medication cocktails should be compounded in a sterile fashion in the pharmacy and be administered with aseptic technique.[45]

Risk Factors

SSI acquisition depends on exposure to bacteria and the host's ability to control the inevitable bacterial contamination of a surgical wound. The likelihood of developing an SSI is a complex interaction among several variables, including overall host characteristics (ie, age, immunosuppression, obesity, diabetes), effectiveness of antimicrobial prophylaxis, surgical site tissue condition and presence of foreign material, and degree of wound contamination.

Table 3 provides a summary of known SSI risk factors, which are also discussed in detail later. Some risk factors that increase risk of SSI are nonmodifiable, such as gender and age. However, other risk factors are modifiable, and their optimization can decrease the likelihood of developing an SSI.

Patient Related, Nonmodifiable

Age

Several studies identify the extremes of age as a risk factor for SSI. The risk of SSI is higher in infants compared with older children and higher among older adults compared

Table 3
Summary of known surgical site infection risk factors

Risk Factor	Pathophysiology
Patient Related, Modifiable	
Diabetes	Hyperglycemia impairs innate immunity mechanism to fight bacteria. In addition, increased glucose level leads to glycosylation of proteins, which in turn slows wound healing[52]
Malnutrition	Poor nutrition leads to poor tissue healing, decreased collagen synthesis, and granuloma formation in surgical wounds. Low albumin level impairs macrophage activation and induces macrophage apoptosis, which decreases innate immunity response. Hypoalbuminemia can lead to tissue edema and leakage of interstitial fluid into the surgical wound[57]
Smoking tobacco	Tobacco smoke impairs wound healing by vasoconstriction, leading to relative ischemia, reduced inflammatory response, and alteration in collagen metabolism[61]
Obesity	Decreased blood flow in adipose tissue leads to less oxygen and antibiotic delivery[64,66,67]
Immunosuppressive medications and conditions	Immunosuppressive medications or clinical conditions blunt the inflammatory phase of wound healing[68,69]
Decreased tissue oxygenation	Decreased tissue oxygenation leads to diminished oxidative killing by neutrophils and impaired tissue healing caused by reduced collagen formation, neovascularization, and epithelialization. Low oxygen levels may decrease the efficacy of perioperative antibiotics[72,73]
Perioperative hypothermia	Perioperative hypothermia impairs host defenses against surgical wound contamination: vasoconstriction causing reduced tissue perfusion to wounded tissue with reduced access for key immune cells, decreased motility of key immune cells, and reduced scar formation[74]
Postoperative hyperglycemia	Cellular functions of leukocyte adherence, chemotaxis, phagocytosis, and bactericidal activity are improved by insulin and better glycemic control, suggesting a direct relation between cellular function deficits and increased blood glucose level[56]
Anticoagulation	Anticoagulants can cause of persistent oozing of the incision, slow wound healing[75]
Blood transfusions	Blood transfusions affect the risk of infection by modulating the immune system[76]

(continued on next page)

Table 3
(continued)

Risk Factor	Pathophysiology
Patient Related, Nonmodifiable	
Age	The skin's dermis and basement membrane thin with increasing age, and the skin loses its supply of cutaneous nerves and blood vessels, which can lead to poor wound healing[46]
History of radiation	Radiation therapy produces underlying tissue damage and contributes to poor wound healing
History of prior SSTI	A prior history of SSTIs may be related to differences in inherent immunity and susceptibility to infection[51]
Exogenous Sources	
Wound contamination from operating room personnel	Transition of skin flora on the hands of health care personnel to the patient and operating room from lack of appropriate hand washing or gloving to surgical sites[23] Movement of microorganisms from surgical staff's hair, mouths, bodies, or shoes to the operating room contaminates surgical wounds[23]
Airborne contamination	Increasing the number of microorganisms in the operating room environment increases opportunity for SSI. Most of the airborne contamination comes from persons present in the operating room and their movements[34,35]
Operation duration	Longer operative duration is associated with increased wound contamination, increased damage to wound cells, and the local environment[28]
Surgical technique	Not maintaining adequate blood supply, not gently handling tissue, inadvertent entry into hollo viscus, leaving behind devitalized tissue, inappropriate use of drains and sutures, and inappropriate postoperative wound management[14]
Foreign material	Foreign material promotes inflammation at the surgical site and increases the risk of SSI[29,30]
Intra-articular steroid injection	Infection may be introduced at the time of injection, especially if rigorous antisepsis is not applied. May decrease the host immune response to the introduction of such bacteria[81]
Periarticular joint injections	Injections are often prepared without the use of a sterile hood; infections can be introduced when these injections are compounded or at the time of infusion,

(continued on next page)

Table 3 (continued)	
Risk Factor	**Pathophysiology**
	because catheters are commonly used to deliver the medications[45]
Wound care	Wounds that remain uncovered after surgery may be subject to environmental contamination or ongoing drainage that decreases the integrity of the surrounding skin[38,39]
Endogenous Sources	
Wound contamination from patient	Shaving creates microscopic cuts in the skin that later serve as niduses for bacteria to multiply[14]
	Absence of appropriate barrier devices and drapes allows bacteria from deeper skin layers and hair follicles to recolonize the surgical site during the operation
	Lack of or inappropriate administration of perioperative antibiotics does not prevent the inevitable burden of microorganisms at surgical site[24]
	Without appropriate surgical site preparation, soil and transient organisms are not removed[117]
	Wound classification delineates the degree of contamination of a surgical wound at the time of the operation[118]

with younger cohorts.[46] With increasing age, the skin's dermis and basement membrane thins. In addition, the skin loses its supply of cutaneous nerves and blood vessels. These physiologic changes contribute to slow or impaired wound healing.[47,48]

However, the risk of SSI may only increase up until a certain age. Kaye and colleagues[49] found that, after age 65 years, the risk of SSI decreased by 1.2% for each additional year of life. Therefore, the risk of SSI may be caused by comorbidities and immunosuppression and not directly by increasing age. Furthermore, this result may indicate a selection bias of healthier older patients for surgery.

History of radiation
History of prior radiation therapy at the site of surgery increases SSI risk because of the risk of underlying tissue damage.[50] Irradiated skin is hypovascular and easily injured with slight trauma. Given the damaged tissue and lack of perfusion, surgical incisions in locations with prior radiation treatment are more likely to develop a wound complication.

History of prior skin and soft tissue infection
History of a prior skin and soft tissue infection (SSTI) is another risk factor for SSI development.[51] Although not fully understood, the increased SSI risk among these patients may reflect differences in inherent immunity and susceptibility to infection.

Patient Related, Modifiable

Diabetes mellitus
Patients with diabetes mellitus are more likely to develop SSIs. In a meta-analysis including 14 prospective studies, patients diagnosed with diabetes were twice as

likely to develop an SSI compared with patients without a diagnosis of diabetes.[52] The increased risk of SSI among patients with diabetes is consistent across multiple surgical procedures and is likely multifactorial.[53] Patients with diabetes have a high incidence of small vessel disease, leading to impaired oxygen and nutrition delivery to peripheral tissues. Hypoxemia and lack of nutritional support reduce the systemic ability to prevent infection.[54] Dronge and colleagues[55] found that patients with a hemoglobin A1c level more than 7% were significantly more likely to develop infectious complications compared with patients with a hemoglobin A1c level less than 7%.

Postoperative hyperglycemia
Postoperative hyperglycemia may increase SSI risk more than a diagnosis of diabetes. Hyperglycemia impairs innate immunity mechanism to fight bacteria. In addition, increased glucose level leads to glycosylation of proteins, which in turn slows wound healing. Latham and colleagues[56] found that hyperglycemia during the immediate postoperative period was an independent risk factor for developing SSI even among patients without a history of diabetes, and the risk of infection correlated with the degree of glucose increase. Patients with blood glucose level of 200 mg/dL or higher within 48 hours after surgery had 2.5 times higher odds of developing an SSI than patients with glucose level less than 200 mg/dL.

Malnutrition
Malnutrition is prevalent among surgical patients. One of the most commonly used markers of malnutrition is albumin, and hypoalbuminemia increases the risk of SSI.[57] Hypoalbuminemia may lead to increased risk of SSI through several mechanisms. First, hypoalbuminemia can lead to poor tissue healing, decreased collagen synthesis, and granuloma formation in surgical wounds.[58] These factors can impair wound healing and predispose the tissue to infection. Second, low albumin level impairs macrophage activation and induces macrophage apoptosis, which decreases innate immunity response.[59] Lastly, hypoalbuminemia can lead to tissue edema and leakage of interstitial fluid into the surgical wound.[60] This fluid can serve as a medium for bacteria to proliferate and ultimately lead to infection.

Smoking
Smoking tobacco is associated with adverse outcomes following surgery, including SSI. Postoperative wound healing complications occur more often in smokers and former smokers compared with those who never smoked. A systematic review identified 4 randomized trials that assessed the effect of preoperative smoking cessation (4-week to 8-week interval of abstinence) on postoperative wound healing. Current or past smokers had an increased risk for postoperative infection (odds ratio [OR], 1.9; CI, 1.0–3.5).[61] Other studies have shown that abstinent smokers have a lower SSI risk than do current smokers.[62]

The many compounds that constitute tobacco smoke impair wound healing and increase SSI risk through several mechanisms.[63] The physiologic mechanisms include vasoconstriction, which causes relative ischemia of operated tissues. Tobacco smoke also leads to a reduced inflammatory response and impaired innate immune system response to bacteria.[63] Lastly, the elements in tobacco smoke can alter collagen metabolism, which is essential for skin and tissue integrity.

Obesity
Obesity is another risk factor associated with developing SSI. One meta-analysis included 20 studies that evaluated SSI outcomes in orthopedic surgeries. The investigators found that the risk of SSI for patients with obesity was almost 2 times the SSI

risk for patients without obesity (risk ratio [RR], 1.915; 95% CI, 1.53–2.40).[64] Studies including colorectal surgery patients (OR, 1.59; 95% CI, 1.32–1.91)[65] and coronary artery bypass surgery patients (OR, 1.8; 95% CI, 1.4–2.3)[66] have reported similar conclusions. An additional recent study also found a trend of increasing risk of SSI for almost all surgery types when body mass index increased from normal to morbidly obese.[67]

Obese patients may be at increased risk for SSI because of depth of adipose tissue, creation of dead space, and decreased blood flow in adipose tissue. Without adequate blood flow reaching the tissues, surgical wounds are less likely to heal. Decreased blood flow may also reduce antibiotic delivery and increase wound tension.[28]

Immunosuppressive medications and conditions
Patients with suppressed immune systems are at increased risk of SSI because the inflammatory phase of wound healing may be blunted. The increase in SSI risk is seen in patients with various levels of immunosuppression, including transplant recipients, patients undergoing chemotherapy, and other patients taking immunosuppressing medications.[68,69] In contrast, glucocorticoids may not affect SSI risk as strongly as other immunosuppressive therapies.[70] Some degree of antiinflammation may prevent wounds from becoming chronically inflamed, whereas significant suppression of inflammation can prevent wound healing.[71]

Decreased tissue oxygenation
Low oxygenation also increases the risk of SSIs. Oxygen tension is often low in wounds and in colorectal anastomoses at the end of surgery, which may reduce bacterial eradication, the body's defenses against bacteria, and tissue healing. Possible mechanisms include diminished oxidative killing by neutrophils and impaired tissue healing caused by reduced collagen formation, neovascularization, and epithelialization.[72] Further, many of the antibiotics used perioperatively for SSI prophylaxis are oxygen dependent in their effect,[73] and low oxygen levels may decrease their effectiveness.

Perioperative hypothermia
Maintaining normal body temperature is vital for the body to maintain its normal function. However, many factors that patients are exposed to in the operating room can cause hypothermia: anesthetic drugs, cold operating room, skin antisepsis, cold irrigation of a patient with the body uncovered, and the use of intravenous solutions. Most cellular functions are temperature dependent, and hypothermia also provokes systemic responses.[74] Several mechanisms help to explain why perioperative hypothermia impairs host defenses against surgical wound contamination, including vasoconstriction and subsequent diminished perfusion, decreased motility of key immune cells, and reduced scar formation, which is necessary to prevent wound dehiscence and recontamination.

Anticoagulation
Although postoperative anticoagulation is an evidence-based practice to prevent deep vein thrombosis in the postoperative period, anticoagulants may increase the risk of SSIs. Several studies have implicated anticoagulation therapy as a cause of persistent oozing of the incision, slow wound healing, and subsequent SSIs.[75]

Blood transfusions
Red blood cell transfusion also increases the risk of SSI.[76] Blood transfusions increase the risk of infection by impairing normal monocyte function and decreasing tumor necrosis α production in response to endotoxin (lipopolysaccharide).[77]

GUIDELINES FOR PREVENTION

Several detailed published guidelines for SSI prevention exist, including the following 4 published primary guideline documents:

1. "Strategies to Prevent Surgical Site Infections in Acute Care Hospitals: 2014 Update."[78] The Society for Healthcare Epidemiology of America (SHEA) sponsored this document, and members of numerous other organizations with SSI prevention expertise also contributed.
2. "Global Guidelines for the Prevention of Surgical Site Infection."[79] The World Health Organization (WHO) published this updated document in 2018.
3. "American College of Surgeons and Surgical Infection Society: Surgical Site Infection Guidelines, 2016 Update."[80]
4. "Centers for Disease Control and Prevention Guideline for the Prevention of Surgical Site Infection, 2017."[81]

Based on these guideline documents, available evidence, and our personal experience, the authors have categorized SSI prevention strategies into 3 categories: best practices that all acute care hospitals should follow, additional interventions with possible benefit, and unproven or controversial interventions.

Recommendations

The authors have identified 9 core best practices that are consistently recommended by SSI prevention experts and guideline documents (**Table 4**). The authors recommend that all acute care hospitals incorporate each of the following SSI prevention measures into surgical protocols:

Preoperative bathing

Preoperative bathing or showering on the night before or day of surgery is a simple, low-risk intervention that decreases bacterial load of the skin, including the surgical site.[82] Many experts strongly recommend this practice as a standard of care for SSI prevention,[81] but definitive reduction in SSI risk has not been proved. Furthermore, for routine preoperative bathing, the ideal soap or antiseptic agent is not known, and many hospitals implement bathing protocols based on local epidemiology and cost considerations (preoperative bathing with chlorhexidine gluconate [CHG] is discussed later).

Antimicrobial prophylaxis

Antimicrobial prophylaxis given shortly before surgical incision is indicated for most clean-contaminated procedures, as well as certain clean procedures with severe consequences of infection (eg, procedures involving implantation of prosthetic implants).[79] Multispecialty consensus guidelines recommend preferred antibiotic agents based on common pathogens known to cause SSI following particular procedures; however, local epidemiology of SSI and hospital antibiograms should also influence antibiotic selection.[83] Antimicrobial prophylaxis protocols should promote optimized timing and dose of antibiotics, including redosing of antibiotics during surgery for prolonged procedures, or when blood loss is excessive. For nonemergent colorectal procedures, oral antibiotics and mechanical bowel preparation should be provided on the day before surgery, in addition to intravenous antibiotic prophylaxis before skin incision.[78–80] Prophylactic antibiotics should be discontinued after closure of incision because of increased risk of adverse events and because no SSI reduction benefit associated with postoperative antibiotic prophylaxis has been shown.[79,81]

Table 4
Summary of surgical site infection primary prevention guidelines, risk factors, and best-practice recommendations

Prevention Guideline	Risk Factor Addressed	Recommendations and Supporting Evidence
Preoperative bathing	Endogenous bacterial contamination of surgical site	• Patients should bathe their full bodies with soap or an antiseptic agent on at least the night before or day of surgery[79,81]
Antimicrobial prophylaxis	Endogenous and exogenous bacterial contamination of surgical site	• Administer prophylactic antibiotics for indicated procedures according to evidence-based guidelines[83] • Select agent based on common pathogens that cause SSI for procedure being performed, published guidelines, and local antibiograms.[83] • Begin antibiotic infusion within 60 min before incision; however, for vancomycin and fluoroquinolones, begin infusion within 120 min before incision[78,80,83] • Adhere to guidelines for antibiotic doses, including weight-based vancomycin dosing and 3-g cefazolin doses for patients with weight >120 kg.[78,83] • Redose antibiotics during surgery for prolonged procedures or for procedures with excessive blood loss[78,83] • Provide oral antibiotics, intravenous antibiotics, and mechanical bowel preparation before nonemergent colorectal procedures[78–80] • Discontinue perioperative antibiotics after closure of surgical incision[79,81]
Perioperative preparation of operative site	Endogenous and exogenous bacterial contamination of surgical site	• Avoid hair removal at operative site unless hair interferes with surgery. If hair must be removed,

(continued on next page)

Table 4
(continued)

Prevention Guideline	Risk Factor Addressed	Recommendations and Supporting Evidence
		remove hair outside of operating room with a clipper or depilatory agent[78,79]
		• Use an alcohol-based antiseptic solution containing chlorhexidine for surgical skin preparation, unless a contraindication exists[79]
		• Use chlorhexidine or povidone-iodine solutions that contain low concentrations (eg, 4%) or no alcohol for vaginal antisepsis before hysterectomy and vaginal procedures, including cesarean section[87,88]
Surgical hand preparation	Exogenous bacterial contamination of surgical site	• Use an appropriate antiseptic agent to perform surgical hand scrub for the length of time recommended by the manufacturer[78,79]
Maintenance of normothermia	Hypothermia-induced vasoconstriction and tissue hypoxia at surgical site	• Use warming devices in the operating room before and during the surgical procedure to maintain body temperature of at least $36.0^\circ C$[78,79]
Hyperoxygenation	Tissue hypoxia at surgical site	• For patients undergoing general anesthesia and tracheal intubation and who have normal pulmonary function, provide 80% Fio_2 intraoperatively and, when possible, for 2–6 h after surgery[78,79,81]
Wound protectors	Endogenous and exogenous bacterial contamination of surgical site	• Use impervious plastic wound protectors for open abdominal surgery, particularly colorectal and biliary tract procedures[78,80]
Glucose control	Hyperglycemia	• Maintain immediate postoperative blood

(continued on next page)

Table 4 (continued)		
Prevention Guideline	Risk Factor Addressed	Recommendations and Supporting Evidence
		glucose of ≤180 mg/dL for diabetic and nondiabetic patients[78–80]
Perioperative checklist	Potential for noncompliance with best practices	• Use a checklist based on the WHO Surgical Safety Checklist[90] to improve compliance with best practices, including SSI prevention strategies[78]

Abbreviation: Fio_2, fraction of inspired oxygen.

Perioperative preparation of operative site

Hair removal should be performed only if hair interferes with surgery.[78,84] When hair removal is necessary, a clipper or depilatory agent should be used outside of the operating room. Hair shaving should not occur. If a clipper is used, a disposable clipper head should be used and changed between patients.

Surgical skin preparation should be performed with an alcohol-containing antiseptic solution, unless a contraindication to the alcohol component exists (eg, procedures involving mucosa, cornea, or ear).[78] Alcohol-based skin preparation agents are flammable, and operating room personnel should take precautions to avoid fires in the operating room, especially for procedures using an electrosurgical device (eg, Bovie).[85] Personnel should allow the skin preparation solution to dry per manufacturer instructions for use and avoid pooling of the solution.

WHO guidelines preferentially recommend the use of CHG-alcohol solutions rather than povidone-iodine-alcohol solutions,[79] whereas other organizations do not make specific recommendations regarding type of alcohol-containing solution. Although few head-to-head studies have been performed to compare efficacy of CHG versus povidone-iodine–containing solutions, CHG alcohol was superior to povidone-iodine alcohol in a randomized controlled trial analyzing SSI prevention following cesarean section.[86] As a result, the authors preferentially recommend use of CHG alcohol for skin antisepsis. Vaginal cleansing with either 4% CHG or povidone-iodine should occur before hysterectomy and vaginal procedures, including cesarean section.[87,88]

Surgical hand preparation

Surgical hand preparation should be performed with either a suitable antimicrobial soap or alcohol-based hand rub.[78,79] Hand preparation should occur for the duration recommended by the manufacturer of the antiseptic agent chosen.

Maintenance of normothermia

Preoperative and intraoperative warming devices should be used in order to maintain temperature of at least 36.0°C.[74,78,84] In addition to decreasing SSI risk, maintenance of normothermia may also decrease blood loss and transfusion requirements.

Hyperoxygenation

Patients who undergo surgery with general anesthesia and tracheal intubation and who have normal pulmonary function should receive 80% fraction of inspired oxygen (Fio_2) intraoperatively and, when feasible, for 2 to 6 hours postoperatively.[78,79] The benefit of hyperoxygenation may be greatest for open colorectal surgery. Updated WHO guidelines continue to recommend hyperoxygenation despite exclusion of 2 studies that showed benefit but have subsequently received scrutiny for possible data integrity breaches.[89]

Glucose control

Blood glucose should be monitored and controlled in the immediate postoperative time period for all surgical patients, including patients with and without a diagnosis of diabetes mellitus.[78–80] Protocols should be used to ensure that postoperative glucose monitoring occurs and that insulin is used to maintain glucose level less than or equal to 180 mg/dL for at least the first 24 hours after surgery. At a minimum, we recommend that all hospitalized postoperative patients without diabetes mellitus have 1 blood glucose value checked in the first 24 hours after surgery.

Perioperative checklist

Acute care hospitals should use surgical safety checklists to improve compliance with best practices for SSI prevention.[78] The authors recommend that hospitals modify the 19-item WHO Surgical Safety Checklist[90] to include additional SSI prevention practices detailed here, as well as other important SSI prevention measures applicable to the specific hospital or procedure.

Considerations

Numerous potentially effective SSI prevention strategies are not included in the 9 core best practices listed earlier. Compared with the core interventions, these additional strategies do not have the same strength of endorsement by SSI prevention guidelines or experts and have fewer data to support universal implementation. However, especially for hospitals, procedures, or patient populations with increased SSI rates despite adherence to core SSI prevention measures, implementation of additional strategies may help to decrease SSI risk.[78] This article discusses the following 4 commonly used auxiliary strategies for SSI prevention.

Staphylococcus aureus screening and decolonization

Patients undergoing high-risk cardiothoracic, orthopedic, or neurosurgical procedures known to be colonized with S aureus should receive preoperative intranasal mupirocin 2% ointment or an alternative intranasal agent with antistaphylococcal activity, as well as CHG bathing for up to 5 days before surgery.[78,84] However, no standardized approach exists for S aureus screening or decolonization, and guideline documents give conflicting recommendations regarding the practice of universal decolonization of patients undergoing high-risk procedures. For example, the WHO strongly recommends against routine decolonization of patients not known to be S aureus carriers, primarily to avoid spread of resistance to mupirocin.[79]

Although optimal strategies for S aureus screening and targeted decolonization versus universal decolonization before high-risk surgical procedures continue to be debated, experts generally agree that routine universal S aureus preoperative screening is not necessary before lower-risk procedures.[78,79] Nevertheless, some hospitals may consider screening and decolonization for certain patients and procedures depending on SSI rates caused by S aureus; patient-specific risk factors for S aureus SSI; and availability of resources to reliably screen, follow up screening results, and implement protocolized decolonization strategies for patients found to have nasal S aureus carriage. In addition, although decolonization protocols typically recommend preoperative application of 2% nasal mupirocin twice daily for several days close to the date of planned surgery,[80] application of intranasal povidone-iodine swabs on the day of surgery shortly before incision may be an effective, more practical, and less expensive alternative that precludes concerns regarding resistance to mupirocin.[91,92]

Colorectal surgery bundles

Multiple studies have shown the potential for implementation of colorectal surgery best-practice bundles to improve outcomes, including SSI rates.[93] Colorectal surgery bundles commonly include elements of the 9 core best practices for SSI prevention detailed in this article, as well as additional, less-proven interventions. Based on success of bundles, theoretic benefit, and low risk of harm, the authors support implementation of additional strategies to be included for bundles for colorectal SSI prevention, such as gown and glove change before fascial and skin closure and use of a dedicated wound closure tray.

Operating room traffic control

Increased operating room foot traffic and door openings can disrupt air quality and flow, potentially increasing microbial concentrations at the surgical site and SSI risk.[36,37] The authors support interventions designed to decrease unnecessary operating room traffic and door openings.

Operating room disinfection

Attention must be paid to operating room maintenance and care, including air handling and disinfection of the environment and equipment.[14,78] Adjunctive disinfection practices, such as use of ultraviolet light in the operating room, might provide additional benefit but require further study.[94]

Controversies

Preoperative chlorhexidine gluconate bathing

Although all patients should receive a bath or shower the night before or evening of surgery, insufficient evidence exists to recommend universal preoperative use of CHG.[79] However, if not cost-prohibitive, CHG is a reasonable agent to use for preoperative bathing. Use of 2% CHG-impregnated cloths may provide greater reduction in SSI risk than use of CHG soap.[95]

Local antibiotics

Local and topical antibiotics are commonly used during surgery for the purpose of decreasing SSI risk. However, in general, high-quality data supporting these practices are sparse. For example, powdered vancomycin is commonly applied to surgical sites, but available data are insufficient to recommend its widespread use for SSI prevention. Furthermore, use of powdered vancomycin could be associated with local adverse effects.[96] Another example is use of gentamicin-collagen sponges to prevent SSI. Single-center trials suggested benefit when these sponges were used in colorectal surgery, but a multicenter randomized trial showed harm.[78,97] Meta-analyses have suggested that gentamicin-collagen sponges might be more successful in decreasing SSI risk following cardiothoracic surgery.[98]

Surgical wound irrigation

Incisional wounds are commonly irrigated with saline, antiseptics, or antibiotics for the purpose of SSI prevention. No consensus exists among best irrigation practices for SSI prevention, and high-quality data are not available to support routine irrigation with antibiotics. Incisional wound irrigation with povidone-iodine might be more effective in decreasing SSI risk than saline irrigation, but this topic requires further study.[79]

Antiseptic drapes

Some surgeons use adhesive plastic incise drapes, often impregnated with an antiseptic agent. These drapes are applied to patient skin after skin antisepsis is performed, and the surgeon cuts through the drape and skin. Available data do not support routine use of antiseptic drapes for SSI prevention.[78,84]

Antiseptic-impregnated sutures

Triclosan-coated sutures are commonly used to decrease SSI risk, but data evaluating this practice are mixed.[99] In addition, limited data have suggested possible negative effect on wound healing.[100] Guideline recommendations regarding triclosan-coated sutures are contradictory and range from a recommendation against routine use[78] to conditional recommendations supporting their use.[79,80]

Advanced dressings

Advanced dressings for primarily closed surgical wounds, such as silver-containing or antimicrobial-impregnated dressings, have not been proved to significantly decrease SSI rates compared with standard dressings.[80,84] Regardless of type of dressing used, dressings should be sterile and be placed and changed using aseptic technique.

Wound protectors

Plastic wound protectors can facilitate retraction of an incision without requiring additional mechanical retractors and can decrease SSI risk after open abdominal surgeries.[78,80] Benefit may be greatest for colorectal and biliary tract procedures.

Prophylactic negative pressure wound therapy

Routine use of prophylactic negative pressure wound therapy has not been shown to decrease SSIs. A recent, large, randomized clinical trial found that there was no significant difference in the risk of SSI after cesarean delivery in obese women with prophylactic negative pressure wound therapy (3.6%) versus standard wound dressing (3.4%).[101] Low-quality evidence suggests that prophylactic negative pressure wound therapy on primarily closed, high-risk surgical wounds decreases SSI risk compared with use of standard wound dressings.[79,80] Examples of high-risk wounds include wounds complicated by surrounding soft tissue damage, poor blood flow, hematoma, or intraoperative contamination. The pressure level or duration of negative pressure therapy needed to maximize SSI risk reduction is not known.

THERAPEUTIC OPTIONS

Surgical debridement and removal of the infected tissue is the most important facet of therapy for many SSIs, with antimicrobial therapy being an important adjunct component.[102] However, the type of debridement and duration of antimicrobial therapy depend on the depth and anatomic site of infection and the presence of prosthetic material. However, deep-incisional and organ/space infections almost universally require operative evacuation of the infected tissue.

Superficial-incisional SSIs can typically be treated with oral antibiotics and without surgical debridement. In contrast, patients with systemic symptoms (temperature >38.5°C, heart rate >110 beats/min) or with suspected deep-incisional or organ/space SSI generally require exploration of the surgical site in addition to antibiotics.[102] The specific antibiotic and duration of therapy are determined by the location of the infection, the depth of infection, the adequacy of surgical debridement, and resistance patterns of the causative pathogens. However, in general, clinicians should initiate systemic antibiotic therapy when a patient has systemic symptoms of infection or a clinician suspects a deep-incision or organ/space SSI. For example, 1 study found that patients with mediastinitis who receive antibiotics active against the identified pathogen within 7 days of debridement had a 60% reduction in mortality compared with patients who did not receive effective antibiotic therapy.[103]

ASSESSMENT

The CDC conducted the Study of the Efficacy of Nosocomial Infection Control (SENIC) to determine the cost-effectiveness of infection prevention activities, including surveillance.[104] These and many subsequent studies concluded that infection surveillance programs and feedback of SSI rates to surgeons decrease overall SSI rates by 32% to 50%.[105,106] These data form the basis for the CDC's recommendation that hospitals routinely perform surveillance for SSIs and report the information back to surgeons.[14]

Surveillance Methodology

Strategies for targeting surveillance by procedure type

Given the significant resources required to perform SSI surveillance, many infection prevention programs focus their SSI surveillance efforts on a subset of patients. Hospitals may determine surgical populations for targeted surveillance in several ways. One strategy is to target high-volume surgical procedures for surveillance, because SSIs related to these procedures would pose risk to a large number of patients. Examples of high-volume procedures include colorectal procedures, abdominal hysterectomies, and hip and knee arthroscopies. Notably, US hospitals are required to publicly report rates of SSI following colorectal and abdominal hysterectomy procedures. Another strategy is to target high-risk procedures for surveillance, because SSIs after these procedures convey high risk of morbidity. Examples of high-risk procedures include spinal fusion and craniotomies. A third strategy is to focus surveillance efforts on surgical procedures that have rates of SSI that are higher than expected at that institution (based on historical comparisons). Typically, infection prevention programs use a combination of these targeting strategies.

Strategies for surgical site infection case finding

Direct prospective case finding through daily chart review and observation of the surgical site by infection prevention personnel is considered the most sensitive and rigorous method to identify patients with SSI.[106] However, direct surveillance is no longer practiced for several reasons. First, daily observation of the wound is resource intensive and impractical for modern infection prevention programs. Second, indirect methods that involve medical record review without direct wound observation have shown sensitivity of 84% to 89% and specificity of 99.8%, and they require fewer resources compared with direct observation.[107,108] In addition, most SSIs occur following discharge from the index hospitalization and can only be detected through postdischarge surveillance methods.[109]

Many infection prevention programs screen records for possible indicators of SSI and proceed with complete chart review only when an indicator is present. NHSN suggests several methods to identify patients with possible SSI, including review of medical records for signs and symptoms of SSI; review of admission, readmission, emergency room visits, and operating room logs; review of laboratory, imaging, or other diagnostic test reports; review of clinician notes; International Classification of Diseases-10 Clinical Modification (ICD-10-CM) Infection Diagnosis codes; surgeon surveys; and patient surveys.[16] However, NHSN states that facilities may use any combination of methods to identify potential patients with SSI. Therefore, considerable variability among case-finding methods across facilities exists.

Microbiology data

Many SSI surveillance programs use positive microbiology results as an indicator of possible SSI. However, microbiology data are not perfect indicators of SSI because cultures or other microbiology studies are not obtained in every case; superficial wound infections are frequently treated with local wound management with or without antibiotics. Studies have shown that surveillance systems that rely solely on microbiologic data only identify 33% to 65% of all SSIs.[110]

Antimicrobial administration

Antibiotic use beyond the expected number of postoperative days (used for perioperative prophylaxis) can be used to predict SSI.[110,111] However, postoperative antibiotic use alone is not sensitive or specific for SSI detection. Some patients continue to receive antibiotics following a surgical procedure for prophylaxis or treatment of a pre-existing infection. In addition, antibiotics are not always required for management of superficial SSIs.[102] Therefore, antibiotics should only be used in combination with other parameters to screen patients for possible SSI.

Administrative claims data

Several studies have evaluated the utility of using administrative billing data as an indicator of SSI.[111–113] Using administrative claims data increases detection of SSIs relative to standard surveillance methods.[114] In addition, studies have found that using administrative data as a flag for further chart review by infection preventionists saves time and significantly decreases the burden of surveillance compared with standard methods.[113,114] In addition, US Centers for Medicare and Medicaid Services (CMS) Medicare claims data can be used to accurately distinguish between hospitals with high and low rates of infection following certain procedure types.

However, several limitations to using administrative data to facilitate surveillance exist. First, billing is performed retroactively. Therefore, surveillance systems that rely on administrative data as the first trigger to review charts for SSI cannot detect SSI in real time and intervene or provide feedback in a timely manner. Second, recent studies of administrative data for SSI surveillance have typically been performed on clean procedures, including cardiac, arthroplasty, vascular, and breast procedures. The utility of administrative billing data as an indicator of SSI following other procedure types is unclear.

Electronic surveillance

With the evolution of the electronic medical record, infection prevention programs and software vendors are exploring automated methods to detect patients with SSI. However, at this time, no single effective SSI prediction tool exists. For example, 1 study of an automated algorithm that used specified laboratory parameters and antimicrobial use to detect SSIs found the model performed poorly, with overall sensitivity of 37.8%, and had poor interhospital ability to generalize.[115] Development of electronic surveillance tools with improved accuracy is an area of ongoing research.

Surgical site infection metrics and data feedback

SSI rates are typically calculated per 100 procedures and may be stratified by procedure type and surgeon. SSI rates should be periodically assessed for trends and reported to surgeons, perioperative services staff, and hospital leaders. Peer-to-peer comparative SSI rate data may be helpful to identify surgeons whose rates are higher than those of peers; however, without adequate adjustment for difference in patient-level or procedure-level risk factors, peer-to-peer comparative data should be used for performance improvement purposes only.

Surveillance systems that detect SSIs in near real time allow for concurrent feedback to surgical and perioperative personnel as SSIs are identified. This type of surveillance allows performance improvement teams to investigate for potential lapses in patient care (eg, missed administration of perioperative antibiotic, failure to maintain postoperative glucose control) and take actions to improve compliance with recommended best practices. Because SSIs are low-frequency events, it can sometimes be difficult for infection prevention and perioperative teams to detect when there is a meaningful increase or cluster of infections over baseline. Use of statistical process control charts to analyze SSI surveillance data and alert staff when a potential cluster has occurred may promote earlier detection of important SSI rate increases.[116]

In summary, surveillance for SSI and data feedback are important functions of infection prevention teams. However, methods for conducting surveillance and the quality of surveillance vary across health care facilities and depend on availability of resources. Infection prevention programs should periodically evaluate their surveillance programs to ensure they are maximally effective and reflect the most recent recommended best practices for SSI prevention.

SUMMARY

SSIs are the most common and costly health care–associated infections in the United States[1,2,7] and lead to significant patient morbidity and mortality.[4,11] However, adhering to evidence-based preventive practices can decrease the rate of SSI. In general, aggressive surgical debridement in addition to appropriate antibiotic therapy is necessary for SSI treatment.

CLINICS CARE POINTS

- Before surgical incision, patients need to receive the appropriate type and dose of antibiotic within the appropriate time frame. Patients may also require additional antibiotic doses for prolonged procedures.

- Perioperative staff should only remove patient hair if it interferes with the surgery, and, even then, hair removal should be done with a clipper or depilatory agent outside of the operating room.

- The skin over the surgical site needs to be cleansed with an alcohol-containing antiseptic solution.

- Providers must perform hand preparation with a suitable antimicrobial soap or alcohol-based hand rub before entering the operating room.

- During the operation, every effort should be made to maintain normothermia, hyperoxygenation, and normal glucose levels.

- Hospitals should use surgical safety checklists to improve compliance with practices for SSI prevention.

DISCLOSURE

Dr Anderson reported grants from CDC Epicenter (U54CK000483) during the conduct of the study; grants from Agency for Healthcare Research and Quality, personal fees from UpToDate, and royalties for authorship outside the submitted work.

REFERENCES

1. Lewis SS, Moehring RW, Chen LF, et al. Assessing the relative burden of hospital-acquired infections in a network of community hospitals. Infect Control Hosp Epidemiol 2013;34(11):1229–30.
2. Zimlichman E, Henderson D, Tamir O, et al. Health care-associated infections: a meta-analysis of costs and financial impact on the US health care system. JAMA Intern Med 2013;173(22):2039–46.
3. Steiner CA, Karaca Z, Moore BJ, et al. STATISTICAL BRIEF# 223. 2017.
4. Agency for Healthcare Research and Quality. Healthcare cost and utilization project - statistics on hospital stays. 2013 web site. Available at: http://hcupnet.ahrq.gov/. Accessed November 17, 2020.
5. Scott RD. The direct medical costs of healthcare-associated infections in US hospitals and the benefits of prevention 2009. Available at: https://www.cdc.gov/hai/pdfs/hai/scott_costpaper.pdf.
6. Allegranzi B, Bagheri Nejad S, Combescure C, et al. Burden of endemic healthcare-associated infection in developing countries: systematic review and meta-analysis. Lancet 2011;377(9761):228–41.
7. Magill SS, O'Leary E, Janelle SJ, et al. Changes in prevalence of health care–associated infections in US Hospitals. N Engl J Med 2018;379(18):1732–44.
8. Geubbels EL, Wille JC, Nagelkerke NJ, et al. Hospital-related determinants for surgical-site infection following hip arthroplasty. Infect Control Hosp Epidemiol 2005;26(5):435–41.
9. Baker AW, Dicks KV, Durkin MJ, et al. Epidemiology of surgical site infection in a community hospital network. Infect Control Hosp Epidemiol 2016;37(5):519–26.
10. Anderson DJ, Hartwig MG, Pappas T, et al. Surgical volume and the risk of surgical site infection in community hospitals: size matters. Ann Surg 2008;247(2):343–9.
11. Anderson DJ, Kaye KS, Chen LF, et al. Clinical and financial outcomes due to methicillin resistant Staphylococcus aureus surgical site infection: a multicenter matched outcomes study. PLoS One 2009;4(12):e8305.
12. Martone WJ, Nichols RL. Recognition, prevention, surveillance, and management of surgical site infections: introduction to the problem and symposium overview. Clin Infect Dis 2001;33(Suppl 2):S67–8.
13. Kirkland KB, Briggs JP, Trivette SL, et al. The impact of surgical-site infections in the 1990s: attributable mortality, excess length of hospitalization, and extra costs. Infect Control Hosp Epidemiol 1999;20(11):725–30.
14. Mangram AJ, Horan TC, Pearson ML, et al. Guideline for prevention of surgical site infection, 1999. Infect Control Hosp Epidemiol 1999;20(4):247–80.
15. Estimating the additional hospital inpatient cost and mortality associated with selected hospital-acquired conditions. Agency for healthcare research and quality. 2017. Available at: https://www.ahrq.gov/hai/pfp/haccost2017-results.html. Accessed October 20, 2019.
16. Centers for Disease Control and Prevention. Surgical Site Infection (SSI) event web site. Available at: https://www.cdc.gove/nhsn/pdfs/pscmanual/9pscssicurrent.pdf. Accessed November 20, 2020.
17. Dicks KV, Lewis SS, Durkin MJ, et al. Surveying the surveillance: surgical site infections excluded by the January 2013 updated surveillance definitions. Infect Control Hosp Epidemiol 2014;35(5):570–3.
18. Wenzel RP. Surgical site infections and the microbiome: an updated perspective. Infect Control Hosp Epidemiol 2019;40(5):590–6.

19. Seidelman JL, Baker AW, Ge M, et al. 905. Surgical site infections following colon surgery in a large network of community hospitals. Open Forum Infect Dis 2020;7(Supplement_1):S486–7.

20. Baker AW, Lewis SS, Alexander BD, et al. Two-phase hospital-associated outbreak of Mycobacterium abscessus: investigation and mitigation. Clin Infect Dis 2017;64(7):902–11.

21. Everett ED, Pearson S, Rogers W. Rhizopus surgical wound infection with elasticized adhesive tape dressings. Arch Surg 1979;114(6):738–9.

22. Wenger PN, Brown JM, McNeil MM, et al. Nocardia farcinica sternotomy site infections in patients following open heart surgery. J Infect Dis 1998;178(5):1539–43.

23. Leaper D, Edmiston C. World Health Organization: global guidelines for the prevention of surgical site infection. J Hosp Infect 2017;95(2):135–6.

24. Lee KY, Coleman K, Paech D, et al. The epidemiology and cost of surgical site infections in Korea: a systematic review. J Korean Surg Soc 2011;81(5):295–307.

25. Fleischmann W, Meyer H, Baer A. Bacterial recolonization of the skin under a Polyurethane drape in hip surgery. J Hosp Infect 1996;34(2):107–16.

26. Seropian R, Reynolds BM. Wound infections after preoperative depilatory versus razor preparation. Am J Surg 1971;121(3):251–4.

27. Ko W, Lazenby WD, Zelano JA, et al. Effects of shaving methods and intraoperative irrigation on suppurative mediastinitis after bypass operations. Ann Thorac Surg 1992;53(2):301–5.

28. Korol E, Johnston K, Waser N, et al. A systematic review of risk factors associated with surgical site infections among surgical patients. PLoS One 2013;8(12):e83743.

29. Berard F, Gandon J. Postoperative wound infections: the influence of ultraviolet irradiation of the operating room and of various other factors. Ann Surg 1964;160(Suppl 2):1–192.

30. Elek SD, Conen PE. The virulence of Staphylococcus pyogenes for man; a study of the problems of wound infection. Br J Exp Pathol 1957;38(6):573–86.

31. Davidson T, Lewandowski E, Smerecki M, et al. Taking your work home with you: potential risks of contaminated clothing and hair in the dental clinic and attitudes about infection control. Can J Infect Control 2017;32(3):137–42.

32. Fagernes M, Lingaas E. Factors interfering with the microflora on hands: a regression analysis of samples from 465 healthcare workers. J Adv Nurs 2011;67(2):297–307.

33. Parry MF, Grant B, Yukna M, et al. Candida osteomyelitis and diskitis after spinal surgery: an outbreak that implicates artificial nail use. Clin Infect Dis 2001;32(3):352–7.

34. Lidwell OM, Lowbury EJ, Whyte W, et al. Airborne contamination of wounds in joint replacement operations: the relationship to sepsis rates. J Hosp Infect 1983;4(2):111–31.

35. Edmiston CE Jr, Seabrook GR, Cambria RA, et al. Molecular epidemiology of microbial contamination in the operating room environment: Is there a risk for infection? Surgery 2005;138(4):573–9 [discussion: 579–582].

36. Roth JA, Juchler F, Dangel M, et al. Frequent door openings during cardiac surgery are associated with increased risk for surgical site infection: a prospective observational study. Clin Infect Dis 2019;69(2):290–4.

37. Andersson AE, Bergh I, Karlsson J, et al. Traffic flow in the operating room: an explorative and descriptive study on air quality during orthopedic trauma implant surgery. Am J Infect Control 2012;40(8):750–5.

38. Manian FA. The role of postoperative factors in surgical site infections: time to take notice. Clin Infect Dis 2014;59(9):1272–6.

39. Dumville JC, Gray TA, Walter CJ, et al. Dressings for the prevention of surgical site infection. Cochrane Database Syst Rev 2016;12:CD003091.

40. Charalambous CP, Tryfonidis M, Sadiq S, et al. Septic arthritis following intra-articular steroid injection of the knee–a survey of current practice regarding anti-septic technique used during intra-articular steroid injection of the knee. Clin Rheumatol 2003;22(6):386–90.

41. McIntosh AL, Hanssen AD, Wenger DE, et al. Recent intraarticular steroid injection may increase infection rates in primary THA. Clin Orthop Relat Res 2006; 451:50–4.

42. Desai A, Ramankutty S, Board T, et al. Does intraarticular steroid infiltration increase the rate of infection in subsequent total knee replacements? Knee 2009;16(4):262–4.

43. Jevsevar DS, Brown GA, Jones DL, et al. The American Academy of Orthopaedic Surgeons evidence-based guideline on: treatment of osteoarthritis of the knee. J Bone Joint Surg Am 2013;95(20):1885–6.

44. Yin JB, Cui GB, Mi MS, et al. Local infiltration analgesia for postoperative pain after hip arthroplasty: a systematic review and meta-analysis. J Pain 2014; 15(8):781–99.

45. Seidelman J, Baker AW, Anderson DJ, et al. Do periarticular joint infections present an increase in infection risk? Infect Control Hosp Epidemiol 2018;39(7): 890–1.

46. Kaye KS, Anderson DJ, Sloane R, et al. The effect of surgical site infection on older operative patients. J Am Geriatr Soc 2009;57(1):46–54.

47. Fore J. A review of skin and the effects of aging on skin structure and function. Ostomy Wound Manage 2006;52(9):24–35, quiz 36–37.

48. Reddy M. Skin and wound care: important considerations in the older adult. Adv Skin Wound Care 2008;21(9):424–36, quiz 437–438.

49. Kaye KS, Schmit K, Pieper C, et al. The effect of increasing age on the risk of surgical site infection. J Infect Dis 2005;191(7):1056–62.

50. Olsen MA, Lefta M, Dietz JR, et al. Risk factors for surgical site infection after major breast operation. J Am Coll Surg 2008;207(3):326–35.

51. Faraday N, Rock P, Lin EE, et al. Past history of skin infection and risk of surgical site infection after elective surgery. Ann Surg 2013;257(1):150–4.

52. Zhang Y, Zheng QJ, Wang S, et al. Diabetes mellitus is associated with increased risk of surgical site infections: a meta-analysis of prospective cohort studies. Am J Infect Control 2015;43(8):810–5.

53. Martin ET, Kaye KS, Knott C, et al. Diabetes and risk of surgical site infection: a systematic review and meta-analysis. Infect Control Hosp Epidemiol 2016;37(1): 88–99.

54. Turina M, Fry DE, Polk HC Jr. Acute hyperglycemia and the innate immune system: clinical, cellular, and molecular aspects. Crit Care Med 2005;33(7): 1624–33.

55. Dronge AS, Perkal MF, Kancir S, et al. Long-term glycemic control and postoperative infectious complications. Arch Surg 2006;141(4):375–80 [discussion: 380].

56. Latham R, Lancaster AD, Covington JF, et al. The association of diabetes and glucose control with surgical-site infections among cardiothoracic surgery patients. Infect Control Hosp Epidemiol 2001;22(10):607–12.

57. Hennessey DB, Burke JP, Ni-Dhonochu T, et al. Preoperative hypoalbuminemia is an independent risk factor for the development of surgical site infection following gastrointestinal surgery: a multi-institutional study. Ann Surg 2010; 252(2):325–9.

58. Testini M, Margari A, Amoruso M, et al. [The dehiscence of colorectal anastomoses: the risk factors]. Ann Ital Chir 2000;71(4):433–40.

59. Rivadeneira DE, Grobmyer SR, Naama HA, et al. Malnutrition-induced macrophage apoptosis. Surgery 2001;129(5):617–25.

60. Runyon BA. Low-protein-concentration ascitic fluid is predisposed to spontaneous bacterial peritonitis. Gastroenterology 1986;91(6):1343–6.

61. Wukich DK, McMillen RL, Lowery NJ, et al. Surgical site infections after foot and ankle surgery: a comparison of patients with and without diabetes. Diabetes Care 2011;34(10):2211–3.

62. Sorensen LT, Karlsmark T, Gottrup F. Abstinence from smoking reduces incisional wound infection: a randomized controlled trial. Ann Surg 2003;238(1):1.

63. Sorensen LT. Wound healing and infection in surgery: the pathophysiological impact of smoking, smoking cessation, and nicotine replacement therapy: a systematic review. Ann Surg 2012;255(6):1069–79.

64. Yuan K, Chen HL. Obesity and surgical site infections risk in orthopedics: a meta-analysis. Int J Surg 2013;11(5):383–8.

65. Wick EC, Hirose K, Shore AD, et al. Surgical site infections and cost in obese patients undergoing colorectal surgery. Arch Surg 2011;146(9):1068–72.

66. Harrington G, Russo P, Spelman D, et al. Surgical-site infection rates and risk factor analysis in coronary artery bypass graft surgery. Infect Control Hosp Epidemiol 2004;25(6):472–6.

67. Meijs AP, Koek MBG, Vos MC, et al. The effect of body mass index on the risk of surgical site infection. Infect Control Hosp Epidemiol 2019;40(9):991–6.

68. Filsoufi F, Rahmanian PB, Castillo JG, et al. Incidence, treatment strategies and outcome of deep sternal wound infection after orthotopic heart transplantation. J Heart Lung Transpl 2007;26(11):1084–90.

69. Payne WG, Naidu DK, Wheeler CK, et al. Wound healing in patients with cancer. Eplasty 2008;8:e9.

70. Corcoran TB, Myles PS, Forbes AB, et al. Dexamethasone and Surgical-Site Infection. N Engl J Med 2021;384(18):1731–41.

71. Bosanquet DC, Rangaraj A, Richards AJ, et al. Topical steroids for chronic wounds displaying abnormal inflammation. Ann R Coll Surg Engl 2013;95(4): 291–6.

72. Hopf HW, Holm J. Hyperoxia and infection. Best Pract Res Clin Anaesthesiol 2008;22(3):553–69.

73. Wetterslev J, Meyhoff CS, Jørgensen LN, et al. The effects of high perioperative inspiratory oxygen fraction for adult surgical patients. Cochrane Database Syst Rev 2015;(6). Available at: https://www.cochranelibrary.com/cdsr/doi/10.1002/14651858.CD008884.pub2/abstract?cookiesEnabled.

74. Kurz A, Sessler DI, Lenhardt R. Perioperative normothermia to reduce the incidence of surgical-wound infection and shorten hospitalization. Study of Wound Infection and Temperature Group. N Engl J Med 1996;334(19):1209–15.

75. Wang Z, Anderson FA Jr, Ward M, et al. Surgical site infections and other post-operative complications following prophylactic anticoagulation in total joint arthroplasty. PLoS One 2014;9(4):e91755.
76. Rohde JM, Dimcheff DE, Blumberg N, et al. Health care-associated infection after red blood cell transfusion: a systematic review and meta-analysis. JAMA 2014;311(13):1317–26.
77. Muszynski J, Nateri J, Nicol K, et al. Immunosuppressive effects of red blood cells on monocytes are related to both storage time and storage solution. Transfusion 2012;52(4):794–802.
78. Anderson DJ, Podgorny K, Berrios-Torres SI, et al. Strategies to prevent surgical site infections in acute care hospitals: 2014 update. Infect Control Hosp Epidemiol 2014;35(Suppl 2):S66–88.
79. Global guidelines for the prevention of surgical site infection, second edition. Geneva: World Health Organization; 2018. Licence: CC BY-NC-SA 3.0 IGO. p. 58–158.
80. Ban KA, Minei JP, Laronga C, et al. American college of surgeons and surgical infection society: surgical site infection guidelines, 2016 update. J Am Coll Surg 2017;224(1):59–74.
81. Berrios-Torres SI, Umscheid CA, Bratzler DW, et al. Centers for disease control and prevention guideline for the prevention of surgical site infection, 2017. JAMA Surg 2017;152(8):784–91.
82. Seal LA, Paul-Cheadle D. A systems approach to preoperative surgical patient skin preparation. Am J Infect Control 2004;32(2):57–62.
83. Bratzler DW, Dellinger EP, Olsen KM, et al. Clinical practice guidelines for antimicrobial prophylaxis in surgery. Am J Health Syst Pharm 2013;70(3):195–283.
84. Global guidelines for the prevention of surgical site infection. Geneva (Switzerland): World Health Organization; 2018. Available at: https://www.ncbi.nlm.nih.gov/books/NBK536404/.
85. Jones EL, Overbey DM, Chapman BC, et al. Operating room fires and surgical skin preparation. J Am Coll Surg 2017;225(1):160–5.
86. Tuuli MG, Liu J, Stout MJ, et al. A randomized trial comparing skin antiseptic agents at cesarean delivery. N Engl J Med 2016;374(7):647–55.
87. Prevention of infection after gynecologic procedures. The American College of Obstetricians and Gynecologists. ACOG practice bulletin. Number 195. 2018. Available at: https://www.acog.org/clinical/clinical-guidance/practice-bulletin/articles/2018/06/prevention-of-infection-after-gynecologic-procedures.
88. Haas DM, Morgan S, Contreras K, et al. Vaginal preparation with antiseptic solution before cesarean section for preventing postoperative infections. Cochrane Database Syst Rev 2018;7:Cd007892.
89. Myles PS, Carlisle JB, Scarr B. Evidence for compromised data integrity in studies of liberal peri-operative inspired oxygen. Anaesthesia 2019;74(5):573–84.
90. Haynes AB, Weiser TG, Berry WR, et al. A surgical safety checklist to reduce morbidity and mortality in a global population. N Engl J Med 2009;360(5):491–9.
91. Phillips M, Rosenberg A, Shopsin B, et al. Preventing surgical site infections: a randomized, open-label trial of nasal mupirocin ointment and nasal povidone-iodine solution. Infect Control Hosp Epidemiol 2014;35(7):826–32.
92. Rezapoor M, Nicholson T, Tabatabaee RM, et al. Povidone-iodine-based solutions for decolonization of nasal staphylococcus aureus: a randomized, prospective, placebo-controlled study. J Arthroplasty 2017;32(9):2815–9.

93. Keenan JE, Speicher PJ, Nussbaum DP, et al. Improving outcomes in colorectal surgery by sequential implementation of multiple standardized care programs. J Am Coll Surg 2015;221(2):404–14.e401.

94. Cook TM, Piatt CJ, Barnes S, et al. The impact of supplemental intraoperative air decontamination on the outcome of total joint arthroplasty: a pilot analysis. J Arthroplasty 2019;34(3):549–53.

95. Graling PR, Vasaly FW. Effectiveness of 2% CHG cloth bathing for reducing surgical site infections. AORN J 2013;97(5):547–51.

96. Baker AW, Chen LF. Letter to the editor regarding: "Effectiveness of local vancomycin powder to decrease surgical site infections: a meta-analysis" by Chiang et al. Spine J 2014;14(6):1092.

97. Bennett-Guerrero E, Pappas TN, Koltun WA, et al. Gentamicin-collagen sponge for infection prophylaxis in colorectal surgery. N Engl J Med 2010;363(11):1038–49.

98. Kowalewski M, Pawliszak W, Zaborowska K, et al. Gentamicin-collagen sponge reduces the risk of sternal wound infections after heart surgery: Meta-analysis. J Thorac Cardiovasc Surg 2015;149(6):1631–40.e1631.

99. Wu X, Kubilay NZ, Ren J, et al. Antimicrobial-coated sutures to decrease surgical site infections: a systematic review and meta-analysis. Eur J Clin Microbiol 2017;36(1):19–32.

100. Deliaert AE, Van den Kerckhove E, Tuinder S, et al. The effect of triclosan-coated sutures in wound healing. A double blind randomised prospective pilot study. J Plast Reconstr Aesthet Surg 2009;62(6):771–3.

101. Tuuli MG, Liu J, Tita ATN, et al. Effect of prophylactic negative pressure wound therapy vs standard wound dressing on surgical-site infection in obese women after cesarean delivery: a randomized clinical trial. JAMA 2020;324(12):1180–9.

102. Stevens DL, Bisno AL, Chambers HF, et al. Practice guidelines for the diagnosis and management of skin and soft tissue infections: 2014 update by the Infectious Diseases Society of America. Clin Infect Dis 2014;59(2):e10–52.

103. Karra R, McDermott L, Connelly S, et al. Risk factors for 1-year mortality after postoperative mediastinitis. J Thorac Cardiovasc Surg 2006;132(3):537–43.

104. Haley RW, Culver DH, White JW, et al. The efficacy of infection surveillance and control programs in preventing nosocomial infections in US hospitals. Am J Epidemiol 1985;121(2):182–205.

105. Cruse PJ, Foord R. The epidemiology of wound infection. A 10-year prospective study of 62,939 wounds. Surg Clin North Am 1980;60(1):27–40.

106. Olson MM, Lee JT Jr. Continuous, 10-year wound infection surveillance. Results, advantages, and unanswered questions. Arch Surg 1990;125(6):794–803.

107. Baker C, Luce J, Chenoweth C, et al. Comparison of case-finding methodologies for endometritis after cesarean section. Am J Infect Control 1995;23(1):27–33.

108. Cardo DM, Falk PS, Mayhall CG. Validation of surgical wound surveillance. Infect Control Hosp Epidemiol 1993;14(4):211–5.

109. Ming DY, Chen LF, Miller BA, et al. The impact of depth of infection and postdischarge surveillance on rate of surgical-site infections in a network of community hospitals. Infect Control Hosp Epidemiol 2012;33(3):276–82.

110. Wenzel RP, Osterman CA, Hunting KJ, et al. Hospital-acquired infections. I. Surveillance in a university hospital. Am J Epidemiol 1976;103(3):251–60.

111. Yokoe DS, Noskin GA, Cunningham SM, et al. Enhanced identification of postoperative infections among inpatients. Emerg Infect Dis 2004;10(11):1924–30.

112. Platt R, Kleinman K, Thompson K, et al. Using automated health plan data to assess infection risk from coronary artery bypass surgery. Emerg Infect Dis 2002;8(12):1433–41.

113. Inacio MC, Paxton EW, Chen Y, et al. Leveraging electronic medical records for surveillance of surgical site infection in a total joint replacement population. Infect Control Hosp Epidemiol 2011;32(4):351–9.

114. Bolon MK, Hooper D, Stevenson KB, et al. Improved surveillance for surgical site infections after orthopedic implantation procedures: extending applications for automated data. Clin Infect Dis 2009;48(9):1223–9.

115. Martin LA, Neighbors HW, Griffith DM. The experience of symptoms of depression in men vs women: analysis of the National Comorbidity Survey Replication. JAMA Psychiatry 2013;70(10):1100–6.

116. Baker AW, Haridy S, Salem J, et al. Performance of statistical process control methods for regional surgical site infection surveillance: a 10-year multicentre pilot study. BMJ Qual Saf 2018;27(8):600–10.

117. Dumville JC, McFarlane E, Edwards P, et al. Preoperative skin antiseptics for preventing surgical wound infections after clean surgery. Cochrane Database Syst Rev 2013;(3):CD003949.

118. McLaws ML, Murphy C, Whitby M. Standardising surveillance of nosocomial infections: the HISS program. Hospital infection standardised surveillance. J Qual Clin Pract 2000;20(1):6–11.

Methicillin-Resistant *Staphylococcus aureus*: An Update on Prevention and Control in Acute Care Settings

Andie S. Lee, MBBS, DTM&H, MSc[a],*, Benedikt D. Huttner, MD, MS[b],
Gaud Catho, MD[c], Stephan Harbarth, MD, MS[c]

KEYWORDS

- Methicillin-resistant *Staphylococcus aureus* • MRSA • Epidemiology
- Infection prevention • Infection control • Active surveillance cultures • Screening
- Decolonization

KEY POINTS

- Methicillin-resistant *Staphylococcus aureus* (MRSA) is an important cause of health-care–associated infections and remains endemic in many health care facilities worldwide.
- Since the 2000s, there has been decreasing clinical and health-economic burden of MRSA compared with multidrug-resistant gram-negative bacteria worldwide, often following implementation of concerted and coordinated multifaceted interventions.
- A change in the epidemiology of MRSA has been noted with increasing introduction of community-associated MRSA into acute care settings (particularly pediatrics), requiring modified infection prevention and control measures (eg, including health care worker screening and contact tracing of household members).
- Despite overall successes in reducing the burden of this multidrug-resistant organism, the optimal approach to MRSA control has been controversial due to limited high-quality evidence to support interventions. However, over the past 15 years, new data from robust large-scale studies have emerged, particularly with regard to MRSA screening and decolonization (targeted and universal) strategies.
- Flexibility to adapt and institute evidence-based measures in the context of local epidemiology, infrastructure, and resources is essential for successful MRSA control.

[a] Departments of Infectious Diseases and Microbiology, Royal Prince Alfred Hospital, University of Sydney, Missenden Road, Camperdown, Sydney, NSW 2050, Australia; [b] Division of Infectious Diseases, University of Geneva Hospitals, University of Geneva, Rue Gabrielle-Perret-Gentil 4, Geneva CH-1205, Switzerland; [c] Infection Control Programme, University of Geneva Hospitals, Rue Gabrielle-Perret-Gentil 4, Geneva CH-1205, Switzerland
* Corresponding author.
E-mail address: andie.lee@health.nsw.gov.au

Infect Dis Clin N Am 35 (2021) 931–952
https://doi.org/10.1016/j.idc.2021.07.001
0891-5520/21/© 2021 Elsevier Inc. All rights reserved.

id.theclinics.com

INTRODUCTION

Methicillin-resistant *Staphylococcus aureus* (MRSA), first described in 1961,[1] has become endemic in health care facilities worldwide. MRSA is a leading cause of skin and soft tissue infections presenting to emergency departments in the United States[2] and in many regions, a significant proportion of invasive infections due to *S aureus* are methicillin resistant (more than 50% in parts of Southern Europe and the Asia-Pacific region).[3,4] The virulence and survival fitness of this pathogen[5] likely contribute to the increased mortality, length of stay, and health care costs associated with MRSA compared with methicillin-sensitive *S aureus* (MSSA).[6] Given its significant impacts on human health, MRSA has been included in the World Health Organization's high priority list of drug-resistant bacteria targeted for the development of new antimicrobials.[7]

Strategies to control MRSA address the reservoir of carriers, routes of transmission, and antibiotic selection pressure (**Fig. 1**). In practice, multiple interventions are often used in an attempt to effectively curb transmission and infection. However, the utility of some control measures is debated due to the inability to eradicate endemic MRSA and the disruption in patient care and costs associated with some strategies.[8,9] Finally, many experts now argue that control of highly resistant gram-negative bacteria, such as carbapenemase-producing Enterobacteriaceae should have higher priority.[7,10,11]

This review provides an update regarding approaches to MRSA control in health care settings with endemic MRSA. Controversies surrounding control measures and recent evidence from rigorously conducted large studies also are discussed. This review does not cover the "search-and-destroy" strategy used in countries with low MRSA prevalence, such as the Netherlands and Denmark (refer to the national policy of the Dutch Working Party on Infection Prevention[12]), or the control of livestock-associated MRSA (see Ref.[13]).

DECLINING METHICILLIN-RESISTANT *STAPHYLOCOCCUS AUREUS* RATES IN MANY REGIONS

MRSA epidemiology exhibits marked geographic variation. It is important to note, however, that data from different regions should be compared with caution due to varying definitions used for data collection, study populations, intensity of surveillance, and duration of follow-up. Prospective surveillance networks now exist in many regions, enabling early detection of increasing MRSA rates and facilitating timely

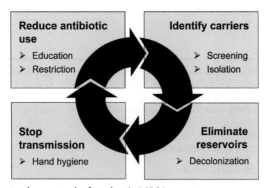

Fig. 1. Approaches to the control of endemic MRSA.

implementation of interventions. These data are also valuable for feedback to institutions, benchmarking and monitoring the success of control strategies.

Trends in Europe

Data from the European Antimicrobial Resistance Surveillance Network (EARS-Net)[3] illustrate the marked variation in Europe in the proportion of *S aureus* isolates that are methicillin resistant. In general, there is an increase in MRSA prevalence from the north to south/east of the continent (**Fig. 2**). These differences are thought to be at least partly explained by varying antibiotic use and infection control practices.[14,15]

It is interesting to note that there have been steady or decreasing MRSA infections rates seen in a number of high-income countries from the early to mid-2000s (see **Fig. 2**). For example, although MRSA rates were high in France in the 1990s, the country subsequently experienced a decline in these rates (**Fig. 3**). This trend seemed to follow a stringent national control program gradually introduced between 1993 and 2004,[16] which included strengthening infection control activities, and mandatory MRSA surveillance and notification of outbreaks.

In the United Kingdom, MRSA bloodstream infections (BSIs) rose during the 1990s, peaking in 2003 with subsequent yearly reduction, then more recent plateauing in rates (**Fig. 4**). As was the case in France, this favorable trend followed implementation of a national strategy, including universal screening on hospital admission.[17] Although the national hand hygiene campaign is considered a major contributor to the decline in MRSA,[18] it is likely that the multifaceted approach, together with a clear target and support from the Department of Health, resulted in the marked improvement.

In addition to France and the United Kingdom, there is now a diverse group of European countries, with varying baseline MRSA prevalence, that have been able to reverse previously increasing trends in MRSA (see **Fig. 2**). Although the proportion of MRSA among *S aureus* isolates decreased in Europe from 27% in 2007 to 17% in 2015, a study of the burden of antibiotic-resistant bacteria in this region has estimated that the incidence of MRSA infections has actually increased by 1.28 times during this period, mainly due to infections in infants and older individuals (>55 years).[11]

Trends in the United States

In the United States, MRSA rates steadily increased from 1998, with MRSA accounting for 53% of *S aureus* clinical isolates in 2005.[19] Since that year, there has been a decrease in hospital-onset BSIs due to MRSA (17% annual reduction between 2005 and 2012, with a slower decline seen between 2013 and 2016).[20] As was the case in parts of Europe, a series of infection control interventions during this period may have contributed to the decline. In 2007, Veterans Affairs hospitals throughout the United States introduced a multimodal strategy involving universal MRSA screening, contact precautions, hand hygiene promotion, and institutional culture change.[21] Between 2005 and 2017, there was a 55% decrease in MRSA infections in Veterans Affairs hospitals.[22] Many US states also mandated specific MRSA control interventions,[23] and in 2008, the Centers for Medicare and Medicaid Services introduced financial penalties, declining additional payment to hospitals for preventable health-care–acquired complications such as health-care–associated infections (HAIs).[24]

Potential Explanations for Declines in Methicillin-Resistant Staphylococcus aureus

It is often difficult to identify the precise determinants of successful MRSA control. Decreasing MRSA rates may reflect improved infection control practices and enhanced antibiotic stewardship. Some argue, however, that widespread declines

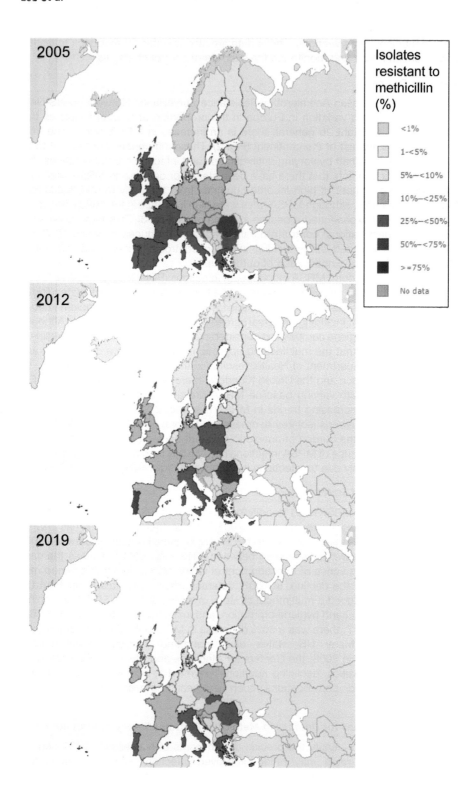

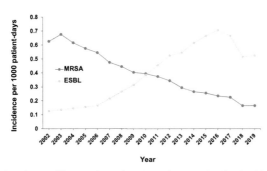

Fig. 3. French national surveillance data showing changes in the incidence of MRSA and extended spectrum beta-lactamase (ESBL)-producing Enterobacteriaceae (2002–2019). (Data *from* Santé publique France. Available at: www.santepubliquefrance.fr. Accessed March 26, 2021)

in MRSA are attributable to changes in the organism itself, including shifts in circulating clones.[25] An observational study in Oxford (United Kingdom) found that MRSA rates fell in line with national trends from 2003, but this decline preceded local roll-out of enhanced infection control interventions in 2006.[26] Typing data showed that the decline was strain-specific, particularly involving ST36. Similarly, areas of France where enhanced interventions were not implemented also experienced decreasing MRSA rates.[27]

Biological factors, such as reduced bacterial fitness manifesting as decreased survival and/or growth rate,[28] could explain the decline in particular strains. A Danish study explored this hypothesis by typing stored isolates from the first MRSA epidemic in Denmark (1957–1980). They found a significant fitness cost associated with multiple antibiotic resistances, which, based on mathematical modeling, could explain declines in phage complex 83A observed in Denmark.[29] The relative contribution of infection control strategies versus biological factors on declining MRSA rates remains an area of debate.

IMPORTATION OF COMMUNITY-ASSOCIATED METHICILLIN-RESISTANT *STAPHYLOCOCCUS AUREUS* INTO HEALTH CARE SETTINGS

The importation of virulent and transmissible community-associated (CA-MRSA) into acute care settings poses challenges around the globe. Indeed, a growing body of evidence suggests that CA-MRSA lineages are increasingly responsible for HAIs.[30] Although no precise international surveillance data are currently available on this worrisome trend, several studies have reported epidemiologic data on CA-MRSA infections among hospitalized patients.

First, several US investigators have found an increase in the relative proportion of MRSA BSIs due to the endemic CA-MRSA USA300 strain, including hospital-onset BSIs, despite overall decreasing trends of MRSA BSI in the United States.[31,32] Second, many nosocomial CA-MRSA outbreaks have been reported, highlighting the

Fig. 2. Proportion of invasive *S aureus* isolates with methicillin resistance from 2005 to 2019 in countries participating in the European Antimicrobial Resistance Surveillance Network (EARS-Net). (*From* EARS-Net data. Available at: http://ecdc.europa.eu/en/activities/surveillance/EARS-Net/Pages/index.aspx. Accessed March 26, 2021; with permission)

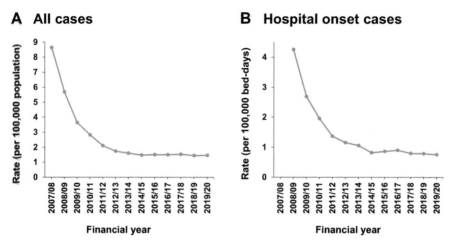

A All cases

B Hospital onset cases

Fig. 4. Trends in rates of MRSA bacteremia in England per 100,000 population (*A*) and hospital-onset cases per 100,000 bed-days (*B*) (2007–2020). (*From* Public Health England. Available at: https://www.gov.uk/government/statistics/mrsa-mssa-and-e-coli-bacteraemia-and-c-difficile-infection-annual-epidemiological-commentary. Accessed March 26, 2021)

epidemic potential of CA-MRSA transmission in acute care settings.[33,34] Finally, mathematical models predict that CA-MRSA strains harboring smaller SCC*mec* elements will eventually displace traditional hospital-acquired MRSA strains in hospitals, with significant clinical and public health implications.[35]

Although this emerging trend is of concern, it does not fundamentally change preventive measures to control MRSA in hospitals, described later in this article in more detail. The only major exception may be the more aggressive staff screening policies implemented in the context of a documented CA-MRSA outbreak in a hospital ward, especially in the absence of an identified reservoir of patients colonized with CA-MRSA.[36]

RECENT EVIDENCE AND CONTROVERSIES REGARDING METHICILLIN-RESISTANT *STAPHYLOCOCCUS AUREUS* CONTROL STRATEGIES

Before discussing research regarding MRSA control, it is important to highlight issues to consider before applying research findings to clinical practice. Studies often report the effect of multiple simultaneously implemented interventions, making it difficult to determine the relative contribution of each intervention. It is also noteworthy that studies have been conducted in the context of varying baseline MRSA prevalence. Thus, results may not be generalizable to all settings. Reporting bias, where negative studies are less likely to be published, must also be considered. In addition, many studies have suboptimal design and analysis. In the past, most studies have been observational or quasi-experimental, with few randomized controlled trials. Fortunately, data from several high-quality intervention studies are now available.

Research concerning MRSA control interventions has resulted in ongoing debate with regard to the utility of MRSA screening, isolation, decolonization, and environmental cleaning. The importance of hand hygiene and antibiotic stewardship is less controversial. The potential advantages and disadvantages of various interventions are summarized in **Table 1** and discussed in the following sections.

Table 1
Advantages and disadvantages of various methicillin-resistant *Staphylococcus aureus* control strategies

Infection Control Measure	Mode of Action	Potential Advantages	Potential Disadvantages/ Barriers to Implementation
Hand hygiene	Reduces cross-transmission	Simple Inexpensive Not organism specific	Requires behavior change Difficult to sustain high hand hygiene compliance rates
MRSA screening of patients	Early identification of carriers	Identifies reservoir Reduces infection risk for the individual patient (eg, appropriate perioperative antibiotic prophylaxis)	Costs Resources MRSA-specific Needs to be linked with other measures (eg, isolation, decolonization) Optimal population and method controversial
MRSA screening and decolonization of health care workers	Reduces reservoir	Complete assessment of reservoir Interruption of MRSA transmission to patients Reduction of infection risk for the individual health care worker Decreased transmission risk to close contacts/ community reservoir	Disruption to patient care False reassurance of noncolonized or nonidentified health care workers Ethical considerations (stigmatization) Costs
Isolation	Increased barrier to cross-transmission	Not organism specific	Costs Potential negative psychological effects Possible decrease in quality of care of patient
Targeted decolonization	Reduces reservoir	Interruption of MRSA transmission to other patients Reduces infection risk for the individual patient	Not feasible for all patients Risk of mupirocin and chlorhexidine resistance Side effects of decolonization treatment
Universal decolonization (routine chlorhexidine bathing)	Reduces reservoir	Reduces infection risk for the individual patient Not organism specific	Risk of chlorhexidine resistance Side effects of decolonization treatment
Antibiotic stewardship	Reduces selection pressure	Not organism specific (includes *Clostridium difficile*)	Opposition from physicians and pharmaceutical industry Most effective interventions unclear Long-term effects unclear
Enhanced environmental cleaning	Reduces environmental reservoir	Not organism specific	Strong evidence for efficacy lacking Best strategy unclear

Abbreviation: MRSA, methicillin-resistant *S aureus*.

Hand Hygiene

As MRSA is most commonly transmitted between patients via the contaminated hands of health care workers (HCWs), a multimodal approach to improving hand hygiene practices is an integral part of standard infection control measures.[37] The effectiveness of hand hygiene promotion has been demonstrated in terms of reductions in MRSA transmission and infections at local and national levels.[18,38–40] Although efforts to improve hand hygiene practices in health care facilities are important, controversy exists regarding the utility of attempts to further increase hand hygiene compliance in settings where baseline compliance is already high (>50%). In this situation, studies, including dynamic modeling, suggest that this intervention alone may not result in further significant reduction in MRSA transmission.[41,42]

Screening for Methicillin-Resistant Staphylococcus aureus

Most MRSA carriage is asymptomatic and therefore not identified using routine clinical cultures. The latter alone may only identify 18% of actual MRSA patient-days.[43] A significant number of colonized patients will subsequently develop infection, with estimates of up to 25% of patients in intensive care units (ICUs).[44] Active MRSA surveillance may identify this large asymptomatic reservoir of transmission and infection risk using screening cultures or more rapid nucleic acid amplification tests (NAATs), which are often polymerase chain reaction (PCR)-based assays. Patients identified to be colonized may then be placed on contact precautions and decolonization treatment, usually in the form of topical antibiotics and antiseptics, may be instituted in an attempt to eradicate carriage and/or reduce risk of MRSA infection.

Active surveillance may be universal, where all patients admitted to hospital are screened, or targeted, where screening is limited to patient groups at increased risk of colonization, such as those with prior antibiotic use, prolonged hospitalization, ICU admission, hemodialysis, or contact with a known MRSA carrier. Risk factors for MRSA colonization may vary in different regions[45,46]; therefore, targeted screening approaches should be tailored to local MRSA epidemiology. HCWs who are MRSA carriers can also act as reservoirs for outbreaks and ongoing transmission within hospitals, especially for CA-MRSA. HCW screening in settings with endemic MRSA is beyond the scope of this review but is discussed elsewhere.[36]

Until recently, universal MRSA screening has been one of the most controversial issues in infection control due to questions about its effectiveness, pathogen-specific approach, and costs, particularly for screening using NAATs.[9] Active surveillance is considered most useful in patients at high risk of MRSA infection, such as in outbreak settings.[47] More recently, studies have focused on universal screening in endemic settings to reduce infection risk, with conflicting results (**Table 2**).

In 2008, a hospital-wide observational study conducted in the United States showed that universal MRSA screening was associated with reduction in MRSA disease.[43] In contrast, a prospective crossover study in surgical wards of a Swiss hospital published the same year did not find a reduction in MRSA infections or acquisition.[48] Other studies have compared molecular-based and culture-based screening, also with varying results.[49,50] A large prospective multicenter study, reported in 2013 in 33 surgical wards in Europe and Israel, did not find that screening was associated with a reduction in MRSA infections overall.[51] However, screening combined with contact precautions and decolonization was associated with decreasing MRSA infection rates in the subgroup of clean surgery wards.

There have been a number of high-quality studies exploring the utility of MRSA screening in ICUs. Previous reports, predominantly retrospective or quasi-

Table 2
Selected studies of universal methicillin-resistant *Staphylococcus aureus* screening

Study, Country	Setting	Design	Control Group	Total Duration (mo)	Rapid Screening	Decolonization[a]	Admission MRSA Prevalence (%)	Baseline MRSA Infection Rate (per 1000 Patient-days)	Additional Interventions	Findings	Primary Outcome
Robicsek et al,[32] 2008, US	Hospital-wide	Before-after	No	45	Molecular (commercial) modified in-house	Targeted (at physician discretion)	6.3	0.89	Staged ICU screening then universal screening	Reduction in MRSA disease	Positive
Harbarth et al,[38] 2008, Switzerland	Surgery	Crossover	Yes	24	Molecular (in-house)	Targeted	5.1	0.91	Modified perioperative prophylaxis	No reduction in MRSA infections	Negative
Jeyaratnam et al,[39] 2008, UK	Geriatrics, Oncology, Surgery	Crossover	Yes	14	Molecular (commercial) vs selective broth/chromogenic agar	Targeted	6.7	1.09	Preemptive isolation if high-risk; discharge screening	No reduction in MRSA transmission	Negative
Hardy et al,[40] 2010, UK	Surgery	Crossover	Yes	16	Molecular (commercial) vs chromogenic agar	Targeted (with naseptin if high-level mupirocin resistance)	3.6	Not stated	Rescreening every 4 d; decolonization in 71% molecular vs 41% culture arms	Reduction in MRSA transmission	Positive
Huskins et al,[44] 2011, US	ICU	Cluster-randomized trial	Yes	17	Selective broth/selective agar (mannitol salt agar with oxacillin)	No (but some targeted use at physician discretion)	9.5–12.4	13.7–13.9 (colonization and infection)	Rescreening weekly and on discharge	No reduction in MRSA transmission or infection	Negative

(continued on next page)

Table 2
(continued)

Study, Country	Setting	Design	Control Group	Total Duration (mo)	Rapid Screening	Decolonization[a]	Admission MRSA Prevalence (%)	Baseline MRSA Infection Rate (per 1000 Patient-days)	Additional Interventions	Findings	Primary Outcome
Lee et al,[41] 2013, Europe and Israel	Surgery	Prospective interventional cohort	Yes	24	Molecular (commercial) and chromogenic agar	Targeted	2.1	0.56	Universal screening vs hand hygiene vs combination	No reduction in MRSA infection (except for clean surgery)	Negative
Huang et al,[45] 2013, US	ICU	Cluster-randomized trial	Yes	33	Not stated	Group 2 – Targeted; Group 3 – Universal	10.2–11.5	3.4–4.3 (MRSA clinical cultures); 0.5–0.6 (bacteremia)	Group 1 – screening, isolation; Group 2 – screening, targeted decolonization; Group 3 – no screening, universal decolonization	No reduction in MRSA infection in Group 1	Negative (for screening without decolonization)
Derde et al,[46] 2014, Europe	ICU	Cluster-randomized trial	Yes	27	Molecular (commercial) vs chromogenic agar	Universal	3.6	Not stated	Hand hygiene and universal decolonization phase followed by screening phase	No reduction in MRSA transmission (for screening)	Negative
Roth et al,[108] 2016, Canada	Hospital-wide	Quasi-experimental	Yes	44	Selective broth/molecular (commercial) with culture (nonselective agar) confirmation	No	2.6	0.47 (colonization and infection)	Nil	No reduction in MRSA transmission	Negative

Abbreviations: ICU, intensive care unit; MRSA, methicillin-resistant *S aureus*.
a Decolonization refers to topical antibiotic and/or antiseptic treatment. Targeted decolonization refers to treatment of known MRSA carriers; universal decolonization refers to treatment of all patients in the study group, regardless of colonization status.

experimental in design, have largely shown that screening was associated with decreased incidence of MRSA BSIs, not only in the ICU but hospital-wide.[52,53] However, 3 more recent robust cluster-randomized controlled trials did not find that screening was associated with a decrease in MRSA transmission or infections.[54–56] It must be noted, however, that the long turnaround time for screening results (mean 5.2 ± SD 1.4 days) in the first study conducted in 19 ICUs in the United States,[54] where all screening swabs were processed at a central laboratory, may have delayed institution of control measures, decreasing the effectiveness of the screening strategy. The second study, also conducted in the United States in 74 ICUs, showed that MRSA screening and isolation without decolonization was only partially effective in reducing the rate of MRSA clinical isolates or MRSA BSIs.[55] The third study involved 13 European ICUs.[56] It compared PCR-based and culture-based screening and found that in the setting of high compliance with hand hygiene and universal chlorhexidine bathing, the addition of screening did not further reduce the acquisition of multiresistant bacteria, including MRSA.

The costs and adverse effects of universal MRSA screening have also prompted much discussion, particularly with regard to laboratory resources, decolonization, and isolation policies. Some argue that resources are better used for "horizontal" strategies that target all HAIs rather than MRSA alone.[57] A study evaluating the costs and benefits of universal MRSA screening in England found that this strategy was not cost-effective due to the fall in MRSA prevalence in the United Kingdom.[58] Screening admissions to high-risk specialties was likely to represent better resource use in terms of cost per quality-adjusted life-year gained.[58]

Although many recent studies cast doubt on the utility of MRSA screening over non–pathogen-specific approaches such as universal decolonization in the ICU setting, changes in practice should be implemented with caution. There are several important considerations at a local level when assessing the need to screen for MRSA (**Fig. 5**). In certain populations, such as patients undergoing clean surgical procedures, preoperative screening linked with targeted decolonization and surgical prophylaxis with MRSA activity is likely to reduce postoperative MRSA infections.[59] Based on the accumulating evidence, mandates for universal MRSA screening introduced in 2009 to 2010 in the United Kingdom have been modified to recommend a targeted risk-based approach.[60] The authors found that such an approach (predominantly using cultures with selective media) is reasonable and should be based on local MRSA prevalence, risk factors for colonization, and the vulnerability of the patient population.

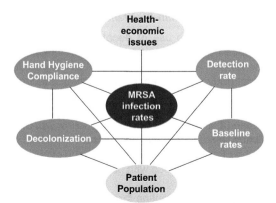

Fig. 5. Important issues to consider when introducing a screening program for MRSA.

Contact Precautions and Isolation

Identifying carriers without additional interventions to reduce the risk of transmission or progression to infection is unlikely to have an impact on MRSA infections. Placing those with MRSA on contact precautions (ie, using gown and gloves for contact with the patient or their environment) may delay colonization of other patients and thereby reduce infection rates.[61] Although studies have found that contact precautions reduce MRSA acquisition, most of these studies are of low quality.[62] A more rigorous cluster-randomized trial in ICUs found that universal glove and gown use did not reduce the overall acquisition of multiresistant gram-positive organisms.[63] There was, however, a small reduction in MRSA acquisition, a secondary outcome of the study.

It is recommended that patients with MRSA are isolated in single rooms or cohorted depending on the availability of single rooms.[64] Where facilities are limited, patients may be isolated based on a risk assessment of the likelihood of transmission and possible impact of MRSA spread to vulnerable patients.[64] Observational studies have shown that single-room isolation reduces MRSA acquisition and infections among hospitalized patients.[65] However, a prospective study of isolation in the ICU did not show a difference in MRSA transmission.[66]

There is debate regarding the utility of contact precautions and isolation.[67] Concerns have been raised about social isolation, feelings of depression, patient satisfaction, and the quality of care provided by HCWs for patients in isolation.[68] It is reassuring to note, however, that an increase in adverse events was not seen in a cluster-randomized controlled ICU trial conducted by Harris and colleagues.[63]

Duration of MRSA colonization in individuals is variable and there is a lack of consensus regarding when contact precautions can be discontinued.[69] A framework guiding discontinuation of contact precautions, including requirements for the number of negative screening cultures over a specified period of time (eg, 3 consecutive negative weekly surveillance cultures), with extension of contact precautions for high-risk patients, including those with chronic wounds or from long-term care facilities, has been suggested.[70]

In view of the limited evidence for isolation of MRSA carriers and potential harms, recommendation of this intervention in all settings may no longer be warranted, particularly where there is good adherence to standard precautions, including hand hygiene, and where MRSA rates are not high or increasing. Experts have called for a review of the necessity of this intervention or, at a minimum, for guidelines to highlight the uncertainties regarding the value of contact precautions and isolation for MRSA control.[9,67]

Targeted Decolonization of Methicillin-Resistant Staphylococcus aureus Carriers

There is increasing interest in the use of decolonization to suppress or eradicate MRSA carriage to reduce transmission and subsequent infection risk.[71] Decolonization is commonly performed with topical intranasal antibiotics (eg, mupirocin) with or without antibacterial body washes (eg, chlorhexidine), although a variety of other agents can been used.[72] Short-term nasal mupirocin is the most effective treatment for eradicating nasal MRSA carriage, with a success rate of up to 90% 1 week after treatment, and between 30% and 60% after longer follow-up, depending on the patient profile and colonization of extranasal body sites.[73,74] It must be noted that eradication of MRSA can be challenging due to the presence of chronic wounds, medical devices, and comorbidities. Compliance with decolonization protocols also influences success rates.[75]

There is insufficient evidence for routine targeted decolonization of all MRSA carriers. Decolonization is often used during MRSA outbreaks, particularly if linked to transmission by HCWs. Data looking specifically at ICUs show that the incidence of MRSA colonization and/or infections was reduced after initiation of decolonization.[76] Other reports have also demonstrated that decolonization of S aureus carriers (including predominantly MSSA carriers) with mupirocin reduces infection rates, particularly in surgical and dialysis patients.[59,77] However, decolonization of MRSA carriers did not reduce infection rates in patients who were predominantly cared for on medical services.[78] As infections may develop after patients leave hospital, a recent study assessed the effectiveness of post-discharge decolonization of MRSA carriers for 5 days twice a month for 6 months and found that it led to a 30% lower risk of MRSA infection at 12 months.[79]

Although there has been demonstrated benefit in some patient groups, the use of decolonization therapy has also raised some concerns. Resistance may emerge with uncontrolled use of mupirocin.[80,81] Treatment failure has been associated with colonization with mupirocin-resistant and/or chlorhexidine-resistant strains at baseline, or recovery of resistant strains after treatment when baseline strains were sensitive.[82,83] Some also question the utility of this intervention due to significant rates of patient recolonization.[72] In health care facilities with high rates of HAIs due to S aureus, it may be reasonable to use decolonization therapy in S aureus carriers who are at high risk of infection, particularly short-term use in those undergoing clean surgical procedures (eg, cardiothoracic and orthopedic surgery) where the evidence for benefit of this intervention is most robust.[59]

Universal Decolonization with Routine Chlorhexidine Bathing

By decreasing the bacterial load on patients' skin, universal decolonization (ie, decolonizing all patients regardless of known MRSA colonization status) with routine chlorhexidine bathing may reduce MRSA transmission and infection. There are several multicenter cluster-randomized controlled trials that have evaluated this intervention in ICU patients.[55,84,85] They have shown that universal decolonization (with chlorhexidine bathing, and the addition of intranasal mupirocin in one study[55]) was effective in reducing acquisition of multidrug-resistant organisms and health-care–associated BSIs.[55,84,86] However, the reduction in BSIs was mostly due to skin commensals, with failure to demonstrate significant decreases in MRSA acquisition or infection.

In contrast, other cluster-randomized controlled trials have failed to reproduce these findings.[85] In addition, a recent study conducted in non–critical care settings showed that universal chlorhexidine bathing and targeted intranasal mupirocin for MRSA carriers did not significantly reduce MRSA or vancomycin-resistant *Enterococcus* clinical cultures or BSIs, except in a post hoc analysis of a subgroup of patients with devices.[87] It is important to bear in mind that chlorhexidine resistance may result in failure of chlorhexidine bathing protocols,[82,88] and chlorhexidine allergy/intolerance and increased costs should also be considered.[89] Thus caution must be exercised with widespread use of chlorhexidine bathing.

Antibiotic Stewardship

Selective pressure from prior antibiotic use is a risk factor for MRSA acquisition.[90] A meta-analysis assessed 76 studies and found a 1.8-fold (95% confidence interval [CI] 1.7–1.9, $P<.001$) increase in the risk of acquiring MRSA in patients with recent antibiotic use, particularly fluoroquinolones (risk ratio 3, 95% CI 2.5–3.5).[90] More recent studies using robust statistical methods have also shown an association between antibiotic use and MRSA incidence at hospital and country levels.[15,91,92]

There is also evidence to suggest that reduction in antibiotic use can result in reduction in MRSA infections.[93] A nonlinear time-series study, conducted across a region in

Scotland, found that a national antibiotic stewardship and infection control program was associated with a reduction in MRSA prevalence density of 50% ($P = .006$) in hospitals as well as a 47% decline ($P<.0001$) in the community over a 16-year period.[94] As antibiotic use is also linked to the incidence of other nosocomial pathogens, the promotion of appropriate antibiotic use should be a priority for all health care facilities.[95]

Environmental Cleaning

MRSA is frequently found in the environment close to colonized patients,[96] with numerous surfaces (eg, keyboards, tourniquets, and files) becoming contaminated. This organism can survive on surfaces for months,[97] acting as an ongoing reservoir for transmission long after a colonized patient has been discharged. Small-scale studies have shown that enhanced cleaning can reduce environmental MRSA contamination.[98,99] Observational studies also suggest that environmental contamination can play a role in MRSA transmission. One such study found that a cleaning intervention was associated with a reduction in MRSA transmission, including from prior room occupants.[100]

Recently, "no touch" cleaning techniques such as ultraviolet (UV) light, hydrogen peroxide, or antibacterial surface materials (such as copper) have been promoted as more efficient and less labor-intensive methods of environmental decontamination.[97] However, most studies evaluating these modalities have been limited to their effect on detectable MRSA contamination of the environment or have used suboptimal study designs that are susceptible to numerous sources of bias when assessing clinical outcomes. Two recent more robust cluster-randomized trials of cleaning interventions, including UV-C[101] and a cleaning bundle,[102] showed a reduction in acquisition of pathogens or HAIs. However, the effects were mainly seen for vancomycin-resistant *Enterococcus* rather than MRSA. Strong clinical evidence correlating cleaning (by any method) or environmental decontamination with a reduction in HAIs due to MRSA remains, therefore, lacking.[103]

Whole Genome Sequencing for Methicillin-Resistant Staphylococcus aureus Control

Whole genome sequencing (WGS) has traditionally been used for demonstrating the population biology of organisms including MRSA.[104] However, over the past decade, this technology has also been a useful tool for investigating MRSA transmission in hospital and community settings.[105–107] The added insights from WGS data, beyond collection of epidemiologic information alone, can assist in refining infection control interventions so they are tailored to local transmission dynamics. However, the lack of widespread and timely access to this technology at present limits its routine clinical use.

SUMMARY

The control of MRSA is paramount in health care settings. Reducing the burden of this pathogen is an important public health priority that has attracted increasing public and political interest. The decline in invasive MRSA infections in many countries seems to correlate with the introduction of multifaceted infection control approaches coupled with strong leadership and administrative support, often at a national level, to facilitate implementation of interventions. With accumulation of high-quality studies evaluating these interventions, flexibility to adapt and institute evidence-based measures in the context of local epidemiology and available resources remains important to optimize MRSA control.

CLINICS CARE POINTS

- Widespread implementation of multifaceted infection prevention and control interventions has been associated with decreases in the clinical burden of MRSA in geographically diverse acute care settings.

- However, there is increasing importation of community-associated MRSA into health care facilities. If associated with hospital outbreaks, additional interventions (eg, health care worker screening and contact tracing of household members) may be required.

- The utility of universal MRSA screening and contact precautions is unclear, particularly when non–pathogen-specific approaches such as universal decolonization are used. Moreover, universal MRSA screening is not cost-effective in low-prevalence settings.

- Screening and targeted decolonization of *S aureus* (including MRSA) carriers can decrease infections in selected high-risk groups, particularly surgical patients undergoing cardiac and orthopedic procedures.

- Universal decolonization using chlorhexidine bathing with or without intranasal mupirocin can reduce acquisition of multidrug-resistant organisms (including MRSA) and health-care–associated BSIs when used in the ICU.

- Local epidemiology, health infrastructure, and available resources are important to consider when developing MRSA control strategies, to ensure that they are optimized and relevant for local needs.

DISCLOSURE

A.S. Lee: Nothing to disclose.

B.D. Huttner: Nothing to disclose.

G. Catho: Nothing to disclose.

S. Harbarth: SH is a member of the scientific advisory board of Sandoz. He has also received financial support for MRSA research activities from the European Commission.

REFERENCES

1. Benner EJ, Kayser FH. Growing clinical significance of methicillin-resistant *Staphylococcus aureus*. Lancet 1968;2:741–4.

2. Talan DA, Krishnadasan A, Gorwitz RJ, et al. Comparison of *Staphylococcus aureus* from skin and soft-tissue infections in US emergency department patients, 2004 and 2008. Clin Infect Dis 2011;53:144–9.

3. European Antimicrobial Resistance Surveillance Network. Available at: https://www.ecdc.europa.eu/en/about-us/partnerships-and-networks/disease-and-laboratory-networks/ears-net. Accessed March 26, 2021.

4. Global Antimicrobial Resistance Surveillance System (GLASS). Available at: https://www.who.int/glass/en/. Accessed March 26, 2021.

5. Lee AS, de Lencastre H, Garau J, et al. Methicillin-resistant *Staphylococcus aureus*. Nat Rev Dis Primers 2018;4:18033.

6. Cosgrove SE, Sakoulas G, Perencevich EN, et al. Comparison of mortality associated with methicillin-resistant and methicillin-susceptible *Staphylococcus aureus* bacteremia: a meta-analysis. Clin Infect Dis 2003;36:53–9.

7. Tacconelli E, Carrara E, Savoldi A, et al. Discovery, research, and development of new antibiotics: the WHO priority list of antibiotic-resistant bacteria and tuberculosis. Lancet Infect Dis 2018;18:318–27.

8. Morgan DJ, Kaye KS, Diekema DJ. Reconsidering isolation precautions for endemic methicillin-resistant *Staphylococcus aureus* and vancomycin-resistant *Enterococcus*. JAMA 2014;312:1395–6.

9. Fatkenheuer G, Hirschel B, Harbarth S. Screening and isolation to control meticillin-resistant *Staphylococcus aureus*: sense, nonsense, and evidence. Lancet 2015;385:1146–9.

10. CDC. Antibiotic resistance threats in the United States, 2019. Atlanta, GA: U.S. Department of Health and Human Services, CDC; 2019.

11. Cassini A, Hogberg LD, Plachouras D, et al. Attributable deaths and disability-adjusted life-years caused by infections with antibiotic-resistant bacteria in the EU and the European Economic Area in 2015: a population-level modelling analysis. Lancet Infect Dis 2019;19:56–66.

12. Dutch Working Party on Infection Prevention (WIP). Policy for methicillin-restistant *Staphylococcus aureus*. 2007. Available at: http://www.wip.nl. Accessed March 26, 2021.

13. Fluit AC. Livestock-associated *Staphylococcus aureus*. Clin Microbiol Infect 2012;18:735–44.

14. Kock R, Becker K, Cookson B, et al. Methicillin-resistant *Staphylococcus aureus* (MRSA): burden of disease and control challenges in Europe. Euro Surveill 2010;15:19688.

15. Borg MA, Camilleri L. What is driving the epidemiology of methicillin-resistant *Staphylococcus aureus* infections in Europe? Microb Drug Resist 2021;27: 889–94.

16. Carlet J, Astagneau P, Brun-Buisson C, et al. French national program for prevention of healthcare-associated infections and antimicrobial resistance, 1992-2008: positive trends, but perseverance needed. Infect Control Hosp Epidemiol 2009;30:737–45.

17. Edgeworth JD, Batra R, Wulff J, et al. Reductions in methicillin-resistant *Staphylococcus aureus*, *Clostridium difficile* infection and intensive care unit-acquired bloodstream infection across the United Kingdom following implementation of a National Infection Control Campaign. Clin Infect Dis 2020;70:2530–40.

18. Stone SP, Fuller C, Savage J, et al. Evaluation of the national cleanyourhands campaign to reduce *Staphylococcus aureus* bacteraemia and *Clostridium difficile* infection in hospitals in England and Wales by improved hand hygiene: four year, prospective, ecological, interrupted time series study. BMJ 2012;344: e3005.

19. Styers D, Sheehan DJ, Hogan P, et al. Laboratory-based surveillance of current antimicrobial resistance patterns and trends among *Staphylococcus aureus*: 2005 status in the United States. Ann Clin Microbiol Antimicrob 2006;5:2.

20. Kourtis AP, Hatfield K, Baggs J, et al. Vital signs: epidemiology and recent trends in methicillin-resistant and in methicillin-susceptible *Staphylococcus aureus* bloodstream infections - United States. MMWR Morb Mortal Wkly Rep 2019;68:214–9.

21. Jain R, Kralovic SM, Evans ME, et al. Veterans Affairs initiative to prevent methicillin-resistant *Staphylococcus aureus* infections. N Engl J Med 2011; 364:1419–30.

22. Jones M, Jernigan JA, Evans ME, et al. Vital signs: trends in *Staphylococcus aureus* infections in Veterans Affairs medical centers - United States, 2005-2017. MMWR Morb Mortal Wkly Rep 2019;68:220–4.

23. Weber SG, Huang SS, Oriola S, et al. Legislative mandates for use of active surveillance cultures to screen for methicillin-resistant *Staphylococcus aureus* and

vancomycin-resistant enterococci: position statement from the Joint SHEA and APIC Task Force. Infect Control Hosp Epidemiol 2007;28:249–60.

24. Lee GM, Kleinman K, Soumerai SB, et al. Effect of nonpayment for preventable infections in U.S. hospitals. N Engl J Med 2012;367:1428–37.

25. Livermore DM. Fourteen years in resistance. Int J Antimicrob Agents 2012;39: 283–94.

26. Wyllie DH, Walker AS, Miller R, et al. Decline of methicillin-resistant *Staphylococcus aureus* in Oxfordshire hospitals is strain-specific and preceded infection-control intensification. BMJ Open 2011;1:e000160.

27. Rolain JM, Abat C, Brouqui P, et al. Worldwide decrease in methicillin-resistant *Staphylococcus aureus*: do we understand something? Clin Microbiol Infect 2015;21:515–7.

28. Touati A, Bellil Z, Barache D, et al. Fitness cost of antibiotic resistance in *Staphylococcus aureus*: a systematic review. Microb Drug Resist 2021. [Epub ahead of print].

29. Nielsen KL, Pedersen TM, Udekwu KI, et al. Fitness cost: a bacteriological explanation for the demise of the first international methicillin-resistant *Staphylococcus aureus* epidemic. J Antimicrob Chemother 2012;67:1325–32.

30. Barcudi D, Sosa EJ, Lamberghini R, et al. MRSA dynamic circulation between the community and the hospital setting: new insights from a cohort study. J Infect 2020;80:24–37.

31. Popovich KJ, Snitkin ES, Hota B, et al. Genomic and epidemiological evidence for community origins of hospital-onset methicillin-resistant *Staphylococcus aureus* bloodstream infections. J Infect Dis 2017;215:1640–7.

32. See I, Mu Y, Albrecht V, et al. Trends in incidence of methicillin-resistant *Staphylococcus aureus* bloodstream infections differ by strain type and healthcare exposure, United States, 2005-2013. Clin Infect Dis 2020;70:19–25.

33. Sax H, Posfay-Barbe K, Harbarth S, et al. Control of a cluster of community-associated, methicillin-resistant *Staphylococcus aureus* in neonatology. J Hosp Infect 2006;63:93–100.

34. Klein S, Hannesen J, Zanger P, et al. Entry of panton-valentine leukocidin-positive methicillin-resistant *Staphylococcus aureus* into the hospital: prevalence and population structure in Heidelberg, Germany 2015-2018. Sci Rep 2020; 10:13243.

35. Di Ruscio F, Guzzetta G, Bjornholt JV, et al. Quantifying the transmission dynamics of MRSA in the community and healthcare settings in a low-prevalence country. Proc Natl Acad Sci U S A 2019;116:14599–605.

36. Albrich WC, Harbarth S. Health-care workers: source, vector, or victim of MRSA? Lancet Infect Dis 2008;8:289–301.

37. World Health Organization (WHO). WHO guidelines on hand hygiene in health care. In: World Alliance for Patient Safety. Geneva, Switzerland: WHO Press Geneva; 2009. p. 1–262.

38. Pittet D, Hugonnet S, Harbarth S, et al. Effectiveness of a hospital-wide programme to improve compliance with hand hygiene. Infection Control Programme. Lancet 2000;356:1307–12.

39. Marimuthu K, Pittet D, Harbarth S. The effect of improved hand hygiene on nosocomial MRSA control. Antimicrob Resist Infect Control 2014;3:34.

40. Luangasanatip N, Hongsuwan M, Limmathurotsakul D, et al. Comparative efficacy of interventions to promote hand hygiene in hospital: systematic review and network meta-analysis. BMJ 2015;351:h3728.

41. Beggs CB, Shepherd SJ, Kerr KG. How does healthcare worker hand hygiene behaviour impact upon the transmission of MRSA between patients?: an analysis using a Monte Carlo model. BMC Infect Dis 2009;9:64.

42. DiDiodato G. Has improved hand hygiene compliance reduced the risk of hospital-acquired infections among hospitalized patients in Ontario? Analysis of publicly reported patient safety data from 2008 to 2011. Infect Control Hosp Epidemiol 2013;34:605–10.

43. Robicsek A, Beaumont JL, Paule SM, et al. Universal surveillance for methicillin-resistant *Staphylococcus aureus* in 3 affiliated hospitals. Ann Intern Med 2008; 148:409–18.

44. Davis KA, Stewart JJ, Crouch HK, et al. Methicillin-resistant *Staphylococcus aureus* (MRSA) nares colonization at hospital admission and its effect on subsequent MRSA infection. Clin Infect Dis 2004;39:776–82.

45. Robicsek A, Beaumont JL, Wright MO, et al. Electronic prediction rules for methicillin-resistant *Staphylococcus aureus* colonization. Infect Control Hosp Epidemiol 2011;32:9–19.

46. Pan A, Lee A, Cooper B, et al. Risk factors for previously unknown meticillin-resistant *Staphylococcus aureus* carriage on admission to 13 surgical wards in Europe. J Hosp Infect 2013;83:107–13.

47. Jernigan JA, Titus MG, Groschel DH, et al. Effectiveness of contact isolation during a hospital outbreak of methicillin-resistant *Staphylococcus aureus*. Am J Epidemiol 1996;143:496–504.

48. Harbarth S, Fankhauser C, Schrenzel J, et al. Universal screening for methicillin-resistant *Staphylococcus aureus* at hospital admission and nosocomial infection in surgical patients. JAMA 2008;299:1149–57.

49. Jeyaratnam D, Whitty CJ, Phillips K, et al. Impact of rapid screening tests on acquisition of meticillin resistant *Staphylococcus aureus*: cluster randomised crossover trial. BMJ 2008;336:927–30.

50. Hardy K, Price C, Szczepura A, et al. Reduction in the rate of methicillin-resistant *Staphylococcus aureus* acquisition in surgical wards by rapid screening for colonization: a prospective, cross-over study. Clin Microbiol Infect 2010;16: 333–9.

51. Lee AS, Cooper BS, Malhotra-Kumar S, et al. Comparison of strategies to reduce meticillin-resistant *Staphylococcus aureus* rates in surgical patients: a controlled multicentre intervention trial. BMJ Open 2013;3:e003126.

52. Huang SS, Yokoe DS, Hinrichsen VL, et al. Impact of routine intensive care unit surveillance cultures and resultant barrier precautions on hospital-wide methicillin-resistant *Staphylococcus aureus* bacteremia. Clin Infect Dis 2006;43: 971–8.

53. Chaberny IF, Schwab F, Ziesing S, et al. Impact of routine surgical ward and intensive care unit admission surveillance cultures on hospital-wide nosocomial methicillin-resistant *Staphylococcus aureus* infections in a university hospital: an interrupted time-series analysis. J Antimicrob Chemother 2008;62:1422–9.

54. Huskins WC, Huckabee CM, O'Grady NP, et al. Intervention to reduce transmission of resistant bacteria in intensive care. N Engl J Med 2011;364:1407–18.

55. Huang SS, Septimus E, Kleinman K, et al. Targeted versus universal decolonization to prevent ICU infection. N Engl J Med 2013;368:2255–65.

56. Derde LP, Cooper BS, Goossens H, et al. Interventions to reduce colonisation and transmission of antimicrobial-resistant bacteria in intensive care units: an interrupted time series study and cluster randomised trial. Lancet Infect Dis 2014; 14:31–9.

57. Wenzel RP, Bearman G, Edmond MB. Screening for MRSA: a flawed hospital infection control intervention. Infect Control Hosp Epidemiol 2008;29:1012–8.
58. Robotham JV, Deeny SR, Fuller C, et al. Cost-effectiveness of national mandatory screening of all admissions to English National Health Service hospitals for meticillin-resistant *Staphylococcus aureus*: a mathematical modelling study. Lancet Infect Dis 2016;16:348–56.
59. Schweizer M, Perencevich E, McDanel J, et al. Effectiveness of a bundled intervention of decolonization and prophylaxis to decrease Gram positive surgical site infections after cardiac or orthopedic surgery: systematic review and meta-analysis. BMJ 2013;346:f2743.
60. Department of Health. Implementation of modified admission MRSA screening guidance for NHS. 2014. Available at: https://www.gov.uk/government/publications/how-to-approach-mrsa-screening. Accessed March 26, 2021.
61. O'Hara LM, Calfee DP, Miller LG, et al. Optimizing contact precautions to curb the spread of antibiotic-resistant bacteria in hospitals: a multicenter cohort study to identify patient characteristics and healthcare personnel interactions associated with transmission of methicillin-resistant *Staphylococcus aureus*. Clin Infect Dis 2019;69:S171–7.
62. Rubin MA, Samore MH, Harris AD. The importance of contact precautions for endemic methicillin-resistant *Staphylococcus aureus* and vancomycin-resistant enterococci. JAMA 2018;319:863–4.
63. Harris AD, Pineles L, Belton B, et al. Universal glove and gown use and acquisition of antibiotic-resistant bacteria in the ICU: a randomized trial. JAMA 2013;310:1571–80.
64. Calfee DP, Salgado CD, Milstone AM, et al. Strategies to prevent methicillin-resistant *Staphylococcus aureus* transmission and infection in acute care hospitals: 2014 update. Infect Control Hosp Epidemiol 2014;35:772–96.
65. Bracco D, Dubois MJ, Bouali R, et al. Single rooms may help to prevent nosocomial bloodstream infection and cross-transmission of methicillin-resistant *Staphylococcus aureus* in intensive care units. Intensive Care Med 2007;33:836–40.
66. Cepeda JA, Whitehouse T, Cooper B, et al. Isolation of patients in single rooms or cohorts to reduce spread of MRSA in intensive-care units: prospective two-centre study. Lancet 2005;365:295–304.
67. Morgan DJ, Wenzel RP, Bearman G. Contact precautions for endemic MRSA and VRE: time to retire legal mandates. JAMA 2017;318:329–30.
68. Nair R, Perencevich EN, Goto M, et al. Patient care experience with utilization of isolation precautions: systematic literature review and meta-analysis. Clin Microbiol Infect 2020;26:684–95.
69. Shenoy ES, Kim J, Rosenberg ES, et al. Discontinuation of contact precautions for methicillin-resistant *Staphylococcus aureus*: a randomized controlled trial comparing passive and active screening with culture and polymerase chain reaction. Clin Infect Dis 2013;57:176–84.
70. Banach DB, Bearman G, Barnden M, et al. Duration of contact precautions for acute-care settings. Infect Control Hosp Epidemiol 2018;39:127–44.
71. Septimus EJ, Schweizer ML. Decolonization in prevention of health care-associated infections. Clin Microbiol Rev 2016;29:201–22.
72. Simor AE. Staphylococcal decolonisation: an effective strategy for prevention of infection? Lancet Infect Dis 2011;11:952–62.
73. Harbarth S, Dharan S, Liassine N, et al. Randomized, placebo-controlled, double-blind trial to evaluate the efficacy of mupirocin for eradicating carriage of

methicillin-resistant *Staphylococcus aureus*. Antimicrob Agents Chemother 1999;43:1412–6.

74. Ammerlaan HS, Kluytmans JA, Wertheim HF, et al. Eradication of methicillin-resistant *Staphylococcus aureus* carriage: a systematic review. Clin Infect Dis 2009;48:922–30.

75. Kluytmans J, Harbarth S. Methicillin-resistant *Staphylococcus aureus* decolonization: "yes, we can," but will it help? Infect Control Hosp Epidemiol 2009;30: 633–5.

76. Ridenour G, Lampen R, Federspiel J, et al. Selective use of intranasal mupirocin and chlorhexidine bathing and the incidence of methicillin-resistant *Staphylococcus aureus* colonization and infection among intensive care unit patients. Infect Control Hosp Epidemiol 2007;28:1155–61.

77. Bode LG, Kluytmans JA, Wertheim HF, et al. Preventing surgical-site infections in nasal carriers of *Staphylococcus aureus*. N Engl J Med 2010;362:9–17.

78. Robicsek A, Beaumont JL, Thomson RB Jr, et al. Topical therapy for methicillin-resistant *Staphylococcus aureus* colonization: impact on infection risk. Infect Control Hosp Epidemiol 2009;30:623–32.

79. Huang SS, Singh R, McKinnell JA, et al. Decolonization to reduce postdischarge infection risk among MRSA carriers. N Engl J Med 2019;380:638–50.

80. Patel JB, Gorwitz RJ, Jernigan JA. Mupirocin resistance. Clin Infect Dis 2009;49: 935–41.

81. Lee AS, Macedo-Vinas M, Francois P, et al. Trends in mupirocin resistance in meticillin-resistant *Staphylococcus aureus* and mupirocin consumption at a tertiary care hospital. J Hosp Infect 2011;77:360–2.

82. Lee AS, Macedo-Vinas M, Francois P, et al. Impact of combined low-level mupirocin and genotypic chlorhexidine resistance on persistent methicillin-resistant *Staphylococcus aureus* carriage after decolonization therapy: a case-control study. Clin Infect Dis 2011;52:1422–30.

83. Poovelikunnel T, Gethin G, Humphreys H. Mupirocin resistance: clinical implications and potential alternatives for the eradication of MRSA. J Antimicrob Chemother 2015;70:2681–92.

84. Climo MW, Yokoe DS, Warren DK, et al. Effect of daily chlorhexidine bathing on hospital-acquired infection. N Engl J Med 2013;368:533–42.

85. Noto MJ, Domenico HJ, Byrne DW, et al. Chlorhexidine bathing and health care–associated infections: a randomized clinical trial. JAMA 2015;313:369–78.

86. Milstone AM, Elward A, Song X, et al. Daily chlorhexidine bathing to reduce bacteraemia in critically ill children: a multicentre, cluster-randomised, crossover trial. Lancet 2013;381:1099–106.

87. Huang SS, Septimus E, Kleinman K, et al. Chlorhexidine versus routine bathing to prevent multidrug-resistant organisms and all-cause bloodstream infections in general medical and surgical units (ABATE Infection trial): a cluster-randomised trial. Lancet 2019;393:1205–15.

88. Batra R, Cooper BS, Whiteley C, et al. Efficacy and limitation of a chlorhexidine-based decolonization strategy in preventing transmission of methicillin-resistant *Staphylococcus aureus* in an intensive care unit. Clin Infect Dis 2010;50:210–7.

89. Pittet D, Angus DC. Daily chlorhexidine bathing for critically ill patients: a note of caution. JAMA 2015;313:365–6.

90. Tacconelli E, De Angelis G, Cataldo MA, et al. Does antibiotic exposure increase the risk of methicillin-resistant *Staphylococcus aureus* (MRSA) isolation? A systematic review and meta-analysis. J Antimicrob Chemother 2008;61:26–38.

91. Vernaz N, Sax H, Pittet D, et al. Temporal effects of antibiotic use and hand rub consumption on the incidence of MRSA and *Clostridium difficile*. J Antimicrob Chemother 2008;62:601–7.

92. Dancer SJ, Kirkpatrick P, Corcoran DS, et al. Approaching zero: temporal effects of a restrictive antibiotic policy on hospital-acquired clostridium difficile, extended-spectrum beta-lactamase-producing coliforms and methicillin-resistant *Staphylococcus aureus*. Int J Antimicrob Agents 2013;41:137–42.

93. Harbarth S, Samore MH. Interventions to control MRSA: high time for time-series analysis? J Antimicrob Chemother 2008;62:431–3.

94. Lawes T, Lopez-Lozano JM, Nebot CA, et al. Effects of national antibiotic stewardship and infection control strategies on hospital-associated and community-associated methicillin-resistant *Staphylococcus aureus* infections across a region of Scotland: a non-linear time-series study. Lancet Infect Dis 2015;15:1438–49.

95. Barlam TF, Cosgrove SE, Abbo LM, et al. Implementing an antibiotic stewardship program: guidelines by the infectious diseases Society of America and the Society for Healthcare Epidemiology of America. Clin Infect Dis 2016;62: e51–77.

96. Chang S, Sethi AK, Eckstein BC, et al. Skin and environmental contamination with methicillin-resistant *Staphylococcus aureus* among carriers identified clinically versus through active surveillance. Clin Infect Dis 2009;48:1423–8.

97. Dancer SJ. Controlling hospital-acquired infection: focus on the role of the environment and new technologies for decontamination. Clin Microbiol Rev 2014;27: 665–90.

98. Goodman ER, Platt R, Bass R, et al. Impact of an environmental cleaning intervention on the presence of methicillin-resistant *Staphylococcus aureus* and vancomycin-resistant enterococci on surfaces in intensive care unit rooms. Infect Control Hosp Epidemiol 2008;29:593–9.

99. Dancer SJ, White LF, Lamb J, et al. Measuring the effect of enhanced cleaning in a UK hospital: a prospective cross-over study. BMC Med 2009;7:28.

100. Datta R, Platt R, Yokoe DS, et al. Environmental cleaning intervention and risk of acquiring multidrug-resistant organisms from prior room occupants. Arch Intern Med 2011;171:491–4.

101. Anderson DJ, Chen LF, Weber DJ, et al. Enhanced terminal room disinfection and acquisition and infection caused by multidrug-resistant organisms and *Clostridium difficile* (the Benefits of Enhanced Terminal Room Disinfection study): a cluster-randomised, multicentre, crossover study. Lancet 2017;389: 805–14.

102. Mitchell BG, Hall L, White N, et al. An environmental cleaning bundle and healthcare-associated infections in hospitals (REACH): a multicentre, randomised trial. Lancet Infect Dis 2019;19:410–8.

103. Han JH, Sullivan N, Leas BF, et al. Cleaning hospital room surfaces to prevent health care-associated infections: a technical brief. Ann Intern Med 2015;163: 598–607.

104. Aanensen DM, Feil EJ, Holden MT, et al. Whole-genome sequencing for routine pathogen surveillance in public health: a population snapshot of invasive *Staphylococcus aureus* in Europe. mBio 2016;7:e00444.

105. Koser CU, Holden MT, Ellington MJ, et al. Rapid whole-genome sequencing for investigation of a neonatal MRSA outbreak. N Engl J Med 2012;366:2267–75.

106. Popovich KJ, Green SJ, Okamoto K, et al. MRSA transmission in ICUs: genomic analysis of patients, their environments and healthcare workers. Clin Infect Dis 2021;72:1879–87.
107. Coll F, Harrison EM, Toleman MS, et al. Longitudinal genomic surveillance of MRSA in the UK reveals transmission patterns in hospitals and the community. Sci Transl Med 2017;9:eaak9745.
108. Roth VR, Longpre T, Taljaard M, et al. Universal vs risk factor screening for methicillin-resistant *Staphylococcus aureus* in a large multicenter tertiary care facility in Canada. Infect Control Hosp Epidemiol 2016;37:41–8.

Vancomycin-Resistant Enterococci
Epidemiology, Infection Prevention, and Control

Seema Joshi, MD[a],*, Anita Shallal, MD[a], Marcus Zervos, MD[b]

KEYWORDS

- VRE • Infection control • Enterococci • Health-care–associated infections
- Antimicrobial stewardship

KEY POINTS

- Due to expanding resistance patterns, VRE infections are becoming more difficult to treat.
- Infection control practices are crucial in management of VRE infections and should be based on patient characteristics, hospital needs, and available resources.
- The use of active surveillance screening and contact precautions has not shown to reduce VRE transmission in endemic settings.
- Measures to interrupt indirect contact transmission, including hand hygiene, chlorhexidine bathing, environmental cleaning, and antimicrobial stewardship, are the main components for prevention and control of VRE.

SIGNIFICANCE OF VANCOMYCIN-RESISTANT ENTEROCOCCI COLONIZATION AND INFECTION

In the United States, enterococci have been ranked as the third most frequently reported pathogen across all types of adult health-care–associated infections in 2015 to 2017.[1] The rising concern for vancomycin-resistant enterococci (VRE) within hospital systems has placed a larger emphasis on revisiting infection control practices, as VRE infection has been known to be associated with excess mortality, prolonged hospitalization, and increased treatment costs.[2] Obtaining source control, and ensuring prompt susceptibility testing and appropriate choice of antimicrobial therapy are key in management of VRE infections.

VRE is defined as having a minimum inhibitory concentration to vancomycin of greater than or equal to 32 mg/mL based on the Clinical and Laboratory Standard Institute guidelines.[3] Enterococci intrinsically have developed a variety of resistance

[a] Division of Infectious Diseases, Henry Ford Hospital, CFP-3, 2799 W Grand Boulevard, Detroit, MI, USA; [b] Wayne State University, CFP-3, 2799 W Grand Boulevard, Detroit, MI, USA
* Corresponding author.
E-mail address: Sjoshi5@hfhs.org

Infect Dis Clin N Am 35 (2021) 953–968
https://doi.org/10.1016/j.idc.2021.07.002
0891-5520/21/© 2021 Elsevier Inc. All rights reserved.
id.theclinics.com

mechanisms. These include penicillin-binding proteins with low affinity to beta-lactams, production of beta-lactamases, and decreased cellular permeability to antibiotics. VRE infections in particular contain plasmid-based genotypes (most common vanA), which encode resistance to glycoproteins.[4] Individuals who are at increased risk for developing infections due to VRE are those with multiple medical comorbidities, those who have received multiple courses of antibiotics in the past, and those who are critically ill. Common VRE infections include urinary tract infections associated with urethral catheters, bacteremia, catheter-related infections, endocarditis, wound infections, and intra-abdominal infections.[5] Enterococci are remarkable in their ability to develop rapid antimicrobial resistance. High-dose daptomycin and linezolid are agents for the treatment of VRE infections; however, emerging antibiotic resistance to these agents limits potential available therapies.[6,7]

EPIDEMIOLOGY

Most enterococci cause infection that originates from the intestinal flora, which can then spread and cause a variety of infections. Colonization with VRE generally precedes infection. There is a 10-fold increased risk of developing a VRE asymptomatic colonization compared with clinically recognized infection. The following individuals are at risk of VRE colonization: health care providers (HCPs), critically ill patients who have received long courses of antibiotics (in particular vancomycin, ceftriaxone, fluoroquinolones, and meropenem), individuals from long-term care facilities, solid-organ transplant patients, and patients with hematological malignancies.[8,9] Colonization can persist for months to years.

Vancomycin-resistant strains of enterococci have been endemic in large hospital settings with epidemics also reported. There is also growing resistance of enterococcus to daptomycin, which is concerning, as this may limit appropriate antibiotic therapy. In 2017, there were an estimated 54,500 patients hospitalized for VRE infections and an estimated 5400 VRE-associated deaths.[10] Enterococcus faecalis remains the most common pathogen; however, rising numbers of Enterococcus faecium have been noted. Not only is there a local concern for rise of VRE, but in 2017 the World Health Organization identified VRE as an important resistant bacteria in their "Global Priority List of Antibiotic-Resistant Bacteria."[11]

TRANSMISSION OF VANCOMYCIN-RESISTANT ENTEROCOCCI

VRE colonization, contact with HCPs, and environmental contamination are all associated with transmission of VRE.[12] Little is known about the dynamics of VRE transfer in hospitals.[13] Recent studies have shown there may be a causal relationship between patient VRE colonization and time-dependent environmental contamination within the hospital.[14] VRE colonization, when compared with vancomycin-susceptible strains, has been shown to be a precursor for developing VRE bloodstream infections (BSIs). The risk of VRE BSIs among colonized patients varies dependent on patient risk factors.[15] VRE is known to survive exposure to heat and certain disinfectants and has been found on numerous inanimate objects within hospitals. HCPs in adjunct with the environment are at the center of enterococcal transmission from patient to patient.

The evolution of antimicrobial resistance in enterococcus is complex. Besides patient characteristics, the spread of vancomycin resistance in Enterococcus occurs through clonal transmission as well as plasmid and transposon dissemination of resistance determinants. There are common issues that exist with regard to prevention, infection control, and management of both VRE and methicillin-resistant Staphylococcus aureus (MRSA) organisms. An investigation completed from a 900-bed tertiary care facility in urban Detroit showed a prevalence rate of almost 20% of coinfection or co-colonization of VRE and MRSA.[16] The study concluded that isolation of vancomycin-resistant *E faecalis* (rather than *E faecium*) and the use of linezolid or clindamycin were risk factors for VRE and MRSA coinfection or co-colonization. In vitro transfer of the *van*A gene from *E faecium* to *S aureus* has been noted, thus making the proximity of VRE and MRSA a risk factor for development of vancomycin-resistant *S aureus*.[17] Vancomycin-resistant *E faecalis* isolates containing Inc18 plasmids and the vancomycin resistance transposon Tn1549 have been identified as precursors for vancomycin resistance in *S aureus*.[16]

ISSUES AND STRATEGIES IN PREVENTION AND CONTROL OF VANCOMYCIN-RESISTANT ENTEROCOCCI INFECTIONS

After understanding the pathogenesis of VRE development, we know that acknowledging risk factors and understanding transmission are keys to prevention. Patient risk factors include prior antimicrobial use, working in health care, admission to the intensive care unit (ICU) with prolonged hospital stay, and being a resident from a long-term care facility. Colonization pressure within hospitals can also lead to contaminated surfaces and increase exposure to other patients. Community-acquired VRE infections are uncommon; however, risk factors for community-acquired VRE include presence of indwelling device, Foley catheter placement, and recent invasive procedures.[18,19]

There is a wide variation in infection control practices for multidrug-resistant organisms (MDROs) by hospitals within the United States and worldwide. Infection prevention and control strategies include hand hygiene, screening for resistance among isolates, surveillance cultures, contact isolation, environmental cleaning, and antimicrobial stewardship. Although infection control guidelines for MDROs from gram-negative organisms are well established, there continues to be varying ideology for infection control practices for gram-positive organisms including VRE and MRSA. The relative impact of the effectiveness of preventive measures for *E faecalis* and *E faecium* is not well established. **Table 1** provides a summary of strategies used in prevention and control of VRE infections.

HAND HYGIENE

Hands are a known major vector of patient-to-patient transmission of VRE. There is a large burden on HCPs to prevent transmission of MDROs; however, recent studies show patient hands while in hospital are just as important a reservoir for transmission within the hospital. This study published in 2019 shows that hand contamination with MDROs, including VRE, is common and has a direct correlation with contamination on high-touch room surfaces in a time-dependent manner.[20] The implementation of hand hygiene (both with soap and water and alcoholic chlorhexidine gel) has been shown to cause a 47% decrease in the acquisition of VRE.[21] Compliance with proper hand hygiene remains an opportunity for improvement, including when to wash hands, what to use to wash hands, and the duration of hand washing. A 30-second wash with soap and water has been shown to eliminate all VRE from hands, whereas a 5-second wash with water had no impact.[22]

COLONIZATION WITH VANCOMYCIN-RESISTANT ENTEROCOCCI

Colonization pressure, which is defined as the proportion of patients colonized with a particular organism during a specified period in a defined geographic area within

Table 1
Summary of strategies in infection prevention and control of VRE infections

Prevention and Control Strategy	What	When	Why
In vitro susceptibility testing	VRE definition are enterococci with MIC to vancomycin ≥32 µg/mL	Always	Early detection of vancomycin resistance is needed to determine appropriate antimicrobial therapy
Hand hygiene	Hand washing before and after contact with the patient and the patient's environment Hand washing with alcohol hand sanitizer Hand washing with soap and water when hands are soiled	Always	VRE has high predisposition to be transmitted through the hands of health care workers
Colonization and decolonization	Colonization occurs in patients with previous antimicrobial therapy	No recommendation	Colonization generally precedes infection Certain patients are high risk for infections and complications
Active surveillance	Use of rectal swabs, perirectal swabs, or stool samples	Not routine May consider if the incidence or prevalence of VRE in the facility is high Always in outbreak situations	To monitor prevalence of colonization and infection May consider in areas of skin breakdown and wounds
Chlorhexidine bathing	Daily bathing with chlorhexidine-impregnated washcloth	Always in patients in intensive care unit Not routine in general medical wards	Daily bathing with chlorhexidine-impregnated washcloths has been shown to decrease the risk of acquisition of MDROs
Environmental cleaning	Adherence to cleaning protocols Monitor effectiveness of routine cleaning	Always May consider novel technologies May consider environmental cultures in outbreak settings	VRE may survive in the environment for up to 1 y

(continued on next page)

Table 1 (continued)			
Prevention and Control Strategy	What	When	Why
Antimicrobial stewardship	Appropriate use of antibiotics to prevent development and spread of resistance	Always	VRE is associated with use of vancomycin, cephalosporin, and antibiotics with anaerobic activity

Abbreviations: MDROs, multidrug-resistant organisms; MIC, minimum inhibitory concentration; VRE, vancomycin-resistant enterococci.

Adapted from Reyes, K., A.C. Bardossy, and M. Zervos, Vancomycin-Resistant Enterococci: Epidemiology, Infection Prevention, and Control. Infect Dis Clin North Am, 2016. 30(4): p. 953-965; with permission.

the hospital, is a crucial factor in VRE acquisition.[23] ICUs, a common reservoir for VRE, showed rates of colonization via rectal swab ranging from 9.7% to 51.9%.[24] Colonization pressure of greater than 50% may outweigh other risk factors. A recent study evaluated 244 hospital rooms that were either hosted by VRE-colonized patients or non–VRE-colonized patients. Of the rooms, 89 were hosting a VRE-colonized patient and 62% (55 rooms) became contaminated with VRE compared with 155 rooms hosting non–VRE colonized patients in which only 28% (43 rooms) became contaminated with VRE.[14] VRE colonization has not only a local, but regional effect, and the presence of VRE in one hospital can have up to a 62% increase in prevalence to another hospital by means of patient transfers or staff working at multiple hospitals.[25]

Fecal burden of enterococci in hospitalized patients are a concern, as VRE often dominates the gut microbiome and is at risk to displace commensal anaerobes.[24] Asymptomatic carriage of VRE in the gastrointestinal tract may be one reason for the persistence of VRE in health care settings. Colonization with VRE, along with bacterial burden, can cause more environmental contamination, particularly in patients with diarrhea, and result in spread to other patients. High bacterial burden is more likely to result in spread.[26]

DECOLONIZATION

Natural clearance of VRE is variable, as colonization has been known to persist from anywhere between 204 and 1371 days.[27] Prolonged asymptomatic colonization of VRE in the gastrointestinal tract can perpetuate endemicity and spread. The modality of VRE decolonization was previously through the use of antibiotics. Newer studies are now evaluating the effectiveness of mechanical decolonization. Ultimately, the method of decolonization to decrease VRE burden is not recommended, as recolonization often occurs within a short time.

Decolonization may, however, be considered in an epidemic or a focused high-risk patient group in which populations are at high risk to develop VRE infections with significant morbidity and mortality. A prospective cohort study conducting active surveillance in a transplant ICU found that liver transplant candidates and recipients colonized with VRE had an increased risk of developing both VRE infection and death compared with noncolonized patients.[28] Among liver transplant patients, active surveillance showed similar VRE isolates suggesting linked transmission during hospital admissions.[29] Among patients about to receive hematopoietic stem cell transplantation, VRE colonization increased the incidence of VRE BSI; however, it was not associated with increased mortality.[30] This occurred despite infection control measures being implemented effectively.

Decolonization protocols consist of antimicrobials, as well as mechanical modalities which are becoming of more common practice. Antibiotics used for decolonization include oral bacitracin, oral absorbable linezolid, and nonabsorbable daptomycin.[31] One decolonization protocol used the administration of polyethylene glycol bowel preparation to wash-out fecal bacterial microbiome and *Lactobacillus rhamnosus* probiotic to maintain colonization resistance after antimicrobial decolonization.[31] A more recent study used a multisystem, mechanical decolonization protocol without antimicrobials and was shown to have high success rates.[32] This included a combination of environmental cleansing, mechanical evacuation with glycerin enemas, replacement of normal gut flora, and nutrition support and skin hygiene cleansing.[32] VRE decolonization is not generally recommended and should be considered only in certain high-risk populations, or in an outbreak situation.[30,32]

ACTIVE SURVEILLANCE FOR VANCOMYCIN-RESISTANT ENTEROCOCCI

Active surveillance has been used to identify VRE-colonized patients in epidemic and outbreak situations. This may benefit patients for targeted antimicrobial prophylaxis in situations such as transplant or nursing home patients, and also enhance infection prevention measures to prevent VRE infection and spread.[33] Obtaining stool cultures, and rectal and perirectal swabs are screening methods to detect VRE. The use of real-time polymerase chain reaction (to detect *van*A and *van*B genes), VRE screening broth, and automated DNA extraction are some methods used to expedite VRE detection.[34] Identifying positive VRE status can result in earlier antibiotic administration in an infected patient, as a delay of more than 2 days in effective antimicrobial therapy for VRE infection can be associated with a threefold increase in 30-day mortality.[35] The sensitivity of first rectal VRE screening can be less than 50%, an important factor to remember when obtaining surveillance cultures.[36]

High-risk patient groups may need screening for VRE, such as those admitted to the ICU, oncology and transplant wards, patients on chronic dialysis, and patients admitted to acute hospitals from long-term facilities. This is because active surveillance within this population may decrease the risk of developing VRE infection and screening may decrease transmission.[33]

The exact frequency of active screening to identify VRE is not well established. Different screening approaches that have been studied include culturing on admission and periodically, assuming a positive culture pending VRE screen and cohorting colonized patients.[37] There are varying data on clinical care and cost-effectiveness of active screening for VRE within the general public. More recent studies have revealed that discontinuation of active surveillance culturing leads to facility cost saving, with no increased harm, including mortality, was observed.[38]

As VRE surveillance culturing is a sensitive detection method, it is important to note that active surveillance cultures may be of benefit during a rare VRE outbreak. In outbreak situations, microbiologic surveillance and prompt contact precautions (CPs) with strict hand hygiene are vital to control VRE spread. Hospitals with high rates of VRE infections may also benefit from surveillance cultures to identify a genetic or clonal link within the reservoir of VRE-colonized patients to prevent an epidemic.

CONTACT PRECAUTIONS

There are a variety of modes of transmission with VRE; however, most infections are felt to be related to indirect contact transmission being spread between a patient and HCPs, or contamination between the patient and the surrounding hospital environment. The Healthcare Infection Control Practices Advisory Committee (HICPAC) and the Centers for Disease Control and Prevention (CDC) recommend CPs for "all patients infected with target MDROs and for patients that have been previously identified as being colonized with target MDROs (eg, patients transferred from other units of facilities who are known to be colonized)" who are admitted to acute care hospitals.[39] Previously, the use of CPs for VRE was a common practice, with up to 90% of acute care hospitals complying with recommendations made by the CDC; with heterogeneity in its practices.[40] As more knowledge has been acquired in approaches to infection prevention, newer studies around the globe have found lacking utility in the use of CPs for VRE and MRSA.[41]

The use of CPs includes the practice of isolated patient rooms, dedicated equipment, and use of gloves and gowns. Dedicated time for training staff and the monetary cost of extra gowns and gloves are needed to achieve high compliance. Considerations for maintaining CP in patients with VRE include known colonization, pending negative stool or rectal swabs to guide discontinuation, and high-risk patients (including those who are immunosuppressed, those receiving broad-spectrum antibiotic therapy without VRE activity, those in high-risk hospital units or hospitals with high rates of VRE infection).[42] The duration of CP for VRE varies widely in hospitals: on a case-by-case basis, indefinitely after a positive culture for VRE, or until repeat cultures have cleared.[43] Within each hospital, discontinuation of CPs for patients with VRE colonization or infection should address laboratory testing and surveillance strategies, VRE CP policy implementation and oversight, and which patients should be included.[42]

From a patient perspective, the impact of isolation due to CPs may have psychological effects, which include increased rates of anxiety, fear, depression, and uncertainty.[44] Direct patient care may be negatively affected by CPs due to decreased health care contact and increased adverse events (such as falls, pressure ulcers, medication administration errors, and deep vein thrombosis).[44–46] Discontinuing CP from a hospital perspective is also associated with increased bed availability and revenue recovery, as well as a reduction in personal protective equipment expenditures with an annual savings of approximately $650,000.[47–49]

CPs have variable effectiveness in different hospital settings. There are some studies that do show a decreased acquisition of VRE that has been associated with CPs.[50–52] Multiple other studies, however, have shown the use of CPs for VRE was not associated with decreased rates of transmission and can have an overall negative impact.[41,46,49,53] A cluster-randomized trial in 20 ICUs across the United States evaluated the use of mandatory gown and gloves for all patient contacts when entering patient rooms to study VRE and MRSA acquisition over a 10-month period.[54] This study concluded there was no statistical significance in the primary outcome of acquisition of VRE and MRSA with the use of CPs.[54]

The use of CPs for VRE has been in place by the CDC since 1970, when compliance was low with hand hygiene, lack of chlorhexidine bathing, and minimal surveillance for health-care–associated infections.[55] Resources at different institutions have now been focusing on horizontal infection control strategies to prevent spread of multiple MDROs rather than a vertical strategy focusing solely on VRE. This includes increased focus on hand hygiene, bare-below-the-elbows, chlorhexidine bathing, environmental cleaning, and care bundles.[4,41,56] These factors should be considered before implementing CP for VRE.

CHLORHEXIDINE BATHING

Chlorhexidine gluconate solution is a safe, effective, and low-cost agent for reducing the risk of health-care–associated infections like VRE.[57] The topical antiseptic solution ranges in concentrations from 0.5% to 4.0%, and daily bathing has been shown to reduce body surface bioburden, thus decreasing the risk of acquisition of MDROs.[58]

Earlier studies revealed universal decolonization reduces health-care–related BSI in ICU patients, particularly device-associated infections, reducing the rate by 28%.[59,60] It has since become standardized practice to bathe ICU patients older than 2 months in chlorhexidine to reduce the rates of central-line–associated BSI.[61] A randomized trial showed decolonization with chlorhexidine bathing did not significantly reduce all-cause BSI in non-ICU medical and surgical ward patients, although post hoc analysis noted significant benefit in those with medical devices such as central lines and lumbar drains, decreasing all-cause bacteremia with MRSA or VRE by 32%.[62] Further study is needed on whether the practice reduces outcomes such as mortality or length of hospital stay.[63]

The implications of chlorhexidine bathing on resistance also remains unclear. A study by Alotaibi and colleagues[64] noted that in hospital environments with increased chlorhexidine use, there was less susceptibility of VRE to chlorhexidine compared with vancomycin-sensitive *E faecium*. Another study noted the gene for *van*A-type vancomycin resistance was upregulated after 15 minutes of exposure to chlorhexidine, although the clinical relevance is unclear.[65]

ENVIRONMENTAL CLEANING

Contact with a contaminated environment can transfer VRE to uncontaminated surfaces. In one study,[20] an estimated 29% of rooms were contaminated with an MDRO within 24 hours of admission, and 10% of patients' hands were colonized with an MDRO at enrollment. Although hands of HCPs are recognized as an important vector for MDRO contamination,[66] equipment (including stethoscopes) can also act as a vector.[67] The estimated proportion for transfer frequency was 33% for HCP hands, 30% for gloves, and 10% for gowns. High-touch surfaces, including bed controls, call buttons, and bedside tray tables are also important locations where MDROs can colonize.[20]

Cleaning of patient care areas is often suboptimal, as one study revealed up to 94% of rooms of patients with VRE colonization or infection had 1 or more positive environmental cultures before cleaning, and 71% were still positive after housekeeping cleaning.[68] Use of bleach on bathroom surfaces, sodium hypochlorite, and alcohol for equipment are typical cleaning protocols.[69] Furthermore, the use of vaporized hydrogen peroxide in room disinfection showed patients were 80% less likely to acquire VRE.[70] Newer technologies, including ultraviolet light, have been shown to result in significant decrease in VRE contamination of frequently handled surfaces,[71] particularly when added to standard protocol.[72] These nontouch cleaning machines have the advantage of not requiring changes to the room's ventilation, not leaving residue after treatment, and having rapid exposure times.[73] However, these machines come with issues including cost, installation, hospital layout, and training.

Based on the results of microbiological screening studies, environmental colonization has been shown to correlate with patient VRE colonization.[74] New acquisition of VRE and new contamination of rooms with VRE were independently associated with increased length of stay in a facility and a higher likelihood of requiring hospitalization.[14] Prior environmental contamination increases the risk of VRE acquisition.[75]

OUTBREAKS OF VANCOMYCIN-RESISTANT ENTEROCOCCI

Outbreaks of VRE are frequently associated with lack of implementation or compliance of infection prevention and control measures.[76] More recently, outbreaks have occurred in solid-organ transplant units,[77] neonatal ICUs,[78,79] and general medical and critical care units.[80,81] Contaminated medical equipment, including rectal thermometers[82] and nonsterile preparation of injectable contrast,[83] have also been implicated as sources for outbreaks.

A multifaceted approach involving infection control specialists, infectious disease physicians, laboratory personnel, and pharmacists is essential in outbreak investigations for VRE.[84] Laboratory testing, including molecular and nucleotide whole genome sequence–based typing, can facilitate the process. Molecular methods should be used only in conjunction with epidemiologic case information. In outbreak settings, a bundle of prevention and control measures are implemented usually simultaneously and are composed of cohorting of patients, active surveillance cultures, environmental culture, extensive environmental cleaning, education, and antimicrobial stewardship.

ANTIMICROBIAL STEWARDSHIP

Inappropriate antibiotic use is associated with the development of antimicrobial resistance. Prior vancomycin or anti-anaerobic antibiotic exposure is a risk factor for VRE infection, and an independent risk factor for mortality in patients with enterococcal bacteremia. The HICPAC guidelines recommend prudent use of vancomycin, third-generation cephalosporins, and anti-anaerobic antimicrobials including metronidazole to prevent VRE infections.[85] More recent studies[9,86] have revealed exposure to fluoroquinolones and carbapenems is also associated with VRE bacteremia. Equally important is the length of antimicrobial therapy, as the risk for VRE increases with longer durations of antibiotic exposure.[9]

Antimicrobial stewardship is particularly challenging in the era of the Coronavirus Disease 2019 (COVID-19) pandemic, when unnecessary antibiotic use is high,[87] with approximately three-quarters of patients with COVID-19 receiving antibiotics.[88] The long-term consequences of increased prescription antibiotic use in both hospitalized and outpatients with COVID-19 is yet to be determined.

The One Health approach focuses on simultaneous protection of humans, animals, and the environment from climate change.[89] Indeed, one key feature that could reduce the burden of disease from antimicrobial resistance is by adopting its public health strategies,[90] including those aimed at reducing antimicrobial use in animals and animal feed.[91]

It is critical for facilities around the globe to implement infectious disease physician-led antimicrobial stewardship programs.[92,93] This multidisciplinary approach optimizes antibiotic choices and discourages antibiotic use when clinically unnecessary.[94] Antimicrobial exposure is an important risk factor for VRE, and stewardship is crucial for infection control.[95] The emergence of resistance of enterococci to newer antimicrobials, including daptomycin, supports the use of antimicrobial stewardship to reduce VRE colonization and infection.[96]

CLINICS CARE POINTS

- VRE is defined as having a minimum inhibitory concentration to vancomycin of greater than or equal to 32 mg/mL based on the Clinical and Laboratory Standard Institute guidelines.
- Risk factors for transmission of VRE include known colonization, contact with HCPs, and environmental contamination.
- Hand hygiene is a key element in decreasing the risk of VRE acquisition.
- Active surveillance and decolonization of VRE carriers is not recommended due to high risk of relapse; however, can be considered in high-risk populations and outbreak situations.
- The use of contact precautions has not been shown to have decreased rates of VRE transmission.
- Chlorhexidine bathing reduces health-care–associated BSIs in ICU patients.
- Environmental cleaning with bleach, sodium hypochlorite, alcohol, vaporized hydrogen peroxide, and ultraviolet light can reduce VRE contamination of surfaces.
- Prudent use and duration of vancomycin, third-generation cephalosporins, and anaerobic antimicrobials can prevent VRE infections.

DISCLOSURE

No disclosures related to present study. Disclosures of Marcus Zervos include grants to institution, Moderna, Johnson & Johnson, Merck, Pfizer, and consultant to Contrafect.

REFERENCES

1. Weiner-Lastinger LM, Abner S, Edwards JR, et al. Antimicrobial-resistant pathogens associated with adult healthcare-associated infections: summary of data reported to the National Healthcare Safety Network, 2015-2017. Infect Control Hosp Epidemiol 2020;41:1–18.
2. Chiang HY, Perencevich EN, Nair R, et al. Incidence and outcomes associated with infections caused by vancomycin-resistant enterococci in the United States: systematic literature review and meta-analysis. Infect Control Hosp Epidemiol 2017;38:203–15.
3. Clinical and Laboratory Standards Institute. Performance standards for antimicrobial susceptibility testing (Supplement M100). 30th edition. Wayne, PA: Clinical and Laboratory Standards Institue; 2020.
4. Vehreschild M, Haverkamp M, Biehl LM, et al. Vancomycin-resistant enterococci (VRE): a reason to isolate? Infection 2019;47:7–11.
5. Olivier CN, Blake RK, Steed LL, et al. Risk of vancomycin-resistant enterococcus (VRE) bloodstream infection among patients colonized with VRE. Infect Control Hosp Epidemiol 2008;29:404–9.
6. Kohinke RM, Pakyz AL. Treatment of vancomycin-resistant enterococci: focus on daptomycin. Curr Infect Dis Rep 2017;19:33.
7. Miller WR, Murray BE, Rice LB, et al. Resistance in vancomycin-resistant enterococci. Infect Dis Clin North Am 2020;34:751–71.
8. Kaya A, Kaya SY, Balkan II, et al. Risk factors for development of vancomycin-resistant enterococcal bacteremia among VRE colonizers: a retrospective case control study. Wien Klin Wochenschr 2020;133(9-10):478–83.

9. Gouliouris T, Warne B, Cartwright EJP, et al. Duration of exposure to multiple antibiotics is associated with increased risk of VRE bacteraemia: a nested case-control study. J Antimicrob Chemother 2018;73:1692–9.

10. Centers for Disease Control and Prevention. Biggest threats and data 2019. Available at: https://www.cdc.gov/DrugResistance/Biggest-Threats.html. Accessed March 25, 2021.

11. World Health Organization. Global priority list of antibiotic-resistant bacteria to guide research, discovery, and development of new antibiotics. 2017. Available at: https://www.who.int/medicines/publications/global-priority-list-antibiotic-resistant-bacteria/en/. Accessed March 25, 2021.

12. McDermott H, Skally M, O'Rourke J, et al. Vancomycin-resistant enterococci (VRE) in the intensive care unit in a nonoutbreak setting: identification of potential reservoirs and epidemiological associations between patient and environmental VRE. Infect Control Hosp Epidemiol 2018;39:40–5.

13. Zhou MJ, Li J, Salmasian H, et al. The local hospital milieu and healthcare-associated vancomycin-resistant enterococcus acquisition. J Hosp Infect 2019; 101:69–75.

14. Cassone M, Zhu Z, Mantey J, et al. Interplay between patient colonization and environmental contamination with vancomycin-resistant Enterococci and their association with patient health outcomes in postacute care. Open Forum Infect Dis 2020;7:ofz519.

15. Salgado CD. The risk of developing a vancomycin-resistant *Enterococcus* bloodstream infection for colonized patients. Am J Infect Control 2008;36:S175.e5–8.

16. Reyes K, Malik R, Moore C, et al. Evaluation of risk factors for coinfection or co-colonization with vancomycin-resistant enterococcus and methicillin-resistant *Staphylococcus aureus*. J Clin Microbiol 2010;48:628–30.

17. Yoon YK, Lee MJ, Ju Y, et al. Determining the clinical significance of co-colonization of vancomycin-resistant enterococci and methicillin-resistant *Staphylococcus aureus* in the intestinal tracts of patients in intensive care units: a case-control study. Ann Clin Microbiol Antimicrob 2019;18:28.

18. Omotola AM, Li Y, Martin ET, et al. Risk factors for and epidemiology of community-onset vancomycin-resistant *Enterococcus faecalis* in southeast Michigan. Am J Infect Control 2013;41:1244–8.

19. Raja NS, Karunakaran R, Ngeow YF, et al. Community-acquired vancomycin-resistant *Enterococcus faecium*: a case report from Malaysia. J Med Microbiol 2005;54:901–3.

20. Mody L, Washer LL, Kaye KS, et al. Multidrug-resistant organisms in hospitals: what is on patient hands and in their rooms? Clin Infect Dis 2019;69:1837–44.

21. De Angelis G, Cataldo MA, De Waure C, et al. Infection control and prevention measures to reduce the spread of vancomycin-resistant enterococci in hospitalized patients: a systematic review and meta-analysis. J Antimicrob Chemother 2014;69:1185–92.

22. Noskin GA, Stosor V, Cooper I, et al. Recovery of vancomycin-resistant enterococci on fingertips and environmental surfaces. Infect Control Hosp Epidemiol 1995;16:577–81.

23. Ajao AO, Harris AD, Roghmann MC, et al. Systematic review of measurement and adjustment for colonization pressure in studies of methicillin-resistant *Staphylococcus aureus*, vancomycin-resistant enterococci, and *Clostridium difficile* acquisition. Infect Control Hosp Epidemiol 2011;32:481–9.

24. Axelrad JE, Lebwohl B, Cuaresma E, et al. Gut colonization with vancomycin-resistant *Enterococcus* and risk for subsequent enteric infection. Gut Pathog 2018;10:28.

25. Lee BY, Yilmaz SL, Wong KF, et al. Modeling the regional spread and control of vancomycin-resistant enterococci. Am J Infect Control 2013;41:668–73.

26. Jackson SS, Harris AD, Magder LS, et al. Bacterial burden is associated with increased transmission to health care workers from patients colonized with vancomycin-resistant *Enterococcus*. Am J Infect Control 2019;47:13–7.

27. Yoon YK, Lee SE, Lee J, et al. Risk factors for prolonged carriage of vancomycin-resistant *Enterococcus faecium* among patients in intensive care units: a case-control study. J Antimicrob Chemother 2011;66:1831–8.

28. Russell DL, Flood A, Zaroda TE, et al. Outcomes of colonization with MRSA and VRE among liver transplant candidates and recipients. Am J Transpl 2008;8:1737–43.

29. Banach DB, Peaper DR, Fortune BE, et al. The clinical and molecular epidemiology of pre-transplant vancomycin-resistant enterococci colonization among liver transplant recipients. Clin Transpl 2016;30:306–11.

30. Ford CD, Gazdik MA, Lopansri BK, et al. Vancomycin-resistant *Enterococcus* colonization and bacteremia and hematopoietic stem cell transplantation outcomes. Biol Blood Marrow Transpl 2017;23:340–6.

31. Cheng VC, Chen JH, Tai JW, et al. Decolonization of gastrointestinal carriage of vancomycin-resistant *Enterococcus faecium*: case series and review of literature. BMC Infect Dis 2014;14:514.

32. Choi E, Lee SJ, Lee S, et al. Comprehensive, multisystem, mechanical decolonization of vancomycin-resistant *Enterococcus* and carbapenem-resistant Enterobacteriacease without the use of antibiotics. Medicine (Baltimore) 2021;100:e23686.

33. Humphreys H. Controlling the spread of vancomycin-resistant enterococci. Is active screening worthwhile? J Hosp Infect 2014;88:191–8.

34. Drews SJ, Johnson G, Gharabaghi F, et al. A 24-hour screening protocol for identification of vancomycin-resistant *Enterococcus faecium*. J Clin Microbiol 2006;44:1578–80.

35. Zasowski EJ, Claeys KC, Lagnf AM, et al. Time is of the essence: the impact of delayed antibiotic therapy on patient outcomes in hospital-onset enterococcal bloodstream infections. Clin Infect Dis 2016;62:1242–50.

36. Kaki R, Yu Y, O'Neill C, et al, Hamilton Health Sciences Infection Prevention and Control Team. Vancomycin-resistant enterococcus (VRE) transmission and risk factors in contacts of VRE carriers. Infect Control Hosp Epidemiol 2014;35:876–9.

37. Pogorzelska M, Stone PW, Larson EL. Wide variation in adoption of screening and infection control interventions for multidrug-resistant organisms: a national study. Am J Infect Control 2012;40:696–700.

38. Payne VC, Clark CC, Turner N. Clinical and financial implications for discontinuing active surveillance culturing (ASC) for methicillin-resistant *Staphylococcus aureus* & vancomycin-resistant *Enterococcus* in community hospitals [abstract]. Am J Infect Control 2020;48:S52–3.

39. Healthcare Infection Control Practices Advisory Committee, Centers for Disease Control and Prevention. Multidrug-resistant organisms (MRO) management 2015. Available at: https://www.cdc.gov/infectioncontrol/guidelines/mdro/index.html. Accessed March 25, 2021.

40. Morgan DJ, Murthy R, Munoz-Price LS, et al. Reconsidering contact precautions for endemic methicillin-resistant *Staphylococcus aureus* and vancomycin-resistant *Enterococcus*. Infect Control Hosp Epidemiol 2015;36:1163–72.

41. Marra AR, Edmond MB, Schweizer ML, et al. Discontinuing contact precautions for multidrug-resistant organisms: a systematic literature review and meta-analysis. Am J Infect Control 2018;46:333–40.

42. Banach DB, Bearman G, Barnden M, et al. Duration of contact precautions for acute-care settings. Infect Control Hosp Epidemiol 2018;39:127–44.

43. Russell D, Beekmann SE, Polgreen PM, et al. Routine use of contact precautions for methicillin-resistant *Staphylococcus aureus* and vancomycin-resistant *Enterococcus*: which way is the pendulum swinging? Infect Control Hosp Epidemiol 2016;37:36–40.

44. Abad C, Fearday A, Safdar N. Adverse effects of isolation in hospitalised patients: a systematic review. J Hosp Infect 2010;76:97–102.

45. Gandra S, Barysauskas CM, Mack DA, et al. Impact of elimination of contact precautions on noninfectious adverse events among MRSA and VRE patients. Infect Control Hosp Epidemiol 2018;39:1272–3.

46. Martin EM, Bryant B, Grogan TR, et al. Noninfectious hospital adverse events decline after elimination of contact precautions for MRSA and VRE. Infect Control Hosp Epidemiol 2018;39:788–96.

47. Schrank GM, Snyder GM, Davis RB, et al. The discontinuation of contact precautions for methicillin-resistant *Staphylococcus aureus* and vancomycin-resistant *Enterococcus*: impact upon patient adverse events and hospital operations. BMJ Qual Saf 2020;29:1–2.

48. Edmond MB, Masroor N, Stevens MP, et al. The impact of discontinuing contact precautions for VRE and MRSA on device-associated infections. Infect Control Hosp Epidemiol 2015;36:978–80.

49. Young K, Doernberg SB, Snedecor RF, et al. Things we do for no reason: contact precautions for MRSA and VRE. J Hosp Med 2019;14:178–80.

50. Cheah ALY, Cheng AC, Spelman D, et al. Mathematical modelling of vancomycin-resistant enterococci transmission during passive surveillance and active surveillance with contact isolation highlights the need to identify and address the source of acquisition. BMC Infect Dis 2018;18:511.

51. Mac S, Fitzpatrick T, Johnstone J, et al. Vancomycin-resistant enterococci (VRE) screening and isolation in the general medicine ward: a cost-effectiveness analysis. Antimicrob Resist Infect Control 2019;8:168.

52. Johnstone J, Shing E, Saedi A, et al. Discontinuing contact precautions for vancomycin-resistant enterococcus (VRE) is associated with rising vre bloodstream infection rates in Ontario hospitals, 2009-2018: a quasi-experimental study. Clin Infect Dis 2020;71:1756–9.

53. Hwang JH, Park JS, Lee E, et al. Active surveillance for carbapenem-resistant Enterobacteriaceae, vancomycin-resistant enterococci and toxigenic clostridium difficile among patients transferred from long-term care facilities in Korea. J Hosp Infect 2018;99:487–91.

54. Harris AD, Pineles L, Belton B, et al. Universal glove and gown use and acquisition of antibiotic-resistant bacteria in the ICU: a randomized trial. JAMA 2013;310:1571–80.

55. Wenzel RP, Edmond MB. Infection control: the case for horizontal rather than vertical interventional programs. Int J Infect Dis 2010;14:S3–5.

56. Haessler S, Martin EM, Scales ME, et al. Stopping the routine use of contact pre-cautions for management of MRSA and VRE at three academic medical centers: an interrupted time series analysis. Am J Infect Control 2020;48:1466–73.

57. Edmiston CE Jr, Bruden B, Rucinski MC, et al. Reducing the risk of surgical site infections: does chlorhexidine gluconate provide a risk reduction benefit? Am J Infect Control 2013;41:S49–55.

58. Gall E, Long A, Hall KK. Chlorhexidine bathing strategies for multidrug-resistant organisms: a summary of recent evidence. J Patient Saf 2020;16:S16–22.

59. Climo MW, Yokoe DS, Warren DK, et al. Effect of daily chlorhexidine bathing on hospital-acquired infection. N Engl J Med 2013;368:533–42.

60. Denny J, Munro CL. Chlorhexidine bathing effects on health-care-associated in-fections. Biol Res Nurs 2017;19:123–36.

61. Marschall J, Mermel LA, Fakih M, et al. Strategies to prevent central line-associated bloodstream infections in acute care hospitals: 2014 update. Infect Control Hosp Epidemiol 2014;35:753–71.

62. Huang SS, Septimus E, Kleinman K, et al. Chlorhexidine versus routine bathing to prevent multidrug-resistant organisms and all-cause bloodstream infections in general medical and surgical units (ABATE Infection trial): a cluster-randomised trial. Lancet 2019;393:1205–15.

63. Lewis SR, Schofield-Robinson OJ, Rhodes S, et al. Chlorhexidine bathing of the critically ill for the prevention of hospital-acquired infection. Cochrane Database Syst Rev 2019;8:CD012248.

64. Alotaibi SMI, Ayibiekea A, Pedersen AF, et al. Susceptibility of vancomycin-resistant and -sensitive enterococcus faecium obtained from Danish hospitals to benzalkonium chloride, chlorhexidine and hydrogen peroxide biocides. J Med Microbiol 2017;66:1744–51.

65. Bhardwaj P, Ziegler E, Palmer KL. Chlorhexidine induces VanA-type vancomycin resistance genes in enterococci. Antimicrob Agents Chemother 2016;60:2209–21.

66. Montoya A, Schildhouse R, Goyal A, et al. How often are health care personnel hands colonized with multidrug-resistant organisms? A systematic review and meta-analysis. Am J Infect Control 2019;47:693–703.

67. Wolfensberger A, Clack L, Kuster SP, et al. Transfer of pathogens to and from pa-tients, healthcare providers, and medical devices during care activity-a system-atic review and meta-analysis. Infect Control Hosp Epidemiol 2018;39:1093–107.

68. Eckstein BC, Adams DA, Eckstein EC, et al. Reduction of *Clostridium difficile* and vancomycin-resistant *Enterococcus* contamination of environmental surfaces af-ter an intervention to improve cleaning methods. BMC Infect Dis 2007;7:61.

69. Grabsch EA, Mahony AA, Cameron DR, et al. Significant reduction in vancomycin-resistant enterococcus colonization and bacteraemia after introduc-tion of a bleach-based cleaning-disinfection programme. J Hosp Infect 2012;82:234–42.

70. Passaretti CL, Otter JA, Reich NG, et al. An evaluation of environmental decon-tamination with hydrogen peroxide vapor for reducing the risk of patient acquisi-tion of multidrug-resistant organisms. Clin Infect Dis 2013;56:27–35.

71. Marra AR, Schweizer ML, Edmond MB. No-touch disinfection methods to decrease multidrug-resistant organism infections: a systematic review and meta-analysis. Infect Control Hosp Epidemiol 2018;39:20–31.

72. Anderson DJ, Chen LF, Weber DJ, et al. Enhanced terminal room disinfection and acquisition and infection caused by multidrug-resistant organisms and

Clostridium difficile (the Benefits of Enhanced Terminal Room Disinfection study): a cluster-randomised, multicentre, crossover study. Lancet 2017;389:805–14.

73. Casini B, Tuvo B, Cristina ML, et al. Evaluation of an ultraviolet C (UVC) light-emitting device for disinfection of high touch surfaces in hospital critical areas. Int J Environ Res Public Health 2019;16:3572.

74. Cassone M, Mantey J, Perri MB, et al. Environmental panels as a proxy for nursing facility patients with methicillin-resistant *Staphylococcus aureus* and vancomycin-resistant *Enterococcus* colonization. Clin Infect Dis 2018;67:861–8.

75. Drees M, Snydman DR, Schmid CH, et al. Prior environmental contamination increases the risk of acquisition of vancomycin-resistant enterococci. Clin Infect Dis 2008;46:678–85.

76. Fossi Djembi L, Hodille E, Chomat-Jaboulay S, et al. Factors associated with vancomycin-resistant enterococcus acquisition during a large outbreak. J Infect Public Health 2017;10:185–90.

77. Kreidl P, Mayr A, Hinterberger G, et al. Outbreak report: a nosocomial outbreak of vancomycin resistant enterococci in a solid organ transplant unit. Antimicrob Resist Infect Control 2018;7:86.

78. Marom R, Mandel D, Haham A, et al. A silent outbreak of vancomycin-resistant enterococcus faecium in a neonatal intensive care unit. Antimicrob Resist Infect Control 2020;9:87.

79. Andersson P, Beckingham W, Gorrie CL, et al. Vancomycin-resistant *Enterococcus* (VRE) outbreak in a neonatal intensive care unit and special care nursery at a tertiary-care hospital in Australia—a retrospective case-control study. Infect Control Hosp Epidemiol 2019;40:551–8.

80. Garcia Martinez de Artola D, Castro B, Ramos MJ, et al. Outbreak of vancomycin-resistant *Enterococcus* on a haematology ward: management and control. J Infect Prev 2017;18:149–53.

81. Kampmeier S, Tonnies H, Correa-Martinez CL, et al. A nosocomial cluster of vancomycin resistant enterococci among COVID-19 patients in an intensive care unit. Antimicrob Resist Infect Control 2020;9:154.

82. Donskey CJ, Chowdhry TK, Hecker MT, et al. Effect of antibiotic therapy on the density of vancomycin-resistant enterococci in the stool of colonized patients. N Engl J Med 2000;343:1925–32.

83. Sundermann AJ, Babiker A, Marsh JW, et al. Outbreak of vancomycin-resistant *Enterococcus faecium* in interventional radiology: detection through whole-genome sequencing-based surveillance. Clin Infect Dis 2020;70:2336–43.

84. Singh A, Goering RV, Simjee S, et al. Application of molecular techniques to the study of hospital infection. Clin Microbiol Rev 2006;19:512–30.

85. Muto CA, Jernigan JA, Ostrowsky BE, et al. SHEA guideline for preventing nosocomial transmission of multidrug-resistant strains of *Staphylococcus aureus* and *Enterococcus*. Infect Control Hosp Epidemiol 2003;24:362–86.

86. Cheah AL, Peel T, Howden BP, et al. Case-case-control study on factors associated with vanB vancomycin-resistant and vancomycin-susceptible enterococcal bacteraemia. BMC Infect Dis 2014;14:353.

87. Lucien MAB, Canarie MF, Kilgore PE, et al. Antibiotics and antimicrobial resistance in the COVID-19 era: perspective from resource-limited settings. Int J Infect Dis 2021;104:250–4.

88. Langford BJ, So M, Raybardhan S, et al. Antibiotic prescribing in patients with COVID-19: rapid review and meta-analysis. Clin Microbiol Infect 2021;27(4):520–31.

89. Rabinowitz PM, Natterson-Horowitz BJ, Kahn LH, et al. Incorporating one health into medical education. BMC Med Educ 2017;17:45.
90. Gudipati S, Zervos M, Herc E. Can the one health approach save us from the emergence and reemergence of infectious pathogens in the era of climate change: implications for antimicrobial resistance? Antibiotics (Basel) 2020;9:599.
91. McEwen SA, Collignon PJ. Antimicrobial resistance: a one health perspective. Microbiol Spectr 2018;6.
92. Rupali P, Palanikumar P, Shanthamurthy D, et al. Impact of an antimicrobial stewardship intervention in India: evaluation of post-prescription review and feedback as a method of promoting optimal antimicrobial use in the intensive care units of a tertiary-care hospital. Infect Control Hosp Epidemiol 2019;40:512–9.
93. Nauriyal V, Rai SM, Joshi RD, et al. Evaluation of an antimicrobial stewardship program for wound and burn care in three hospitals in Nepal. Antibiotics (Basel) 2020;9:914.
94. Crnich CJ, Jump R, Trautner B, et al. Optimizing antibiotic stewardship in nursing homes: a narrative review and recommendations for improvement. Drugs Aging 2015;32:699–716.
95. Contreras GA, Munita JM, Arias CA. Novel strategies for the management of vancomycin-resistant enterococcal infections. Curr Infect Dis Rep 2019;21:22.
96. Lee CR, Lee JH, Park KS, et al. Quantitative proteomic view associated with resistance to clinically important antibiotics in gram-positive bacteria: a systematic review. Front Microbiol 2015;6:828.

Multidrug-Resistant Gram-Negative Bacteria
Infection Prevention and Control Update

John P. Mills, MD[a],*, Dror Marchaim, MD[b,c]

KEYWORDS

- Gram-negative bacteria • MDR-GNB • CRE • Nosocomial infections
- ESKAPE pathogens • Infection control

KEY POINTS

- Multidrug-resistant Gram-negative bacteria (MDR-GNB) infections constitute a great threat to human health because of their propensity for human-to-human spread and limited therapeutic options
- The lack of standardized microbiological definitions of resistance among certain Gram-negative bacteria (GNB) leads to nonuniformity in infection control established recommendations
- Infection control interventions should be implemented in parallel in both acute-care hospitals and connected long-term care facilities (LTCFs) to maximize the effectiveness of prevention interventions among high-risk patients across the continuum of care
- Clinical cultures only identify a minority of patients colonized with MDR-GNB; active surveillance is necessary to detect asymptomatic MDR-GNB carriage
- Screening methods for active surveillance of extended-spectrum β-lactamases (ESBL) and carbapenem-resistant Enterobacterales (CRE) colonization are more sensitive than methods for the detection of carbapenem-resistant *A. baumannii* (CRAB) and carbapenem-resistant *Pseudomonas aeruginosa* (CRPA)
- Hand hygiene (HH), contact precautions (CPs), and cohorting are key containment measures for MDR-GNB prevention
- CPs are recommended for all carriers of CRE, CRPA, and CRAB
- In settings of high endemic rates, cohorting with dedicated staff is recommended for carbapenemase-producing CRE carriers. It is also recommended for CRAB (or *A. baumannii* in general) prevention, depending on local endemicity
- Cohorting carriers of different MDR-GNB together may result in cross-transmission of resistance elements and adversely impact antimicrobial resistance in a facility

Continued

[a] Division of Infectious Diseases, University of Michigan Medical School, F4177 University Hospital South, 1500 E. Medical Center Dr, Ann Arbor, MI 48109-5226, USA; [b] Sackler School of Medicine, Tel-Aviv University, Tel-Aviv, Israel; [c] Division of Infectious Diseases, Shamir (Assaf Harofeh) Medical Center, Zerifin, Israel
* Corresponding author.
E-mail address: millsjo@med.umich.edu

Infect Dis Clin N Am 35 (2021) 969–994
https://doi.org/10.1016/j.idc.2021.08.001
id.theclinics.com
0891-5520/21/© 2021 Elsevier Inc. All rights reserved.

Continued

- The environment likely plays a role in MDR-GNB acquisitions. Establishing strict terminal cleaning protocols and regular monitoring of the effectiveness of cleaning are important components of successful prevention programs. The use of advanced "no-touch" technologies [automated ultraviolet C (UV-C)–emitting and H2O2-based devices] with terminal room cleaning may provide additional benefits
- Endoscopes, particularly duodenoscopes and bronchoscopes, have been associated with multiple MDR-GNB outbreaks; appropriate reprocessing of these devices is crucial to prevent the transmission of MDR-GNB and serious infections
- Antimicrobial stewardship (AMS) programs must be part of all infection control programs in all facilities and in community health settings; they have been associated with a 50% reduction in MDR-GNB incidence in hospital settings
- Selective oral and digestive decontamination are not recommended for MDR-GNB prevention. The use of colistin for these purposes could be hazardous. Chlorhexidine gluconate bathing reduces MDR-GNB incidence. Fecal microbiota transplantation (FMT) may play a future role in CRE prevention

PEARLS

- Performance of active surveillance for carbapenem-resistant Enterobacterales (CRE) among high-risk populations can facilitate early detection and cohorting of cases, limiting the risk of transmission
- Identifying high-risk populations based on local/regional epidemiology is crucial to determining what patients warrant active surveillance for CRE
- *Acinetobacter baumannii* is notorious for widespread environmental contamination. Enhanced environmental cleaning and use of novel "no-touch" technologies can reduce the risk of environmental persistence and potentially transmission
- Consider endoscopes and environmental water sources as potential reservoirs of multidrug-resistant Gram-negative bacteria (MDR-GNB) during outbreak investigations

PITFALLS

- Active surveillance for carbapenem-resistant *Pseudomonas aeruginosa* (CRPA) and carbapenem-resistant *A. baumannii* (CRAB) is challenging because of the low sensitivity of cultures from any single anatomic site. Multiple sites may need to be cultured to optimize detection.
- Reliance on phenotypic testing alone to detect carbapenem-resistant Enterobacterales (CRE) may fail to detect epidemiologically important resistance genes
- Cohorting patients colonized with different MDR-GNB can potentially result in patient-to-patient cross-transmission of genetic resistance elements
- Data do not support the use of contact precautions (CPs) for patients colonized with extended-spectrum β-lactamases–producing GNB. High utilization of CPs is associated with lower health care worker adherence.
- The use of colistin for selective digestive decontamination (SDD) has the potential to promote colistin resistance

MULTIDRUG-RESISTANT GRAM-NEGATIVE BACTERIA: NOMENCLATURE

Multidrug-resistant Gram-negative bacteria (MDR-GNB) comprise many of the urgent threats identified by the Centers for Disease Control and Prevention (CDC)'s 2019 Antibiotic Resistance report.[1] Most of the "ESKAPE" pathogens[2], which cause a large preponderance of hospital infections although effectively "escaping" the effects of most available therapeutics, are Gram-negative bacteria (GNB), including *Klebsiella pneumoniae, Acinetobacter baumannii, Pseudomonas aeruginosa, Enterobacter* species, and *Escherichia coli*. In this review, MDR Gram-negative ESKAPE bacteria will be referred to as MDR-GNB, although these isolates are frequently extensively drug resistant (XDR), or even pan-drug resistant.[3]

Although antimicrobial resistance among GNB includes many classes of antibiotics, this review will focus specifically on β-lactam resistance.[4] Beta-lactam agents are among the oldest, safest, and cheapest therapeutic options[5] and are bactericidal with an established track record against the most common infectious syndromes.[6] This review will summarize evidence-based infection control measures aimed at halting the emergence and spread of 4 resistance phenotypes among the ESKAPE MDR-GNBs (**Table 1**): (1) Enterobacterales resistant to extended-spectrum cephalosporins: such as pathogens expressing various types of β-lactamases, including the Ambler-A extended-spectrum β-lactamases (ESBL) and the Ambler-C bla_{AmpC} (AmpC); (2) carbapenem-resistant Enterobacterales (CRE); (3) carbapenem-resistant *P. aeruginosa* (CRPA); and (4) *A. baumannii* [including but not solely limited to carbapenem-resistant *A. baumannii* (CRAB)].

MICROBIOLOGICAL DEFINITIONS AND MECHANISMS OF β-LACTAM RESISTANCE

Surveillance of β-lactam resistance among GNB is challenging because of a lack of standardized definitions for MDR-GNB. Different antimicrobial susceptibility testing breakpoints have been set by different international committees (Clinical and Laboratory Standards Institute vs European Committee on Antimicrobial Susceptibility Testing), and these breakpoints have changed over time to optimize the detection of β-lactam resistance.

CRE can be detected either phenotypically by MIC breakpoints or by molecular detection of carbapenemases. Both the Israeli Ministry of Health and the US CDC recommend carbapenemase production testing on all CRE isolates because results can inform local CRE epidemiology and guide appropriate infection control measures.[7,8]

Resistance to extended-spectrum cephalosporins among Enterobacterales can also be detected by either phenotypic third-generation cephalosporin resistance or ESBL production testing.[9,10] There are other prevalent resistance mechanisms to third-generation cephalosporins, most notably bla_{AmpC}.[11] ESBLs are encoded on transmissible mobile genetic elements, whereas AmpC is frequently encoded on chromosomal genes that are upregulated in the setting of antibiotic exposure.[12] Although ESBLs may be acquired in hospitals by patient-to-patient transmission[13], among AmpC, the most common mode of acquisition is by the emergence of resistance due to antimicrobial selective pressure, which might influence the bundle of infection control measures that should be used.

MODES OF MULTIDRUG-RESISTANT GRAM-NEGATIVE BACTERIA ACQUISITION

Prevention tool kits for the acquisition of MDR-GNBs address 2 modes of resistance acquisition: (1) patient-to-patient transmission of MDR-GNB and/or their mobile

Table 1
Multidrug-resistant gram-negative bacteria nomenclature and abbreviations

	Abbreviation	Definition	Examples
Multidrug-Resistant Gram-Negative Bacteria	MDR-GNB	Gram-negative bacteria nonsusceptible to ≥3 classes of antimicrobials	
Extensively Resistant Gram-Negative Bacteria	XDR-GNB	Gram-negative bacteria nonsusceptible to ≥1 agent in all but ≤2 antimicrobial classes	
Enterobacterales			
Carbapenem-Resistant Enterobacterales	CRE	Enterobacterales phenotypically resistant to ≥1 carbapenem -OR- detection of carbapenemase	
Nonfermenting Gram-Negative Bacteria	NF-GNB	Gram-negative bacteria incapable of fermenting glucose	*P. aeruginosa,* *A. baumannii,* *S. maltophilia,* *Burkholderia cepacia* complex
Carbapenem-Resistant *P. aeruginosa*	CRPA	*P. aeruginosa* phenotypically resistant to ≥1 carbapenem	
Carbapenem-Resistant *A. baumannii*	CRAB	*A. baumannii* phenotypically resistant to ≥1 carbapenem	
Beta-Lactamases			
Extended-Spectrum Beta-Lactamases	ESBLs	Enzymes capable of hydrolyzing third- and 4th-generation cephalosporins in addition to penicillin agents	CTX-M, TEM, SHV
AmpC Beta-Lactamases	AmpC	Inducible enzymes (usually chromosomal) that when upregulated confer resistance to first- to third-generation cephalosporins & BL/BLIs	Frequently found in: *E. cloacae,* *C. freundii,* *S. marcescens,* *P. aeruginosa,* *A. baumanii*
Carbapenemase-Producing Organisms	CPOs	Gram-negative bacteria that produce enzymes capable of hydrolyzing carbapenems	KPC, NDM, OXA, VIM

S. maltophilia, Stenotrophomonas maltophilia; Burkholderia cepacia, B. cepacia; C. freundii, Citrobacter freundii; S. marcescens, Serratia marcescens; E. cloacae, Enterobacter cloacae. KPC, Klebsiella pneumoniae carbapenemase; NDM, New Delhi metallo-beta-lactamase; OXA, oxacillinase; VIM, Verona integron-encoded metallo-beta-lactamase.

genetic elements (eg, carbapenemases) (often through an intermediary such as health care staff, the proximal environment, or shared equipment) or (2) *de novo* evolution of resistance, in which susceptible isolates, under antibiotic selective pressure, newly express an MDR phenotype, often mediated by the upregulation of chromosomal gene expression (eg, AmpC) or alterations in outer membrane porin channels or efflux pumps due to certain stressors.[5,14]

Infection control measures in hospitals that address patient-to-patient transmission include (1) hand hygiene (HH), (2) contact isolation precautions, (3) patient cohorting and dedicated staff, (4) environmental cleaning, (5) active surveillance programs to identify asymptomatic carriage, and (6) decolonization protocols. In contrast, tackling *de novo* emergence of resistance requires enforcing adherence to effective antimicrobial stewardship (AMS) policies.[14]

MULTIDRUG-RESISTANT GRAM-NEGATIVE BACTERIA EPIDEMIOLOGY
Acute-care hospitals

ESBL-producing GNB were first described in acute-care facilities, specifically in intensive care units (ICUs), in the 1980s.[15,16] By the mid to late 1990s, ESBL-producing strains had become prevalent in outpatient settings.[17,18] This rapid global dissemination has been largely driven by the clonal expansion of *E. coli* sequence type 131, which frequently harbors the CTX-M beta-lactamase.[19] ESBL colonization prevalence ranges from 2% to 56% among patients admitted to ICUs, depending on the geographic region.[20–22]

Infections due to the nonfermenting MDR-GNB CRAB and CRPA primarily affect patients with prolonged and complicated stays in acute-care hospitals.[23–25] Prolonged prior hospital or ICU stay, recent surgery/procedures, presence of invasive devices, and recent exposure to antibiotics all serve as independent predictors for the acquisition of CRE, CRPA, or CRAB.[23–27]

Long-term care facilities

Long-term care facilities (LTCFs) became a pivotal part of the health care system over the past 3 decades and are now providing more complex post–acute-care management to greater numbers of patients.[28] Today, elderly patients with multiple risk factors for MDR-GNB acquisition, such as multiple comorbidities, indwelling devices, recent exposure to hospitals, and broad-spectrum antibiotics, are frequently managed in LTCFs.[23,24,29,30] Moreover, patients from LTCFs frequently cycle back and forth from acute-care facilities, resulting in additional complexities in terms of transmission and spread.[29,31] Above all, lower adherence with HH and barrier precautions in LTCFs, along with a paucity of infection control resources and expertise, can facilitate the spread of MDR-GNB.[32]

The first reported outbreak of bacteria resistant to ceftazidime in the United States occurred among patients in a chronic-care facility in Massachusetts in 1990.[33] Since that time, ESBL-producing Enterobacterales have become endemic in LTCFs throughout most of the world. Risk factors for ESBL colonization in LTCFs include (1) poor functional status, (2) percutaneous endoscopic gastrostomy tube placement, (3) pressure ulcers, (4) use of ciprofloxacin and/or trimethoprim-sulfamethoxazole (TMP-SMZ), and (5) increased length of stay.[34,35]

CRE have also been identified among LTCF patients, and risk factors for acquisition include the prolonged length of stay in acute care, sharing rooms with known carriers, and the degree of colonization pressure on certain wards.[8]

Resistant *P. aeruginosa* infections, particularly CRPA catheter-associated urinary tract infections (UTIs) and skin and soft-tissue infections, were identified in LTCFs more than 2 decades ago.[8] CRPA infections in this setting have been associated with intermittent urethral catheterization, chronic indwelling urinary catheters, and postsurgical drains.[36,37] CRAB have been detected among ventilated patients in long-term acute-care hospitals (LTACHs) and also in LTCFs in general.[38,39] Importantly, *Acinetobacter* spp. may persist on dry inanimate surfaces for days to months.[40]

Community settings

MDR-GNB infections are considered community acquired (CA) if they occur outside of the hospital or LTCFs or are diagnosed within the first 72 hours of hospitalization. However, the boundary between community settings and health care–associated settings may be blurred as patients with recent health care exposure often resemble patients in acute-care hospitals and LTCFs.[41] Cases of CRE, CRPA, and *A. baumannii* present or incubating at the time of hospital admission were previously termed CA although they often occurred among a population with heavy recent prior exposure to health care.[25] Exclusively CA infections caused by CRE, CRPA, or CRAB remain very rare in most countries.[42]

In contrast to carbapenem-resistant pathogens, CA-ESBL infections have become relatively commonplace in many parts of the world.[5] The community prevalence of ESBL colonization is highly variable. The community prevalence of ESBLs is as high as 46% to 63% in parts of Asia and Africa and as low as 2% in North America.[43] Although the role of patient-to-patient transmission in ESBL acquisition in the community is unclear[13], ESBL infections are clearly associated with worse outcomes,[44] mainly because of the frequent delays in initiating appropriate therapy (DAAT).[11]

Infection control measures to curb the continued emergence and spread of ESBLs in the community are speculative. Developing robust AMS programs in outpatient ambulatory settings, for example, targeting fluoroquinolones, might reduce the emergence and spread of ESBLs in the community.[45,46] In addition, restricting antimicrobial usage in agriculture and food industries is a critical measure.[45]

Table 2
Epidemiologic and biological characteristics of colonization by MDR-GNB

	Anatomic Locations for Screening	Duration of Colonization	Risk for Transmission	Risk of Clinical Infection
ESBL & CRE	Rectum, inguinal, urine.	144 d 50% positivity rate by 3–6 mo, 25% by 6–24 mo in *K. pneumoniae*[162]	Health care acquisition/ community onset ratio 59/52 in *E. coli*[50]; 37/35 in *K. pneumoniae*[163]	44/520 (8.8%)[164] and 42/464 (9%)[165] in *K. pneumoniae*
CRAB	Rectum, respiratory tract, skin, urine[48,49]	20 mo[48]	Health care acquisition/ community onset ratio 32/16	Bacteremia in 108/200 (54%)[166]
CRPA	Rectum, oropharynx, urine, sputum		Health care acquisition/ community onset ratio 70/46[167]	Clinical infection in 41/213 (19.2%)

Abbreviations: CRE, carbapenem-resistant Enterobacterales; CRAB, carbapenem-resistant *Acinetobacter baumannii*; CRPA, carbapenem-resistant *Pseudomonas aeruginosa*; ESBL, extended-spectrum β-lactamase-producing Enterobacterales; GNB, Gram-negative bacteria; MDR, multidrug-resistant.

THE "ICEBERG PHENOMENON": THE ROLE OF COLONIZATION IN THE EPIDEMIOLOGY AND PREVENTION OF MULTIDRUG-RESISTANT GRAM-NEGATIVE BACTERIA TRANSMISSION

Asymptomatic colonization of humans occurs among almost all of the MDR-GNB, and several studies have determined the anatomic locations of colonization, duration of colonization, and the relationship with transmission and clinical infection (**Table 2**).

Anatomic locations of colonization

The colon is the natural habitat of Enterobacterales, and sampling colonic content by rectal (or less preferably perirectal) cultures is the most sensitive and efficient method for identifying CRE and ESBL carriers.[47]

There is less certainty regarding the optimal screening location for CRAB and CRPA.[48] Sampling of several anatomic sites, including the rectum, pharyngeal/respiratory tract, and skin sampling, may increases the yield[48,49] and also the labor and cost burden of surveillance.

Risk of transmission and clinical infection among colonized patients

Surveillance cultures of patients during their hospital stay combined with molecular analysis have traced the clonal transmission of ESBL-producing E. coli in only 50% of ESBL acquisitions (see **Table 2**).[50]

The risk of overt clinical infection for carriers varies tremendously between CRE (~9%) and CRAB (54%) (see **Table 2**). Although this difference may be related to virulence potential, it is also a reflection of differences in the patient population of carriers (eg, ICU patients with CRAB vs the general wards with CRE) and the possible lower detection of CRAB colonization than CRE based on surveillance cultures.

MULTIDRUG-RESISTANT GRAM-NEGATIVE BACTERIA CONTAINMENT
Hand hygiene

HH is a principal component of standard precautions and the cornerstone of infection prevention (**Table 3**).[51] Many studies have demonstrated isolation of the same MDR-GNB from patients and the hands of the health care workers caring for them.[52–54] Therefore, investing in HH compliance among staff is an important intervention to control outbreaks of MDR-GNB.[55–57] Although the isolated impact of improving MDR-GNB acquisition is difficult to quantify,[58] HH is efficacious, inexpensive, and easy to perform. Following the performance of HH either with water and antiseptic soaps or with alcohol-based hand rub, there are significant reductions in the inoculums of MDR-GNB.[59] A recent modeling analysis in the ICU setting demonstrated that HH is the most efficient measure in controlling ESBL acquisitions. This model showed that improving HH compliance from 55% before patient contact and 60% after patient contact to 80% before and after patient contact would reduce the proportion of patients who acquire ESBLs within 90 days by 91%.[60]

Although simple and fundamental to good patient care, compliance with HH is often suboptimal[58] and further interventions need to be implemented to increase compliance among staff, including the use of advanced technologies.[61,62] HH compliance among staff is a core performance measure of every infection control program and it is important to recruit leaders to invest and allocate preventive resources to this task.[63]

Contact precautions

Contact precautions (CPs) include wearing a gown and gloves on entry into the patient environment and removing the gown and gloves before exiting the patient's immediate

Table 3
Evidence-based MDR-GNB infection prevention and control measures

IPC Intervention	Definition	Comments
Hand Hygiene	Washing or sanitizing hands before and after patient care	Highly effective but adherence is often suboptimal. Monitoring and feedback are essential to maintaining high HCW adherence
Contact Precautions	Gown and glove use for all patient care	Data supporting use in endemic settings are strongest for CRE and *A. baumannii*. Data do not support the use of CPs for ESBL prevention.
Environmental Cleaning	Surface disinfection of patient environment and equipment	Crucial to monitor compliance. Consider potential water sources (eg, sinks) in MDR-GNB outbreaks, particularly *P. aeruginosa* and *A. baumannii*. No-touch terminal room technology can reduce the risk of MDRO infection in subsequent room occupant.
Medical Device Reprocessing	HLD/sterilization of invasive medical devices	Duodenoscopes associated with CRE transmission even when following the manufacturer's IFU
Antimicrobial Stewardship	System to limit inappropriate use & optimize antimicrobial prescribing	Associated with 50% absolute risk reduction in MDR-GNB infection/colonization. Most effective when combined with infection control measures.
Active Surveillance	Screening cultures (eg, rectal/perirectal swab) to detect asymptomatic MDR-GNB colonization	Universal vs targeted. Effective in reducing CRE transmission in epidemic and some endemic settings. Unclear role in the prevention of NF-GNB.
Patient and HCP Cohorting	Segregating MDR-GNB–infected or MDR-GNB–colonized patients in one geographic location with the use of dedicated HCP	Effective for epidemic CRE control when bundled with other interventions. Low HCP morale has been reported.
Patient Decolonization	Topical CHG cutaneous decolonization or SDD/SOD	CHG data are strong for MRSA/VRE but more limited for MDR-GNB. Utility of SDD/SOD depends on baseline antibiotic resistance prevalence and carries the risk of increased drug resistance. FMT for this purpose is still experimental.
Interfacility Collaboration	Enhanced communications between facilities regarding patient MDR-GNB status & coordination with state health authorities	Improves early detection of silent MDR-GNB carriers. Strong data supporting a coordinated approach to epidemic CRE control. Crucial to incorporate acute-care hospitals and LTCFs.

environment (see **Table 3**). CPs are preferably used for patients in single rooms. Performing HH before wearing gloves and after removing them is a mandatory part of CPs. Most supportive studies for the prevention of the spread of MDR-GNB include the use of CPs in combination with other infection control strategies and measures.[64,65] Universal use of CPs in ICU patients does not seem to be more effective than targeted CP for MDR-GNB–positive patients. A large cluster-randomized trial of universal gowns and glove use versus standard hospital policies for CPs among ICU patients found a nonstatistically significant 10% reduction in the incidence of MDR-GNB acquisition [risk ratio (RR) = 0.90, confidence interval (CI) = 0.71–1.12, $P = .34$].[66] In addition to being an important component of bundled interventions to limit the epidemic spread of MDR-GNB, CPs are simple and inexpensive and are one of the only tools available in the hospital, other than HH, to reduce the pathogen inoculum and limit transmission of pathogens from patient to patient.

Patients colonized or infected with CRE should always be subjected to CPs[47,67] per CDC recommendations. Current guidelines do not differentiate between carbapenemase-producing CRE and non–carbapenemase-producing CRE in terms of applying CPs (as opposed to cohorting and dedicated staff).

Limited data exist examining the role of CP in the prevention of the spread of nonfermenting MDR-GNB. The use of CPs is recommended for all patients infected or colonized with CRAB or CRPA by the World Health Organization.[68] A. baumanii is notorious for causing widespread environmental contamination and has been associated with higher rates of health care worker acquisition on gowns and gloves than P. aeruginosa.[69] Furthermore, one quasi-experimental study in a French hospital found an increase in the annual incidence of A. baumannii infections after discontinuing their CP policy, with a subsequent reduction after reinstituting the CP policy.[70] Controversy exists over whether CPs should be used for all A. baumannii or only cases of CRAB. For P. aeruginosa, carbapenem resistance occurs through de novo evolution and patient-to-patient transmission. Most facilities subject only patients with CRPA to CPs because carbapenems are regarded as such an important cornerstone antibiotic in the hospital and widespread carbapenem resistance throughout the hospital could be catastrophic.[71]

Although still used in many American hospitals, accumulated data suggest that CPs for ESBL are ineffective in preventing transmission, likely related to the high incidence of undetected CA colonization with these endemic organisms.[72,73] In a US study involving 11 teaching hospitals, as the proportion of patients on CPs exceeded 40% of the unit's occupancy, the compliance with CP and HH recommendations decreased dramatically, and only 5 of these 11 centers continued to implement CP for ESBL carriers following the study.[74] In a controlled study conducted at 2 hospitals in France, the rate of ESBL acquisitions was not associated with CP implementation.[75] However, some national guidelines (eg, in Switzerland) recommend CPs for hospitalized ESBL carriers; and during outbreaks or among high-risk populations (eg, neonates, severely immunosuppressed), CPs may still play a role in preventing ESBL acquisition.[76–78]

Overuse of CPs has the potential to cause harm. Prior studies have found that isolated patients receive less frequent personal contact from health care workers because of the additional effort required in adhering with CPs.[79,80] CPs may be stressful for patients and their families, and isolated patients are prone to higher rates of anxiety, depression, adverse events, and medical errors.[81]

ACTIVE SURVEILLANCE

The use of surveillance cultures to identify asymptomatically colonized patients has become an essential tool in infection prevention and control programs, not only during outbreaks but also as a routine measure for some endemic MDR-GNB.[8] Active surveillance, paired with preemptive contact isolation, reduces colonization pressure, risk of patient-to-patient transmission, and DAAT.[8,82,83] As the reliance on clinical cultures alone has been found to significantly underestimate CRE prevalence, the use of active surveillance cultures will more accurately estimate the colonization pressure of a given health system or unit.[83,84]

In many regions, the endemic prevalence of ESBL colonization in the community is so high that active surveillance is considered of questionable benefit. Efficacy data pertaining to the utility and yield of screening for ESBLs are derived primarily from outbreak settings or from certain high-risk populations such as in the neonatal ICU[85] or among immunosuppressed individuals. A recent large European cluster-randomized trial of ICU infection prevention strategies failed to find benefit of ESBL active surveillance in reducing the incidence of ESBL-producing E coli infections in the context of high compliance with hand hygiene and CHG bathing.[86] Moreover, as not all ESBL acquisitions are associated with patient-to-patient transmission, we believe that active surveillance should be limited only to situations in which its benefit outweighs the burden, such as in outbreak settings. In countries where ESBLs are endemic in community settings, the role of ESBL screening before elective abdominal surgery, to direct the presurgical prophylactic regimen for certain surgical procedures, can be considered.[87]

Screening for CRE among high-risk populations is a practice recommended in some scenarios by most of the national and international bodies.[8,47] As with any screening policy, local policies of which patients to screen should be based if possible on regional epidemiology and risk factor stratification.[47] Populations that may be targeted[25–27] include patients admitted directly from LTACs, patients from other LTCFs with known endemicity, patients with prior travel to foreign countries with high endemic rates, or those transferred directly from another hospital. Both the CDC and Israel Ministry of Health recommend screening close contacts of known CRE carriers.[7,88] Recent hospital stay (in the previous 6 mo) and functional dependency are additional screening candidates. Additional periodic screening policies (eg, weekly) for hospitalized patients in certain high-risk units (eg, ICUs) may be considered during periods of epidemic spread.[47]

The role of active surveillance to prevent spread of nonfermenting MDR-GNB such as CRAB and CRPA is unclear and is not currently recommended by the WHO guidelines for the prevention and control of MDR-GNB.[68] Screening for A. baumannii has 2 major limitations: (1) the best anatomic site for colonization detection has not yet been established (especially among nonventilated patients) and (2) the sensitivity of the diagnostic methods, by using traditional microbiologic methodologies, is known to be low.[48,82] In a study that prospectively screened proven A. baumannii carriers from 6 different anatomic sites, using routine conventional methods, the sensitivity of identifying carriers was only 55% after combining all 6 sites.[48] Because of the poor sensitivity and unclear benefit, most institutions do not screen routinely for A. baumannii carriage. However, there are multiple quasi-experimental studies supporting active surveillance (typically using sputum or rectal cultures) to reduce the incidence of CRAB in endemic or epidemic settings.[89,90] In a Monte Carlo simulation analysis, even with a sensitivity of 55%, active screening reduced A. baumannii transmissions, infections, and deaths by 48%. As screening sensitivity approached 90%, the reduction in transmissions, infections, and deaths reached 78%. For all simulations, active surveillance was also cost-saving, except when carrier prevalence was equal or less than 2% and the sensitivity of the screening test was less than 55%.[82] Recent publications report higher performances for screening the skin with specified sponges and simple sampling procedure.[91]

Cohorting and dedicated staff

Physically cohorting patients infected or colonized with MDR-GNB in a contained area and using dedicated staff to treat only these patients during any given shift may reduce the risk of transmission (see **Table 3**).[67] The resource expenditure required to implement these measures is substantial, and supportive evidence for these practices for MDR-GNB prevention exists primarily in the control of CRE outbreaks and, to a lesser extent CRAB, largely as part of multifaceted bundles that also included active surveillance and additional interventions.[92,93]

Modeling has shown that cohorting was the second most effective intervention in reducing ESBL acquisition in the endemic ICU setting, following HH.[60] In Israel, the establishment of dedicated CRE cohort units with dedicated nursing staff nationwide curbed the emergence and spread of new CRE acquisitions.[67] Cohort units for CRE patients are also common in many facilities in the US and in other countries.[94]

Extrapolation of this practice led Detroit Medical Center to establish a "united cohort unit," in one of its facilities, for all patients with carbapenem-resistant GNB in 2008.[95] Soon thereafter, it became evident that the cocolonization of CRE with *A. baumannii* or *P. aeruginosa* was significantly associated with increased antimicrobial resistance (particularly to colistin and increased MICs to carbapenems[95]) and increased overall mortality.[94] Mobile genetic elements are easily transferrable in these settings and can cross the interspecies barriers.[96,97] This concept of cross-contamination of carbapenemases has also been demonstrated in shared room cohorting of CRE in LTACs.[98] In Israel, even inside the CRE cohort units, patients are separated based on the type of carbapenemse, that is, a carrier of bla_{KPC} is separated from a carrier of bla_{NDM}.

As with CPs, the possible negative psychological impact of cohorting must be considered and quantified longitudinally.[81]

THE ROLE OF THE ENVIRONMENT AND SHARED EQUIPMENT
Environmental contamination

MDR-GNB environmental contamination can occur on virtually any hospital surface, including the floor, the bed frame, the furniture, monitor screens and cables, the various pumps from which parenteral fluids and diet products are administered, the patients' clothes, and the bedsheets (see **Table 3**).[99,100] This most commonly occurs by a colonized patient shedding into his/her immediate vicinity.[100,101] This can result in patient-to-patient transmission primarily through health care workers, whose hands come in contact with the contaminated environment, particularly when HH is suboptimal. The non–glucose-fermenting GNB *A. baumannii* and *P. aeruginosa* have historically been associated with environmental reservoirs.[100,102] Both pathogens survive prolonged periods in low-nutrient environments and are relatively more resistant to some routine cleaning and disinfection products. CRAB can easily be cultured from every high-touch surface surrounding a CRAB carrier in acute-care settings.[103,104]

CRE have been found to contaminate the immediate vicinity of colonized patients as well, with the toilet and the floor around the toilet most frequently testing positive.[105,106] Water sources have also been increasingly implicated in the transmission of MDR-GNB in recent years, with sinks being recognized as a frequent source of hospital-acquired infections.[107] A recent systematic review of MDR-GNB outbreaks originating from water sources found *P. aeruginosa* most commonly implicated, followed by *K. pneumoniae*, *A. baumannii*, and *Enterobacter* spp.[108] Drains, sink surfaces, and faucets were implicated as environmental sources by molecular techniques in the vast majority of cases.

Environmental cleaning

In many outbreak investigation reports of MDR-GNB, preventive bundles applied to successfully contain the outbreak included environmental cleaning, sanitation, and disinfection.[109–112] The CDC recommends that hospitals optimize baseline institutional policies relating to environmental cleaning.[113] Such policies must ensure the adequacy of cleaning and define responsibility for and frequency of cleaning and disinfection of equipment and surfaces and adequate training and retraining of all staff members that have responsibilities for cleaning and disinfection.

Rooms occupied by patients with MDR-GNB should be cleaned and disinfected at least once per day, and dedicated or single-use equipment should be used when possible. Cleaning policies should include the use of an Environmental Protection Agency–registered hospital-approved disinfectant.[113,114] Such surface disinfectant cleaners have been found to be effective against MDR-GNB.[115] Automated "no-touch" technologies such as automated ultraviolet C–emitting (UV-C) and H2O2-based devices are increasingly used for terminal room cleaning after discharge and as part of bundled response to new MDR-GNB outbreaks.[114,116] A recent cluster-randomized trial of standard quaternary ammonium terminal room disinfection versus bleach versus UV-C found that UV-C resulted in a lower incidence of MDRO infection or colonization among the subsequent occupants of the studied rooms.[117] Limited data exist for the prevention of MDR-GNB specifically; however, one study did find that UV-C resulted in less *A. baumannii* surface contamination after a terminal room clean than quaternary ammonium alone.[118]

Following the discharge or transfer of MDR-GNB–colonized patients, formal cleaning and disinfection of the room, its contents, and bathroom should be completed including the laundering of privacy curtains, cleaning, and disinfection of mattresses. Many facilities create specific terminal cleaning protocols for this purpose. Standard precautions do however apply for management of linen and waste from patients with MDR-GNB.[119,120]

Monitoring of cleaning

Monitoring of compliance with environmental cleaning via audits or other measures and distribution of regular cleaning audit reports[113,121] are now fundamental requirements in hospitals.[122] Invisible fluorescent marker or adenosine triphosphate (ATP) bioluminescence can be used to objectively evaluate the thoroughness of cleaning activities in patient rooms by confirming that surface cleaning or disinfection involves contact with all contaminated surfaces. Using ATP bioluminometers has provided quantitative evidence of improved cleanliness of high-touch surfaces after the implementation of an intervention program.[123,124] However, the general utility of ATP monitors is unclear in the absence of validated cleaning benchmark values.[124] Data connecting the level of cleaning to clinical outcomes including the acquisition of MDR-GNB are only recently starting to evolve.[125] Quantifying the exact contribution of improved cleaning on MDR-GNB acquisition will enable stakeholder administrators to weigh the benefits associated with investments aimed at improving the level of cleanliness.

Shared medical equipment

Shared equipment should be minimized in hospitals, particularly among patients with epidemiologically significant pathogens such as the MDR-GNB. Private phones, pens, and computer keyboards are all established vectors for MDR-GNB transmission.[126]

Various types of endoscopes, in particular, duodenoscopes and bronchoscopes, have been linked to multiple outbreaks of CRE and MDR *P. aeruginosa.*[127,128] Appropriate reprocessing of these devices is crucial to prevent the transmission of MDR-GNB. High-level disinfection (HLD) or sterilization should be performed by trained personnel and include visual inspection, manual cleaning, and leak inspection. Pathogen transmission has been described even when following the manufacturer's instructions for reprocessing; enhanced cleaning and reprocessing may be required in some instances and can include a double HLD process or liquid chemical sterilization and/or periodic performance of surveillance microbiologic cultures.[129]

Protocols for cleaning, disinfecting, and sterilizing shared equipment should be established and audited for compliance. Although single-patient-use stethoscopes and blood pressure cuffs are advocated for use among patients with MDR-GNB and in dedicated cohort units, evidence for the benefit of these items is lacking.[130,131]

THE ROLE OF ANTIMICROBIAL STEWARDSHIP

AMS is the core measure in the prevention of MDR-GNB[132] and is a core recommendation of the WHO Antimicrobial Resistance strategy (see **Table 3**).[133] AMS includes not only limiting inappropriate use but also optimizing antimicrobial selection, dosing, route, and duration of therapy administration, to maximize clinical cure or prevention of infection while limiting unintended consequences such as the emergence of resistance. The ultimate goal of AMS is to improve patient care and health care outcomes.[134]

The rationale for AMS programs is that when properly implemented, they can result in large reductions in the overall use of some antimicrobials[135,136] and reductions in MDR-GNB colonization or infection, both by decreasing the risk of *de novo* resistance evolution and reducing the likelihood of exogenous acquisition.[137,138] The benefit of hospital-based AMS has been replicated in many studies. A meta-analysis of 32 studies of the effect of AMS on infection or colonization with MDROs found an overall risk reduction of 51% for MDR-GNB acquisition (incidence ratio = 0.49, 95% CIs = 0.35–0.68).[139] An AMS program in China with restriction of broad-spectrum beta-lactams significantly reduced ceftazidime resistance among *P. aeruginosa* and *A. baumannii* and ciprofloxacin resistance among *P. aeruginosa.*[140] Similarly, in Denmark, the restriction of cephalosporins, fluoroquinolones, and carbapenems has resulted in a sustained reduction in the incidence of both colonization and infections caused by ESBL-producing GNBs.[141]

Hospital-based AMS strategies to reduce the risk of MDR-GNB are described in-depth in the chapter (Chapter 11: Antimicrobial Stewardship and the Infection Control Practitioner: A Natural Alliance. Available at: https://pubmed.ncbi.nlm.nih.gov/34362543/). LTCFs represent a particularly high-yield target because of high rates of antibiotic overuse and high MDRO colonization rates among residents.[142] Barriers to AMS in LTCFs include limited expertise and resources. Successful programs historically have included education campaigns, collaboration with local academic health systems or infectious disease physician groups, and buy-in from LTCF administrative leadership.[143,144]

THE ROLE OF DECOLONIZATION

Therapeutic options to treat and eradicate XDR-GNB (CRE, CRAB, and CRPA) are scarce with very few options available for decolonizing patients (see **Table 3**).[145] Selective digestive tract decontamination (SDD) and selective oropharyngeal decontamination (SOD) are measures that have been shown to reduce rates of ventilator-associated pneumonia and mortality among ICU patients in studies performed in low-MDRO prevalence settings in Holland.[146] Typical agents used for SDD and SOD include colistin, aminoglycosides, and amphotericin B. Evidence that the use of colistin as SOD[147,148] or SDD[149] can lead to the emergence of colistin resistance among human pathogens has limited use of this practice to a handful of countries including the Netherlands, where the rates of CRPA and CRAB are known to be low.[150]

In a small randomized, double-blind, placebo-controlled trial of SDD using oral gentamicin and oral colistin for the eradication of CRE carriage, the percentages of rectal cultures positive for CRE were significantly reduced at 2 weeks following the SDD regimen compared with the placebo arm [odds ratio (OR) = 0.13, $P<.01$].[151] The authors concluded that this SDD regimen could be a suitable decolonization therapy for selected patients colonized with CRE, such as transplant recipients or immunocompromised patients undergoing chemotherapy and patients who require major intestinal or oropharyngeal surgery.[151] A larger randomized trial with 8000 patients in European ICUs with a high prevalence of antimicrobial resistance did not find that SOD or SDD (colistin, tobramycin, and nystatin) reduced the risk of MDR-GNB bloodstream infections compared with daily CHG bathing.[152] We believe it could be potentially hazardous to administer colistin for decolonization purposes because it remains an essential therapeutic option for the treatment of invasive XDR-GNB bloodstream infections[153] and resistance to colistin is emerging in many parts of the world.[95,154]

The use of daily bathing with CHG 4% solution among functionally dependent (bathed in bed) or ICU patients may reduce the risk of MDR-GNB spread and new acquisitions, and it has shown efficacy in preventing additional HAIs (predominantly CLABSI).[155,156] This is a sensible infection prevention strategy for endemic units, among functionally dependent, mechanically intubated patients or patients with central lines.[157]

Fecal microbiota transplantation (FMT) could impact the prevention of CRE and ESBL infections and acquisitions because it has a track record of proven efficacy in *Clostridium difficile* infection.[158] Early trials of FMT for the decolonization of MDR-GNB have shown promise in reducing MDR-GNB colonization.[159] Efficacy and safety data on larger cohorts of carriers, for prolonged periods, will inform whether FMT should be recommended for reducing colonization with MDR-GNB, particularly considering recent reports of donor-to-recipient ESBL transmissions that have highlighted the importance of screening FMT donors for MDR-GNB colonization.[160]

COLLABORATION WITH LONG-TERM CARE FACILITIES

Because of the interconnectedness of hospitals and LTCFs, infection control interventions should ideally be implemented in parallel in both settings to maximize the effectiveness of prevention interventions among high-risk patients across the continuum of care.

In the Israeli nationwide CRE epidemic from 2006 to 2007, a stable decrease in new acquisitions was only evident after broadening the national prevention plan to include LTCFs.[8,67] This experience highlights the importance of close collaboration and communication between infection control programs in acute-care hospitals and surrounding LTCFs. Restrictions put in place to halt patient-to-patient transmission in

LTCFs should ideally be tailored to a facility, based on its structure, its residents' characteristics, the local colonization pressure, and the overall level of care provided in the facility. Sharing of resources, standardizing education and training, and improving interfacility communication regarding MDRO colonization status can allow for a more integrated infection prevention approach across different health care settings.[161]

SUMMARY

Antimicrobial resistance is a global iatrogenic complication of modern medical care. MDR-GNB are prevalent in most facilities, and their containment and treatment pose an enormous challenge. The authors' suggestions are as follows:

1. Active surveillance: screening to detect asymptomatic colonization
   a. ESBL: not routinely recommended
   b. CRE: establish populations who warrant screening based on local and regional CRE epidemiology. We also recommend using molecular assays to determine the presence and type of carbapenemases.
   c. CRAB: should be considered in endemic ICUs, on admission to the unit, and periodically thereafter. Respiratory samples (only from ventilated patients) and skin samples (from wide areas using designated sponges or wipes according to established methodology) are the basic body sites to target.
   d. CRPA: not routinely recommended
2. Containment
   a. HH is a core component in the prevention of MDR-GNB spread
   b. Contact isolation precautions
      i. ESBL: not routinely recommended
      ii. CRE: recommended for carbapenemase-producing and non–carbapenemase-producing CRE isolates
      iii. *A. baumannii*: recommended for all CRAB. Consider use for carbapenem-susceptible isolates in outbreaks or endemic settings
      iv. CRPA: recommended for all carriers
   c. Cohorting with dedicated staff
      i. Avoid "united cohort units" for more than a single MDR-GNB
      ii. ESBL: not routinely recommended
      iii. CRE: recommended for carbapenemase-producing CRE during epidemic spread and in hyperendemic regions.
      iv. CRAB: not routinely recommended, unless during outbreaks or high endemic states in ICU settings or LTACs.
      v. CRPA: not routinely recommended, unless during outbreaks.
3. Environmental cleaning and shared equipment
   a. Establish unit-specific cleaning protocols for units with unique features (eg, hemodialysis, operating rooms, certain outpatient clinics).
   b. Establish strict protocols for terminal cleaning following discharge of an MDR-GNB carrier.
   c. Regularly monitor the level of cleaning (preferably by quantitative processes) and disseminate the results for quality improvement purposes.
   d. Audit compliance with protocols for HLD or sterilization of high-risk shared medical devices such as duodenoscopes and bronchoscopes
4. AMS
   a. Establish an institutional AMS program, monitor adherence, and provide feedback to prescribing providers at regular intervals

5. Decolonization of MDR-GNB carriage
   a. SDD and SOD are not recommended for the routine prevention of MDR-GNB infections among ICU patients
   b. Daily bathing with topical CHG is recommended for functionally dependent patients bathed in bed, mechanically intubated patients, patients with central lines, and ICU patients in general, although efficacy data pertaining specifically to MDR-GNB prevention are limited

DISCLOSURE

This study was not supported financially by any external source. D. M. has received payments previously for lectures and research grants from Merck and GAMA Health care (unrelated to this study). J. P. M. has no potential conflicts of interest.

ACKNOWLEDGMENTS

None.

REFERENCES

1. CDC. Antibiotic resistance threats in the United States, 2019. Atlanta, GA: US Department of Health and Human Services, CDC; 2019.
2. Boucher HW, Talbot GH, Bradley JS, et al. Bad bugs, no drugs: no ESKAPE! An update from the Infectious Diseases Society of America. Clin Infect Dis 2009; 48(1):1–12.
3. Magiorakos AP, Srinivasan A, Carey RB, et al. Multidrug-resistant, extensively drug-resistant and pandrug-resistant bacteria: an international expert proposal for interim standard definitions for acquired resistance. Clin Microbiol Infect 2012;18(3):268–81.
4. Tacconelli E, Cataldo MA, Dancer SJ, et al. ESCMID guidelines for the management of the infection control measures to reduce transmission of multidrug-resistant gram-negative bacteria in hospitalized patients. Clin Microbiol Infect 2014;20(Suppl 1):1–55.
5. Tal Jasper R, Coyle JR, Katz DE, et al. The complex epidemiology of extended-spectrum beta-lactamase-producing enterobacteriaceae. Future Microbiol 2015;10(5):819–39.
6. Tal-Jasper R, Katz DE, Amrami N, et al. Clinical and epidemiological significance of carbapenem resistance in acinetobacter baumannii infections. Antimicrob Agents Chemother 2016;60(5):3127–31.
7. Centers for Disease Control and Prevention. Facility guidance for control of carbapenem-resistant enterobacteriaceae (CRE). November 2015 update - CRE toolkit. 2015. Available at: https://wwwcdcgov/hai/pdfs/cre/CRE-guidance-508pdf.
8. Schwaber MJ, Carmeli Y. An ongoing national intervention to contain the spread of carbapenem-resistant enterobacteriaceae. Clin Infect Dis 2014;58(5): 697–703.
9. Rodriguez-Bano J, Picon E, Navarro MD, et al. Impact of changes in CLSI and EUCAST breakpoints for susceptibility in bloodstream infections due to extended-spectrum beta-lactamase-producing Escherichia coli. Clin Microbiol Infect 2012;18(9):894–900.
10. Marchaim D, Sunkara B, Lephart PR, et al. Extended-spectrum beta-lactamase producers reported as susceptible to piperacillin-tazobactam, cefepime, and

cefuroxime in the era of lowered breakpoints and no confirmatory tests. Infect Control Hosp Epidemiol 2012;33(8):853–5.

11. Marchaim D, Gottesman T, Schwartz O, et al. National multicenter study of predictors and outcomes of bacteremia upon hospital admission caused by Enterobacteriaceae producing extended-spectrum beta-lactamases. Antimicrob Agents Chemother 2010;54(12):5099–104.

12. Endimiani A, Doi Y, Bethel CR, et al. Enhancing resistance to cephalosporins in class C beta-lactamases: impact of Gly214Glu in CMY-2. Biochemistry 2010; 49(5):1014–23.

13. Harris AD, Kotetishvili M, Shurland S, et al. How important is patient-to-patient transmission in extended-spectrum beta-lactamase Escherichia coli acquisition. Am J Infect Control 2007;35(2):97–101.

14. Bogan C, Marchaim D. The role of antimicrobial stewardship in curbing carbapenem resistance. Future Microbiol 2013;8(8):979–91.

15. Babini GS, Livermore DM. Antimicrobial resistance amongst Klebsiella spp. collected from intensive care units in Southern and Western Europe in 1997-1998. J Antimicrob Chemother 2000;45(2):183–9.

16. Bradford PA. Extended-spectrum beta-lactamases in the 21st century: characterization, epidemiology, and detection of this important resistance threat. Clin Microbiol Rev 2001;14(4):933–51, table of contents.

17. Mirelis B, Navarro F, Miro E, et al. Community transmission of extended-spectrum beta-lactamase. Emerg Infect Dis 2003;9(8):1024–5.

18. Goldstein FW. Antibiotic susceptibility of bacterial strains isolated from patients with community-acquired urinary tract infections in France. Multicentre Study Group. Eur J Clin Microbiol Infect Dis 2000;19(2):112–7.

19. Nicolas-Chanoine MH, Bertrand X, Madec JY. Escherichia coli ST131, an intriguing clonal group. Clin Microbiol Rev 2014;27(3):543–74.

20. Emmanuel Martinez A, Widmer A, Frei R, et al. ESBL-colonization at ICU admission: impact on subsequent infection, carbapenem-consumption, and outcome. Infect Control Hosp Epidemiol 2019;40(4):408–13.

21. Assawatheptawee K, Kiddee A, Na-Udom A, et al. Acquisition of extended-spectrum β-lactamase-producing Escherichia coli and Klebsiella pneumoniae in intensive care units in Thailand. J Infect Chemother 2021;27(2):401–5.

22. Mulki SS, Ramamurthy K, Bhat S. Fecal carriage of extended-spectrum beta-lactamase-producing enterobacteriaceae in intensive care unit patients. Indian J Crit Care Med 2017;21(8):525–7.

23. Abbo A, Navon-Venezia S, Hammer-Muntz O, et al. Multidrug-resistant Acinetobacter baumannii. Emerg Infect Dis 2005;11(1):22–9.

24. Aloush V, Navon-Venezia S, Seigman-Igra Y, et al. Multidrug-resistant Pseudomonas aeruginosa: risk factors and clinical impact. Antimicrob Agents Chemother 2006;50(1):43–8.

25. Marchaim D, Chopra T, Bhargava A, et al. Recent exposure to antimicrobials and carbapenem-resistant Enterobacteriaceae: the role of antimicrobial stewardship. Infect Control Hosp Epidemiol 2012;33(8):817–30.

26. Schwaber MJ, Carmeli Y. Carbapenem-resistant Enterobacteriaceae: a potential threat. JAMA 2008;300(24):2911–3.

27. Schwaber MJ, Klarfeld-Lidji S, Navon-Venezia S, et al. Predictors of carbapenem-resistant Klebsiella pneumoniae acquisition among hospitalized adults and effect of acquisition on mortality. Antimicrob Agents Chemother 2008;52(3):1028–33.

28. Munoz-Price LS. Long-term acute care hospitals. Clin Infect Dis 2009;49(3): 438–43.

29. Marchaim D, Chopra T, Bogan C, et al. The burden of multidrug-resistant organisms on tertiary hospitals posed by patients with recent stays in long-term acute care facilities. Am J Infect Control 2012;40(8):760–5.

30. Mills JP, Talati NJ, Alby K, et al. The epidemiology of carbapenem-resistant klebsiella pneumoniae colonization and infection among long-term acute care hospital residents. Infect Control Hosp Epidemiol 2016;37(1):55–60.

31. Won SY, Munoz-Price LS, Lolans K, et al. Emergence and rapid regional spread of Klebsiella pneumoniae carbapenemase-producing Enterobacteriaceae. Clin Infect Dis 2011;53(6):532–40.

32. Bonomo RA. Multiple antibiotic-resistant bacteria in long-term-care facilities: an emerging problem in the practice of infectious diseases. Clin Infect Dis 2000; 31(6):1414–22.

33. Rice LB, Willey SH, Papanicolaou GA, et al. Outbreak of ceftazidime resistance caused by extended-spectrum beta-lactamases at a Massachusetts chronic-care facility. Antimicrob Agents Chemother 1990;34(11):2193–9.

34. Wiener J, Quinn JP, Bradford PA, et al. Multiple antibiotic-resistant Klebsiella and Escherichia coli in nursing homes. JAMA 1999;281(6):517–23.

35. Muder RR, Brennen C, Drenning SD, et al. Multiply antibiotic-resistant gram-negative bacilli in a long-term-care facility: a case-control study of patient risk factors and prior antibiotic use. Infect Control Hosp Epidemiol 1997;18(12): 809–13.

36. Terpenning MS, Bradley SF, Wan JY, et al. Colonization and infection with antibiotic-resistant bacteria in a long-term care facility. J Am Geriatr Soc 1994; 42(10):1062–9.

37. Eberle CM, Winsemius D, Garibaldi RA. Risk factors and consequences of bacteriuria in non-catheterized nursing home residents. J Gerontol 1993;48(6): M266–71.

38. Furuno JP, Hebden JN, Standiford HC, et al. Prevalence of methicillin-resistant Staphylococcus aureus and Acinetobacter baumannii in a long-term acute care facility. Am J Infect Control 2008;36(7):468–71.

39. Sengstock DM, Thyagarajan R, Apalara J, et al. Multidrug-resistant Acinetobacter baumannii: an emerging pathogen among older adults in community hospitals and nursing homes. Clin Infect Dis 2010;50(12):1611–6.

40. Webster C, Towner KJ, Humphreys H. Survival of Acinetobacter on three clinically related inanimate surfaces. Infect Control Hosp Epidemiol 2000;21(4):246.

41. Friedman ND, Kaye KS, Stout JE, et al. Health care–associated bloodstream infections in adults: a reason to change the accepted definition of community-acquired infections. Ann Intern Med 2002;137(10):791–7.

42. van Duin D, Paterson DL. Multidrug-resistant bacteria in the community: an update. Infect Dis Clin North Am 2020;34(4):709–22.

43. Karanika S, Karantanos T, Arvanitis M, et al. Fecal colonization with extended-spectrum beta-lactamase-producing enterobacteriaceae and risk factors among healthy individuals: a systematic review and metaanalysis. Clin Infect Dis 2016;63(3):310–8.

44. Schwaber MJ, Carmeli Y. Mortality and delay in effective therapy associated with extended-spectrum beta-lactamase production in Enterobacteriaceae bacteraemia: a systematic review and meta-analysis. J Antimicrob Chemother 2007; 60(5):913–20.

45. Adler A, Katz DE, Marchaim D. The continuing plague of extended-spectrum beta-lactamase-producing enterobacteriaceae infections. Infect Dis Clin North Am 2016;30(2):347–75.

46. Sarma JB, Marshall B, Cleeve V, et al. Effects of fluoroquinolone restriction (from 2007 to 2012) on resistance in Enterobacteriaceae: interrupted time-series analysis. J Hosp Infect 2015;91(1):68–73.

47. Guidance for control of infections with carbapenem-resistant or carbapenemase-producing Enterobacteriaceae in acute care facilities. MMWR Morb Mortal Wkly Rep 2009;58(10):256–60.

48. Marchaim D, Navon-Venezia S, Schwartz D, et al. Surveillance cultures and duration of carriage of multidrug-resistant Acinetobacter baumannii. J Clin Microbiol 2007;45(5):1551–5.

49. Doi Y. [Antimicrobial resistance testing in clinical practice]. Nihon Rinsho 2012; 70(2):272–5.

50. Adler A, Gniadkowski M, Baraniak A, et al. Transmission dynamics of ESBL-producing Escherichia coli clones in rehabilitation wards at a tertiary care centre. Clin Microbiol Infect 2012;18(12):E497–505.

51. Camins BC, Fraser VJ. Reducing the risk of health care-associated infections by complying with CDC hand hygiene guidelines. Jt Comm J Qual Patient Saf 2005;31(3):173–9.

52. Pittet D, Dharan S, Touveneau S, et al. Bacterial contamination of the hands of hospital staff during routine patient care. Arch Intern Med 1999;159(8):821–6.

53. Guenthner SH, Hendley JO, Wenzel RP. Gram-negative bacilli as nontransient flora on the hands of hospital personnel. J Clin Microbiol 1987;25(3):488–90.

54. Mills JP, Zhu Z, Mantey J, et al. The devil is in the details: factors influencing hand hygiene adherence and contamination with antibiotic-resistant organisms among healthcare providers in nursing facilities. Infect Control Hosp Epidemiol 2019;40(12):1394–9.

55. Trick WE, Vernon MO, Welbel SF, et al. Multicenter intervention program to increase adherence to hand hygiene recommendations and glove use and to reduce the incidence of antimicrobial resistance. Infect Control Hosp Epidemiol 2007;28(1):42–9.

56. Larson EL, Cimiotti JP, Haas J, et al. Gram-negative bacilli associated with catheter-associated and non-catheter-associated bloodstream infections and hand carriage by healthcare workers in neonatal intensive care units. Pediatr Crit Care Med 2005;6(4):457–61.

57. Waters V, Larson E, Wu F, et al. Molecular epidemiology of gram-negative bacilli from infected neonates and health care workers' hands in neonatal intensive care units. Clin Infect Dis 2004;38(12):1682–7.

58. CDC/WHO hand hygiene guidelines crosswalk. Jt Comm Perspect 2008; 28(2):4–7.

59. Montville R, Schaffner DW. A meta-analysis of the published literature on the effectiveness of antimicrobial soaps. J Food Prot 2011;74(11):1875–82.

60. Pelat C, Kardas-Sloma L, Birgand G, et al. Hand hygiene, cohorting, or antibiotic restriction to control outbreaks of multidrug-resistant enterobacteriaceae. Infect Control Hosp Epidemiol 2016;37(3):272–80.

61. Boyce JM. Hand hygiene compliance monitoring: current perspectives from the USA. J Hosp Infect 2008;70(Suppl 1):2–7.

62. Pittet D, Allegranzi B, Sax H, et al. Evidence-based model for hand transmission during patient care and the role of improved practices. Lancet Infect Dis 2006; 6(10):641–52.

63. Erasmus V, Daha TJ, Brug H, et al. Systematic review of studies on compliance with hand hygiene guidelines in hospital care. Infect Control Hosp Epidemiol 2010;31(3):283–94.

64. Chitnis AS, Caruthers PS, Rao AK, et al. Outbreak of carbapenem-resistant enterobacteriaceae at a long-term acute care hospital: sustained reductions in transmission through active surveillance and targeted interventions. Infect Control Hosp Epidemiol 2012;33(10):984–92.

65. Gregory CJ, Llata E, Stine N, et al. Outbreak of carbapenem-resistant Klebsiella pneumoniae in Puerto Rico associated with a novel carbapenemase variant. Infect Control Hosp Epidemiol 2010;31(5):476–84.

66. Harris AD, Morgan DJ, Pineles L, et al. Acquisition of antibiotic-resistant gram-negative bacteria in the Benefits of Universal Glove and Gown (BUGG) cluster randomized trial. Clin Infect Dis 2021;72(3):431–7.

67. Schwaber MJ, Lev B, Israeli A, et al. Containment of a country-wide outbreak of carbapenem-resistant Klebsiella pneumoniae in Israeli hospitals via a nationally implemented intervention. Clin Infect Dis 2011;52(7):848–55.

68. Guidelines for the prevention and control of carbapenem-resistant Enterobacteriaceae, Acinetobacter baumannii and Pseudomonas aeruginosa in health care facilities. Geneva, Switzerland: World Health Organization; 2017.

69. Morgan DJ, Liang SY, Smith CL, et al. Frequent multidrug-resistant Acinetobacter baumannii contamination of gloves, gowns, and hands of healthcare workers. Infect Control Hosp Epidemiol 2010;31(7):716–21.

70. Lefebvre A, Gbaguidi-Haore H, Bertrand X, et al. Impact of barrier precautions and antibiotic consumption on the incidence rate of acquired cases of infection or colonization with Acinetobacter baumannii: a 10-year multi-department study. Am J Infect Control 2011;39(10):891–4.

71. Johnson JK, Smith G, Lee MS, et al. The role of patient-to-patient transmission in the acquisition of imipenem-resistant Pseudomonas aeruginosa colonization in the intensive care unit. J Infect Dis 2009;200(6):900–5.

72. Ben-Ami R, Rodriguez-Bano J, Arslan H, et al. A multinational survey of risk factors for infection with extended-spectrum beta-lactamase-producing enterobacteriaceae in nonhospitalized patients. Clin Infect Dis 2009;49(5):682–90.

73. Rodriguez-Bano J, Alcala JC, Cisneros JM, et al. Community infections caused by extended-spectrum beta-lactamase-producing Escherichia coli. Arch Intern Med 2008;168(17):1897–902.

74. Dhar S, Marchaim D, Tansek R, et al. Contact precautions: more is not necessarily better. Infect Control Hosp Epidemiol 2014;35(3):213–21.

75. Zahar JR, Poirel L, Dupont C, et al. About the usefulness of contact precautions for carriers of extended-spectrum beta-lactamase-producing Escherichia coli. BMC Infect Dis 2015;15:512.

76. Cantey JB, Sreeramoju P, Jaleel M, et al. Prompt control of an outbreak caused by extended-spectrum beta-lactamase-producing Klebsiella pneumoniae in a neonatal intensive care unit. J Pediatr 2013;163(3):672–9, e671–3.

77. Guyot K, Biran V, Doit C, et al. Raman spectroscopic analysis of the clonal and horizontal spread of CTX-M-15-producing Klebsiella pneumoniae in a neonatal intensive care unit. Eur J Clin Microbiol Infect Dis 2012;31(10):2827–34.

78. Kristof K, Szabo D, Marsh JW, et al. Extended-spectrum beta-lactamase-producing Klebsiella spp. in a neonatal intensive care unit: risk factors for the infection and the dynamics of the molecular epidemiology. Eur J Clin Microbiol Infect Dis 2007;26(8):563–70.

79. Kirkland KB, Weinstein JM. Adverse effects of contact isolation. Lancet 1999; 354(9185):1177–8.
80. Saint S, Higgins LA, Nallamothu BK, et al. Do physicians examine patients in contact isolation less frequently? A brief report. Am J Infect Control 2003; 31(6):354–6.
81. Stelfox HT, Bates DW, Redelmeier DA. Safety of patients isolated for infection control. JAMA 2003;290(14):1899–905.
82. Coyle JR, Kaye KS, Taylor T, et al. Effectiveness and cost of implementing an active surveillance screening policy for Acinetobacter baumannii: a Monte Carlo simulation model. Am J Infect Control 2014;42(3):283–7.
83. Bonten MJ. Colonization pressure: a critical parameter in the epidemiology of antibiotic-resistant bacteria. Crit Care 2012;16(4):142.
84. Lee BY, Bartsch SM, Wong KF, et al. Tracking the spread of carbapenem-resistant Enterobacteriaceae (CRE) through clinical cultures alone underestimates the spread of CRE even more than anticipated. Infect Control Hosp Epidemiol 2019;40(6):731–4.
85. Rybczynska H, Melander E, Johansson H, et al. Efficacy of a once-a-week screening programme to control extended-spectrum beta-lactamase-producing bacteria in a neonatal intensive care unit. Scand J Infect Dis 2014;46(6):426–32.
86. Derde LPG, Cooper BS, Goossens H, et al. Interventions to reduce colonisation and transmission of antimicrobial-resistant bacteria in intensive care units: an interrupted time series study and cluster randomised trial. Lancet Infect Dis 2014; 14(1):31–9.
87. Nutman A, Temkin E, Harbarth S, et al. Personalized Ertapenem Prophylaxis for Carriers of Extended-spectrum β-Lactamase-producing Enterobacteriaceae Undergoing Colorectal Surgery. Clin Infect Dis 2020;70(9):1891–7.
88. Solter E, Adler A, Rubinovitch B, et al. Israeli national policy for carbapenem-resistant enterobacteriaceae screening, carrier isolation and discontinuation of isolation. Infect Control Hosp Epidemiol 2018;39(1):85–9.
89. Yamamoto N, Hamaguchi S, Akeda Y, et al. Rapid screening and early precautions for carbapenem-resistant Acinetobacter baumannii carriers decreased nosocomial transmission in hospital settings: a quasi-experimental study. Antimicrob Resist Infect Control 2019;8:110.
90. Valencia-Martín R, Gonzalez-Galan V, Alvarez-Marín R, et al. A multimodal intervention program to control a long-term Acinetobacter baumannii endemic in a tertiary care hospital. Antimicrob Resist Infect Control 2019;8:199.
91. Nutman A, Temkin E, Lellouche J, et al. Detecting carbapenem-resistant Acinetobacter baumannii (CRAB) carriage: which body site should be cultured? Infect Control Hosp Epidemiol 2020;41(8):965–7.
92. Abad CL, Barker AK, Safdar N. A systematic review of the effectiveness of cohorting to reduce transmission of healthcare-associated C. difficile and multidrug-resistant organisms. Infect Control Hosp Epidemiol 2020;41(6): 691–709.
93. Alon D, Mudrik H, Chowers M, et al. Control of a hospital-wide outbreak of carbapenem-resistant Acinetobacter baumannii (CRAB) using the Israeli national carbapenem-resistant Enterobacteriaceae (CRE) guidelines as a model. Infect Control Hosp Epidemiol 2020;41(8):926–30.
94. Marchaim D, Perez F, Lee J, et al. "Swimming in resistance": co-colonization with carbapenem-resistant Enterobacteriaceae and Acinetobacter baumannii or Pseudomonas aeruginosa. Am J Infect Control 2012;40(9):830–5.

95. Marchaim D, Chopra T, Pogue JM, et al. Outbreak of colistin-resistant, carbapenem-resistant Klebsiella pneumoniae in metropolitan Detroit, Michigan. Antimicrob Agents Chemother 2011;55(2):593–9.

96. Doi Y, Adams-Haduch JM, Peleg AY, et al. The role of horizontal gene transfer in the dissemination of extended-spectrum beta-lactamase-producing Escherichia coli and Klebsiella pneumoniae isolates in an endemic setting. Diagn Microbiol Infect Dis 2012;74(1):34–8.

97. Sidjabat HE, Silveira FP, Potoski BA, et al. Interspecies spread of Klebsiella pneumoniae carbapenemase gene in a single patient. Clin Infect Dis 2009; 49(11):1736–8.

98. Hawken SE, Hayden MK, Lolans K, et al. Cohorting KPC+ Klebsiella pneumoniae (KPC-Kp)-positive patients: a genomic exposé of cross-colonization hazards in a long-term acute-care hospital (LTACH). Infect Control Hosp Epidemiol 2020;41(10):1162–8.

99. Talon D. The role of the hospital environment in the epidemiology of multi-resistant bacteria. J Hosp Infect 1999;43(1):13–7.

100. Munoz-Price LS, Namias N, Cleary T, et al. Acinetobacter baumannii: association between environmental contamination of patient rooms and occupant status. Infect Control Hosp Epidemiol 2013;34(5):517–20.

101. Tran HH, Ehsani S, Shibayama K, et al. Common isolation of New Delhi metallo-beta-lactamase 1-producing Enterobacteriaceae in a large surgical hospital in Vietnam. Eur J Clin Microbiol Infect Dis 2015;34(6):1247–54.

102. Nseir S, Blazejewski C, Lubret R, et al. Risk of acquiring multidrug-resistant Gram-negative bacilli from prior room occupants in the intensive care unit. Clin Microbiol Infect 2011;17(8):1201–8.

103. Weber DJ, Rutala WA, Miller MB, et al. Role of hospital surfaces in the transmission of emerging health care-associated pathogens: norovirus, Clostridium difficile, and Acinetobacter species. Am J Infect Control 2010;38(5 Suppl 1): S25–33.

104. Weber DJ, Anderson D, Rutala WA. The role of the surface environment in healthcare-associated infections. Curr Opin Infect Dis 2013;26(4):338–44.

105. Weber DJ, Rutala WA, Kanamori H, et al. Carbapenem-resistant Enterobacteriaceae: frequency of hospital room contamination and survival on various inoculated surfaces. Infect Control Hosp Epidemiol 2015;36(5):590–3.

106. Lerner A, Adler A, Abu-Hanna J, et al. Environmental contamination by carbapenem-resistant Enterobacteriaceae. J Clin Microbiol 2013;51(1):177–81.

107. Kanamori H, Weber DJ, Rutala WA. Healthcare outbreaks associated with a water reservoir and infection prevention strategies. Clin Infect Dis 2016;62(11): 1423–35.

108. Kizny Gordon AE, Mathers AJ, Cheong EYL, et al. The hospital water environment as a reservoir for carbapenem-resistant organisms causing hospital-acquired infections-A systematic review of the literature. Clin Infect Dis 2017; 64(10):1435–44.

109. Dancer SJ. The role of environmental cleaning in the control of hospital-acquired infection. J Hosp Infect 2009;73(4):378–85.

110. Chang HL, Tang CH, Hsu YM, et al. Nosocomial outbreak of infection with multidrug-resistant Acinetobacter baumannii in a medical center in Taiwan. Infect Control Hosp Epidemiol 2009;30(1):34–8.

111. Chan PC, Huang LM, Lin HC, et al. Control of an outbreak of pandrug-resistant Acinetobacter baumannii colonization and infection in a neonatal intensive care unit. Infect Control Hosp Epidemiol 2007;28(4):423–9.

112. Fournier PE, Richet H. The epidemiology and control of Acinetobacter baumannii in health care facilities. Clin Infect Dis 2006;42(5):692–9.

113. CDC. Options for evaluating environmental cleaning. 2010. Available at: https://www.cdc.gov/hai/toolkits/Evaluating-Environmental-Cleaning.html.

114. Carling PC, Huang SS. Improving healthcare environmental cleaning and disinfection: current and evolving issues. Infect Control Hosp Epidemiol 2013;34(5): 507–13.

115. Rogers BA, Aminzadeh Z, Hayashi Y, et al. Country-to-country transfer of patients and the risk of multi-resistant bacterial infection. Clin Infect Dis 2011; 53(1):49–56.

116. Anderson DJ, Gergen MF, Smathers E, et al. Decontamination of targeted pathogens from patient rooms using an automated ultraviolet-C-emitting device. Infect Control Hosp Epidemiol 2013;34(5):466–71.

117. Anderson DJ, Chen LF, Weber DJ, et al. Enhanced terminal room disinfection and acquisition and infection caused by multidrug-resistant organisms and Clostridium difficile (the Benefits of Enhanced Terminal Room Disinfection study): a cluster-randomised, multicentre, crossover study. Lancet 2017; 389(10071):805–14.

118. Rutala WA, Kanamori H, Gergen MF, et al. Enhanced disinfection leads to reduction of microbial contamination and a decrease in patient colonization and infection. Infect Control Hosp Epidemiol 2018;39(9):1118–21.

119. England PH. Carbapenemase-producing Enterobacteriaceae: early detection, management and control toolkit for acute trusts. Available at: https://www.gov.uk/government/publications/carbapenemase-producing-enterobacteriaceae-early-detection-management-and-control-toolkit-for-acute-trusts.   Accessed May 22, 2016.

120. Canada PHAo. Guidance: infection prevention and control measures for health workers in all health settings. Carbapenem-resistant Gram-negative bacilli. 2010. Available at: http://www.phac-aspc.gc.ca/nois-sinp/guide/ipcm-mpci/ipcm-mpci-eng.php. Accessed May 22, 2016.

121. CDPH. Carbapenem-resistant enterobacteriaceae. Available at: www.cdph.ca.gov/programs/hai/Pages/Carbapenem-ResisantEnterobacteriaceae.aspx. Accessed November 25, 2015.

122. Miller BA, Sexton DJ. Shedding light on new methods to improve hospital cleanliness: the use of ultraviolet monitors as surrogate markers for bacterial contamination. Crit Care Med 2010;38(4):1212–4.

123. Boyce JM, Havill NL, Dumigan DG, et al. Monitoring the effectiveness of hospital cleaning practices by use of an adenosine triphosphate bioluminescence assay. Infect Control Hosp Epidemiol 2009;30(7):678–84.

124. Chow A, Arah OA, Chan SP, et al. Alcohol handrubbing and chlorhexidine handwashing protocols for routine hospital practice: a randomized clinical trial of protocol efficacy and time effectiveness. Am J Infect Control 2012;40(9):800–5.

125. Chia PY, Sengupta S, Kukreja A, et al. The role of hospital environment in transmissions of multidrug-resistant gram-negative organisms. Antimicrob Resist Infect Control 2020;9(1):29.

126. Borer A, Gilad J, Smolyakov R, et al. Cell phones and Acinetobacter transmission. Emerg Infect Dis 2005;11(7):1160–1.

127. O'Horo JC, Farrell A, Sohail MR, et al. Carbapenem-resistant Enterobacteriaceae and endoscopy: an evolving threat. Am J Infect Control 2016;44(9): 1032–6.

128. Mehta AC, Muscarella LF. Bronchoscope-related "Superbug" infections. Chest 2020;157(2):454–69.

129. Rutala WA, Weber DJ. Outbreaks of carbapenem-resistant Enterobacteriaceae infections associated with duodenoscopes: What can we do to prevent infections? Am J Infect Control 2016;44(5 Suppl):e47–51.

130. Tschopp C, Schneider A, Longtin Y, et al. Predictors of heavy stethoscope contamination following a physical examination. Infect Control Hosp Epidemiol 2016;37(6):673–9.

131. Youngster I, Berkovitch M, Heyman E, et al. The stethoscope as a vector of infectious diseases in the paediatric division. Acta Paediatr 2008;97(9):1253–5.

132. Siegel JD, Rhinehart E, Jackson M, et al. 2007 guideline for isolation precautions: preventing transmission of infectious agents in health care settings. Am J Infect Control 2007;35(10 Suppl 2):S65–164.

133. WHO. Evolving threat of antimicrobial resistance: options for action. 2012. Available at: http://apps.who.int/iris/bitstream/10665/44812/1/9789241503181_eng.pdf.

134. Dellit TH, Owens RC, McGowan JE Jr, et al. Infectious Diseases Society of America and the Society for Healthcare Epidemiology of America guidelines for developing an institutional program to enhance antimicrobial stewardship. Clin Infect Dis 2007;44(2):159–77.

135. Paterson DL. The role of antimicrobial management programs in optimizing antibiotic prescribing within hospitals. Clin Infect Dis 2006;42(Suppl 2):S90–5.

136. Gross R, Morgan AS, Kinky DE, et al. Impact of a hospital-based antimicrobial management program on clinical and economic outcomes. Clin Infect Dis 2001;33(3):289–95.

137. Pate PG, Storey DF, Baum DL. Implementation of an antimicrobial stewardship program at a 60-bed long-term acute care hospital. Infect Control Hosp Epidemiol 2012;33(4):405–8.

138. Schwartz DN, Abiad H, DeMarais PL, et al. An educational intervention to improve antimicrobial use in a hospital-based long-term care facility. J Am Geriatr Soc 2007;55(8):1236–42.

139. Baur D, Gladstone BP, Burkert F, et al. Effect of antibiotic stewardship on the incidence of infection and colonisation with antibiotic-resistant bacteria and Clostridium difficile infection: a systematic review and meta-analysis. Lancet Infect Dis 2017;17(9):990–1001.

140. Guo W, He Q, Wang Z, et al. Influence of antimicrobial consumption on gram-negative bacteria in inpatients receiving antimicrobial resistance therapy from 2008-2013 at a tertiary hospital in Shanghai, China. Am J Infect Control 2015;43(4):358–64.

141. Knudsen JD, Andersen SE. A multidisciplinary intervention to reduce infections of ESBL- and AmpC-producing, gram-negative bacteria at a University Hospital. PLoS One 2014;9(1):e86457.

142. Jump RLP, Gaur S, Katz MJ, et al. Template for an antibiotic stewardship policy for post-acute and long-term care settings. J Am Med Directors Assoc 2017;18(11):913–20.

143. Adre C, Jump RLP, Spires SS. Recommendations for improving antimicrobial stewardship in long-term care settings through collaboration. Infect Dis Clin North Am 2020;34(1):129–43.

144. Jump RL, Olds DM, Seifi N, et al. Effective antimicrobial stewardship in a long-term care facility through an infectious disease consultation service: keeping a LID on antibiotic use. Infect Control Hosp Epidemiol 2012;33(12):1185–92.

145. Tacconelli E, Mazzaferri F, de Smet AM, et al. ESCMID-EUCIC clinical guidelines on decolonization of multidrug-resistant Gram-negative bacteria carriers. Clin Microbiol Infect 2019;25(7):807–17.

146. Plantinga NL, de Smet A, Oostdijk EAN, et al. Selective digestive and oropharyngeal decontamination in medical and surgical ICU patients: individual patient data meta-analysis. Clin Microbiol Infect 2018;24(5):505–13.

147. Halaby T, Al Naiemi N, Kluytmans J, et al. Emergence of colistin resistance in Enterobacteriaceae after the introduction of selective digestive tract decontamination in an intensive care unit. Antimicrob Agents Chemother 2013;57(7): 3224–9.

148. Heininger A, Meyer E, Schwab F, et al. Effects of long-term routine use of selective digestive decontamination on antimicrobial resistance. Intensive Care Med 2006;32(10):1569–76.

149. Oostdijk EA, Smits L, de Smet AM, et al. Colistin resistance in gram-negative bacteria during prophylactic topical colistin use in intensive care units. Intensive Care Med 2013;39(4):653–60.

150. Kaiser AM, Schultsz C, Kruithof GJ, et al. Carriage of resistant microorganisms in repatriates from foreign hospitals to The Netherlands. Clin Microbiol Infect 2004;10(11):972–9.

151. Saidel-Odes L, Polachek H, Peled N, et al. A randomized, double-blind, placebo-controlled trial of selective digestive decontamination using oral gentamicin and oral polymyxin E for eradication of carbapenem-resistant Klebsiella pneumoniae carriage. Infect Control Hosp Epidemiol 2012;33(1):14–9.

152. Wittekamp BH, Plantinga NL, Cooper BS, et al. Decontamination strategies and bloodstream infections with antibiotic-resistant microorganisms in ventilated patients: a randomized clinical trial. JAMA 2018;320(20):2087–98.

153. Peleg AY, Hooper DC. Hospital-acquired infections due to gram-negative bacteria. N Engl J Med 2010;362(19):1804–13.

154. Qureshi ZA, Hittle LE, O'Hara JA, et al. Colistin-resistant Acinetobacter baumannii: beyond carbapenem resistance. Clin Infect Dis 2015;60(9):1295–303.

155. Climo MW, Yokoe DS, Warren DK, et al. Effect of daily chlorhexidine bathing on hospital-acquired infection. N Engl J Med 2013;368(6):533–42.

156. Afonso E, Blot K, Blot S. Prevention of hospital-acquired bloodstream infections through chlorhexidine gluconate-impregnated washcloth bathing in intensive care units: a systematic review and meta-analysis of randomised crossover trials. Euro Surveill 2016;21(46):30400.

157. Patel A, Parikh P, Dunn AN, et al. Effectiveness of daily chlorhexidine bathing for reducing gram-negative infections: a meta-analysis. Infect Control Hosp Epidemiol 2019;40(4):392–9.

158. Bilinski J, Grzesiowski P, Muszynski J, et al. Fecal microbiota transplantation inhibits multidrug-resistant gut pathogens: preliminary report performed in an immunocompromised host. Arch Immunol Ther Exp (Warsz) 2016;64(3):255–8.

159. Steed DB, Wang T, Raheja D, et al. Gram-negative taxa and antimicrobial susceptibility after fecal microbiota transplantation for recurrent clostridioides difficile infection. mSphere 2020;5(5):e00853.

160. DeFilipp Z, Bloom PP, Torres Soto M, et al. Drug-Resistant E. coli bacteremia transmitted by fecal microbiota transplant. N Engl J Med 2019;381(21):2043–50.

161. Mody L, Washer L, Flanders S. Can infection prevention programs in hospitals and nursing facilities be integrated?: from silos to partners. JAMA 2018; 319(11):1089–90.

162. Feldman N, Adler A, Molshatzki N, et al. Gastrointestinal colonization by KPC-producing Klebsiella pneumoniae following hospital discharge: duration of carriage and risk factors for persistent carriage. Clin Microbiol Infect 2013;19(4): E190–6.

163. Harris AD, Perencevich EN, Johnson JK, et al. Patient-to-patient transmission is important in extended-spectrum beta-lactamase-producing Klebsiella pneumoniae acquisition. Clin Infect Dis 2007;45(10):1347–50.

164. Schechner V, Kotlovsky T, Kazma M, et al. Asymptomatic rectal carriage of blaKPC producing carbapenem-resistant Enterobacteriaceae: who is prone to become clinically infected? Clin Microbiol Infect 2013;19(5):451–6.

165. Borer A, Saidel-Odes L, Eskira S, et al. Risk factors for developing clinical infection with carbapenem-resistant Klebsiella pneumoniae in hospital patients initially only colonized with carbapenem-resistant K pneumoniae. Am J Infect Control 2012;40(5):421–5.

166. Jung JY, Park MS, Kim SE, et al. Risk factors for multi-drug resistant Acinetobacter baumannii bacteremia in patients with colonization in the intensive care unit. BMC Infect Dis 2010;10:228.

167. Thuong M, Arvaniti K, Ruimy R, et al. Epidemiology of Pseudomonas aeruginosa and risk factors for carriage acquisition in an intensive care unit. J Hosp Infect 2003;53(4):274–82.

Prevention of Infection due to *Clostridium* (*Clostridioides*) *difficile*

Amar Krishna, MD[a],*, Teena Chopra, MD, MPH[b]

KEYWORDS

- *Clostridium* (*Clostridioides*) *difficile* • Prevention • Hand hygiene
- Contact precautions • Environmental decontamination • Antibiotic stewardship
- Infection control • Diagnostic stewardship

KEY POINTS

- Preventing *Clostridium* (*Clostridioides*) *difficile* infection is difficult and typically requires a multifaceted bundled approach.
- Prevention strategies fall into two broad categories: infection control and prevention and risk factor reduction.
- Hand hygiene, contact precautions, patient isolation, and environmental decontamination are cornerstones of infection control and prevention. Supplemental strategies include no-touch disinfection technology and detection and isolation of asymptomatic carriers.
- Risk factor reduction should focus on antibiotic stewardship to reduce unnecessary antibiotic use.
- Facilities with significant amount of inappropriate *C. difficile* testing should consider implementing diagnostic stewardship programs to address this issue.

INTRODUCTION

Clostridium (*Clostridioides*) *difficile* is a spore-forming, anaerobic, gram-positive bacillus. It accounts for 10%-20% of episodes of antibiotic-associated diarrhea and the most cases of antibiotic-associated colitis.[1] The Centers for Disease Control and Prevention categorizes *Clostridium difficile* as an urgent threat responsible for significant morbidity and mortality in the United States every year.[2] Prevention of *C difficile* infection (CDI) is especially difficult because of the durability of the spores and requires implementation of multipronged strategies. Useful methods to prevent *C difficile* spread include increased hand hygiene, use of contact precautions, and

[a] Internal Medicine, Norther Light AR Gould Hospital, 140 Academy Street, Presque Isle, ME 04769, USA; [b] Infectious Diseases, Wayne State University/Detroit Medical Center, UHC-2B, 4201 St Antoine, Detroit, MI 48201, USA
* Corresponding author.
E-mail address: akrishna@emhs.org

Infect Dis Clin N Am 35 (2021) 995–1011
https://doi.org/10.1016/j.idc.2021.07.009
0891-5520/21/© 2021 Elsevier Inc. All rights reserved.
id.theclinics.com

environmental decontamination. In addition, a focus on effective antibiotic steward-ship can significantly decrease the burden of disease. The focus of this article is on preventative strategies to reduce CDI frequency.

PATHOGENESIS

C.difficile causes a spectrum of disease with symptoms ranging from diarrhea to toxic megacolon and death. Acquisition occurs through spore ingestion. The pathogenesis centers on the disruption of the indigenous intestinal microbiome. The most common cause of this is systemic antibiotic administration. In individuals with an intact gut microbiome, the spores are unable to find an ecological niche. However, in people with a disrupted gut microbiome, ingested spores are able to germinate and multiply.[3] After germination, the bacterium begins secreting a pair of exotoxins, toxin A and toxin B, which disrupts the cytoskeleton of colonic mucosal epithelium and ultimately leads to a disease state.[4]

The spore represents a reservoir for the organism. Spores are able to resist extreme environmental conditions and are capable of persisting for months in the environ-ment.[5,6] *C difficile* spores are difficult to remove from environmental surfaces and from health care worker hands via routine infection control measures. People with CDI shed spores onto their skin and into the environment. Following successful treat-ment of an episode of symptomatic CDI, people may become asymptomatic carriers of *C difficile*. These individuals continue to shed *C difficile* spores into the environment and can serve as a source of dissemination of spores to others.[7,8]

EPIDEMIOLOGY

CDI has developed into an enormous burden on society. In 2017, *C difficile* was responsible for 365,200 infections and 20,000 deaths.[9] Community-associated CDI constituted about 50% of the cases in 2017. Even though the incidence of health care–associated CDI decreased in 2017 compared with 2011, the burden of community-associated infections remained unchanged.[9] About 18% of patients with community-acquired CDI have no recent outpatient health care exposures.[10] These patients could be acquiring *C difficile* from household exposures or contact with domestic and farm animals.[11,12] CDI imposes major costs on hospital systems, insurance providers, and society as a whole. In the United States, the estimated attrib-utable cost was $11,285 per case, and the total annual economic costs in 2014 were approximately 5.4 billion US dollars.[13,14]

The discovery of strain North American pulsed-field type 1, restriction endonuclease analysis group BI, and PCR ribotype 027 (BI/NAP1/027) occurred in Pittsburgh, during the year 2000. Reports of outbreaks in Canada and other regions of the United States soon followed. Outbreaks due to BI/NAP1/O27 strain were also noted in the United Kingdom and other European countries.[15] This strain exhibits enhanced toxin produc-tion and fluoroquinolone resistance. Importantly, infection due to this strain is associ-ated with more severe disease and increased mortality.[15] Lately from 2011 through 2017, infections due to this strain decreased significantly in the United States which has been attributed to widespread decrease in fluoroquinolone use.[9]

The principal risk factor is antibiotic exposure, both the number of antibiotics and duration of therapy increase the CDI risk; however, symptoms have developed even after exposure to a single antibiotic dose.[16,17] The risk seems to persist for as long as 3 months after antibiotic discontinuation.[18] Recent exposure to inpatient or outpa-tient health care setting also increases CDI risk.[10,18] Among patients who develop CDI during hospitalization, the risk increases with increasing duration of hospital stay.[16]

Other factors also increase the risk of infection, including advanced age, gastric acid suppression, chemotherapy, and chronic disease states.[16,18]

PREVENTION

As stated earlier, CDI prevention generally requires several different interventions. These strategies fall into the broad categories of infection control and prevention as well as risk factor reduction.

INFECTION CONTROL AND PREVENTION

Disease transmission occurs through ingestion of *C difficile* spores, which are the organism's dormant form. The degree of *C difficile* colonization increases at a steady rate and approaches 50% after a month of hospitalization.[19] Colonization can occur either by exposure to a contaminated environment or through contact with health care workers.[7] Infection control and prevention practices seek to reduce transmission of spores to uncolonized individuals. This strategy uses a combination of contact precautions, environmental disinfection, and hand decontamination. Newer approaches include no-touch disinfection technology and detection and isolation of asymptomatic carriers.

Hand Hygiene

Hand hygiene, a fundamental component of infection control, is the most important aspect of preventing *C difficile* transmission. Contamination of a health care worker's hands with *C difficile* occurs regularly when caring for a person with CDI, with rates of contamination of up to 59%.[7,20] In fact, touching the patient is not even required; hand contamination can happen just as often after touching "high-touch" surfaces in the room.[20] Unfortunately, adherence to routine hand hygiene by health care personnel is poor in many settings.[21]

In recent years, use of alcohol-based hand rubs (ABHRs) has gained popularity. Hand hygiene rates are higher with the use of ABHRs.[22] Implementing ABHR decreases the frequencies of both methicillin-resistant *Staphylococcus aureus* (MRSA) and vancomycin-resistant Enterococcus (VRE) infections in the hospital.[23] However, *C difficile* spores are extremely resistant to destruction by alcohol. In fact, the ethanol shock method is used in laboratories to assist in isolating *C difficile* from stool samples.[24] Consequently, health care workers who use ABHRs to decontaminate their hands may simply be moving spores around the skin and not inactivating them.

Conversely, it is hypothesized that using soap and water physically removes the spores from the skin. Several laboratory studies have compared various forms of hand hygiene. Washing with soap and water was superior to ABHRs for spore removal. Soap and water use may lead to a greater than 90% decrease in spore contamination; however, alcohol-based interventions do not reduce the amount of spore contamination.[25] Other studies have analyzed the benefit of chlorhexidine with mixed results. One study found that the efficacy of chlorhexidine antiseptic exceeded plain soap at removing *C difficile*.[7] However, other studies failed to show any benefit to chlorhexidine washes over plain soap.[25]

Consequently, there is a hypothetical risk that widespread implementation of ABHRs could increase CDI incidence. However, no clinical studies have demonstrated this. In an observational study conducted at Veterans Administration Hospital, the CDI rate remained unchanged after implementation of ABHRs. However, there was a 21% reduction in health care–acquired MRSA and a 41% reduction in VRE.[23] Another study analyzed the association between hospital procurement rates of soap and ABHRs with rates of nosocomial infection.[26] They found that increased hospital ordering of soap was independently associated with decreased CDI. Conversely, there was an independent correlation between obtaining elevated quantities of ABHR and decreased MRSA bacteremia.

Based on this evidence, the current Society for Healthcare Epidemiology of America (SHEA)–Infectious Diseases Society of America (IDSA) guidelines recommend, "During outbreaks or in settings with hyperendemic CDI, it is recommended to preferentially use soap and water over alcohol-based products alone before and after providing care for a patient with CDI."[27] In addition, handwashing with soap and water is preferred if there is direct contact with feces or an area where fecal contamination is likely. However, in routine or endemic CDI settings, one can use either soap and water or alcohol-based hand hygiene products along with glove use.

Contact Precautions

Another important aspect to preventing horizontal transfer of spores is instituting isolation procedures. Isolation procedures include contact precautions, individual rooms, and dedicated patient equipment.

Contact precautions refer to the donning of gowns and gloves on room entry and removal before exiting the room.[27] The use of these methods centers on the idea that individuals with active CDI are the main source of disease dissemination. *C difficile* spores frequently contaminate a health care worker's hands, during the routine care of individuals with CDI.[7,20] Recommended hand hygiene practices (noted earlier) must be included as part of contact precautions, and hand hygiene should be practiced before donning gloves and after they are removed. The routine use of gloves may help reduce hand contamination and subsequent transmission to other patients. One prospective study analyzed use of vinyl gloves to interrupt transmission. The interventions included reminder signs and making gloves available in every patient's room. This intervention resulted in a drop in the CDI cases from 7.7 to 1.5 per 1000 patient discharges. The asymptomatic carriage rate also decreased during this intervention.[28] Gown use is also recommended due to potential soiling of health care worker clothing. Nurses' clothes have been documented to become contaminated with *C difficile* during routine clinical duties. However, a study demonstrating this did not specifically assess if the contamination was linked to patient acquisitions or transmissions.[29] Importantly, in a randomized controlled trial of intensive care patients, adverse events including preventable noninfectious events were not increased for patients on contact precautions compared with patients without contact precautions.[30]

Current guidelines recommend continuing contact precautions until 48 hours after diarrhea resolution. However, in situations where the spread of CDI is difficult to control, special contact precautions may need to be implemented, including empiric placement of patients with diarrhea in contact precautions while waiting for the results of *C difficile* testing and continuing precautions of patients with CDI until the time of discharge.[27]

Contamination of a patient's skin and environmental contamination usually occurs before diagnostic tests for *C difficile* are even ordered.[8,31] Therefore, test ordering should occur as soon as there is a suspicion of CDI, and the patient should be placed on contact precautions. This practice allows people to be isolated while results are pending, and once the result finalizes, management can be adjusted appropriately. Unfortunately, a delay in diagnosis of several days frequently occurs. This delay is often attributable to lack of prompt stool sample collection. In addition, using off-site laboratories may further contribute to a delay.[31]

Furthermore, environmental contamination with *C difficile* continues to occur at the time of diarrhea resolution and at the end of treatment, with frequencies of 37% and 14%, respectively. Moreover, 1 to 4 weeks after treatment is completed, rates of *C difficile* colonization are often high, with asymptomatic carriage occurring in 56% of patients and environmental contamination in 50% of rooms in one study.[8] As a result, in the acute care setting, extended contact procedures have a role in preventing spore transmission.

In addition, patients experiencing CDI should have a private room with dedicated toileting facilities to limit interaction with other susceptible individuals. Colonization is more likely among patients exposed to a roommate with *C difficile*.[7] *C difficile* has been discovered on surfaces throughout the room of patients with CDI, including toilets, commodes, privacy curtains, call buttons, bedside tables, and floors.[6,7,20] One intensive care unit compared their rates of *C difficile* acquisition before and after converting their rooms from multibed to single bed. The transmission rate of CDI decreased by 43%.[32] Unfortunately, not all institutions have the ability to support single isolation rooms. If a single room is not available, then cohorting with other infected patients is considered acceptable.[27] Nevertheless, cohorted patients should have dedicated bedside commodes.[6,27] Notably, one institution demonstrated that admission to a *C difficile* cohort ward was independently associated with CDI recurrence.[33]

Furthermore, single-use medical device utilization should be implemented whenever feasible for patients with CDI. If disposable equipment is not available, then the patients should have dedicated equipment left in their rooms. It is also important to ensure proper disinfection of all reusable equipment between patients.[27] CDI spread has been associated with both contaminated electronic rectal thermometers and blood pressure cuffs.[34–36] *C difficile* spores can contaminate electronic thermometer handles. Spore transfer to the disposable probe cover may occur during routine use.[34] In a randomized trial, the CDI rate was lower with single-use disposable thermometers compared with electronic thermometers (relative risk: 0.44%; $P = .026$).[35] Stethoscopes are another possible transmission vector. *C difficile* spore acquisition and transfer by stethoscopes were found to occur as readily as with gloved hands during simulated physical examinations.[37]

An often overlooked facet of infection control is care transitions. It is critical that hospitals and long-term care facilities effectively communicate because patients continue to shed spores for a prolonged duration.[8] Effective handoffs allow the receiving facility to properly prepare and implement precautions, such as isolation procedures.[38] Regrettably, care transitions are often poorly coordinated. Inadequate communication is a major barrier to implementing appropriate prevention procedures.[38]

Environmental Decontamination

Adequate environmental cleaning practices aid in CDI prevention efforts. *C difficile* is regularly recovered throughout an infected patient's rooms.[20] The amount of environmental shedding correlates with the degree of a patient's symptoms.[7,8] Assignment to a room where the previous occupant had CDI predisposes the new occupant to developing CDI. A study showed that CDI was 2.35 times more likely if the room's previous occupant had CDI, even after controlling for age, disease severity, proton pump inhibitor (PPI) use, and antibiotic administration.[39]

Problematically, the spores are incredibly resilient, which makes decontamination extremely challenging. Environmental persistence has been demonstrated for 5 months following intentional inoculation of the floor of a hospital room.[6] Spores are resistant to heat (>80°C), acid (pH <2), and a variety of disinfectants, including the quaternary ammonium compounds typically used in health care environments.[5,40,41]

Chlorine-containing products have been demonstrated to inactivate the spores in vitro.[40] Studies conducted in CDI outbreaks or hyperendemic settings support the use of hypochlorite-based solutions.[42,43] In one study, CDI outbreaks in 2 intensive care units ended when environmental disinfection with hypochlorite solution was instituted. In one unit, hypochlorite disinfection was used in all patient rooms, whereas in the other unit, it was used only in rooms of patients with CDI. Both strategies were successful in reducing CDI rates.[42] In another study, a hospital switched their standard disinfectant to clean rooms of patients with CDI from a quaternary ammonium disinfectant to a 1:10 hypochlorite solution in an attempt to lower their CDI rate.[43] The bone marrow transplant unit experienced a decrease in their CDI rate from 8.6 cases/1000 patient days to 3.3 cases/1000 patient days. In addition, there was a rebound to 8.1 cases/1000 patient days after changing back to a quaternary ammonium solution. Conversely, despite using a hypochlorite-based disinfectant, there was no CDI reduction in 2 other units where the baseline CDI rate was lower.[43] This indicates that when baseline CDI rates are low, environmental contamination is not as great a risk for CDI transmission. Therefore, current guidelines from SHEA and IDSA recommend using sporicidal agents during CDI outbreaks, when CDI rates are hyperendemic and when there is evidence of repeated cases of CDI in the same patient room.[27] Despite these recommendations, use of sporicidal disinfectant to clean CDI rooms might be a common practice in US hospitals even in the absence of an outbreak or hyperendemic CDI.[44,45] Hypochlorite-containing agents also have disadvantages that limit routine use. They are corrosive to metals, have a strong odor, and may be irritating to the skin and respiratory tract.[43,46]

Another obstacle to *C difficile* prevention is that cleaning by environmental service workers is frequently inadequate, and there is often substantial variation in cleaning practices between individual environmental service workers.[47–49] A survey of environmental service workers identified several barriers to effective room cleaning, including lack of time, insufficient supplies, lack of notification when rooms needed to be cleaned, and lack of training. Only 15% of workers identified that bleach is necessary to kill *C difficile*.[50] Therefore, several studies have used interventions aimed at environmental service workers to improve cleaning/disinfection practice.[47,49,51] These interventions have included education, monitoring the thoroughness of cleaning with feedback of performance, and use of cleaning checklists and have resulted in improvement of cleaning practice and reduction of environmental contamination including due to *C difficile*.[47,49,51] Several organizations currently recommend monitoring of cleaning practice.[27] Monitoring by visual inspection is not reliable.[52] Using fluorescent markers or adenosine triphosphate (ATP) bioluminescent assays provides a more objective measure of cleaning practice. Fluorescent marker and ATP bioluminescent application should occur before cleaning, and after cleaning, it should be assessed whether it was removed during cleaning.

Despite improvement in cleaning/disinfection practices with the use of fluorescent markers and ATP bioluminescent assays, studies assessing the impact on reduction in CDI incidence have been contradictory. A multicenter randomized control trial compared standard cleaning with enhanced cleaning which involved monitoring of thoroughness of cleaning based on fluorescent marker removal from high-touch surfaces coupled with feedback on performance to environmental service workers in rooms of patients with and without CDI.[53] Environmental cultures for *C difficile* were also used to evaluate the effectiveness of disinfection. Despite increased marker removal and decreased recovery of *C difficile* from the environment, this did not translate to lower incidence of health care–associated CDI during the intervention or postintervention periods. On the contrary, a quasi-experimental study demonstrated that implementation of an audit and feedback program using fluorescent marking resulted in improved thoroughness of room cleaning and appeared to result in downward trend in CDI incidence.[54]

Formation of dedicated housekeeping teams can markedly improve cleaning/disinfection of rooms in addition to reducing CDI incidence. One study noted that use of fluorescent markers for monitoring and feedback regarding cleaning thoroughness only decreased the rate of positive cultures from CDI rooms from 67% to 57%.[49] However, after implementing daily cleaning by a dedicated disinfection team and requiring supervisor evaluation of rooms at time of discharge through direct observation and/or ATP bioluminescence, the rate of positive CDI room cultures decreased to 7%. This study also noted reduced incidence of health care–associated CDI during the period when cleaning was performed by a dedicated disinfection team and a standardized process was used to clear CDI rooms.[49]

No-Touch Disinfection Technologies

Several studies have noted that environmental cleaning and disinfection of patient rooms is suboptimal.[47,49] Although interventions aimed at environmental service workers can improve cleaning practices, it is unclear if high rates of cleaning can be sustained in the long term.[47,51,55] As a result, there is growing interest in using no-touch disinfection technologies to supplement environmental cleaning. These technologies use either ultraviolet-C (UV-C) light or hydrogen peroxide. Studies indicate these methods can effectively reduce surface microbial contamination including contamination with C difficile.[56,57]

A cluster randomized study at 9 hospitals by Anderson and colleagues[58] showed that enhanced terminal disinfection with UV-C and quaternary ammonium disinfectant of rooms from which a patient colonized/infected with MRSA, VRE, C difficile, and multidrug-resistant Acinetobacter (target organisms) was discharged resulted in decreased incidence of infection/colonization with target organisms in patients subsequently admitted to these rooms. The other two enhanced disinfection methods (bleach only and bleach + UV-C) did not result in decreased incidence when compared with standard cleaning with quaternary ammonium. Terminal disinfection of rooms of discharged patients infected/colonized with C difficile was conducted with one of two disinfection methods (bleach only or bleach + UV-C). When the incidence of C difficile was individually evaluated, no significant difference was noted with or without UV-C. However, a secondary analysis of this study noted a significant decrease in hospital-wide incidence of C difficile in the UV-C and quaternary ammonium disinfectant group.[59] Similarly, a systematic review and meta-analysis by Marra and colleagues[60] which included 13 studies including the aforementioned cluster randomized trial showed that UV-C disinfection can decrease CDI especially in hospitals with high baseline CDI rates. This review also analyzed studies using hydrogen peroxide for environmental disinfection. Meta-analysis of the 5 studies showed nonsignificant reduction in CDI rates with hydrogen peroxide technology.

If using no-touch disinfection technology, rooms should still be cleaned of dust and debris before using the no-touch technology. Both these technologies have substantial capital equipment costs and can be used most practically for terminal disinfection due to the need to remove patients and personnel from the room before their use. Sporicidal efficacy of UV-C decreases in areas that are outside of the direct line of light from the device.[56,60] Although hydrogen peroxide systems show improved sporicidal activity compared with UV-C, they require longer decontamination time. In addition, hydrogen peroxide decontamination requires the heating, ventilation, and air conditioning system to be disabled and the doors and windows be sealed.[55] Therefore, facilities planning to use these technologies should consider these issues in addition to determining which rooms should be disinfected (eg, all patient rooms vs contact precaution rooms only).

Detection and Isolation of Asymptomatic Carriers

Studies using molecular techniques (including whole genome sequencing) indicate that symptomatic patients with CDI contribute to only about one-third of C difficile transmission in the health care setting.[61,62] Other CDI cases might be transmitted by asymptomatic carriers. With regards to transmission by asymptomatic carriers, a genotyping study using multilocus variable number of tandem repeats analysis showed that carriers identified by screening were identified as the sources of 29% of hospital-associated CDI cases.[62] Furthermore, patients colonized with toxigenic C difficile at admission had an almost 6 times higher risk of developing CDI compared with non-colonized patients.[63] Based on these findings, admission screening to identify C difficile carriers has been proposed by some as a measure to prevent nosocomial CDI.

A single center quasi-experimental study by Longtin and colleagues[64] reported a significant decrease (3 per 10,000 patient days vs 6.9 per 10,000 patient days preintervention, P <.001) in incidence of health care–associated CDI with universal admission screening for C difficile coupled with modified contact precautions (glove use only) for carriers. No decrease in CDI incidence was noted in a group of comparator local hospitals over the same time period. Some of the limitations of this study include that it was conducted in a single center and that the study did not assess compliance with contact precautions, effect of environmental cleaning, and knowledge of carrier status on patient management. Another study conducted in an outbreak setting noted decrease in CDI rates with ward-based admission screening for C difficile followed by isolation of carriers.[65] Despite these studies noting benefit of screening and isolation, more evidence from similar or more rigorous trials performed in multiple centers are needed before this costly and resource-intensive intervention can be widely adopted.

RISK FACTOR REDUCTION

Some CDI risk factors, such as advanced age and comorbid conditions, are not modifiable. Reducing unnecessary antibiotic exposure, through antimicrobial stewardship, and avoiding unnecessary gastric acid suppression are both modifiable risk factors that can help protect patients from becoming infected with C difficile. Likewise, probiotic administration may be a potentially beneficial strategy. Finally, vaccines against C difficile are currently in development.

Antibiotic Stewardship

The greatest risk factor for CDI acquisition is prior antibiotic exposure. CDI development has been linked with nearly all antibiotics, although the risk varies significantly between different antimicrobial classes.[16,18] Administration of fluoroquinolones is a key risk factor influencing the spread of the hypervirulent strain BI/NAP1/027.[15] Other high-risk antibiotics include cephalosporins, carbapenems, and clindamycin.[18,66]

Restricting high-risk antibiotics controls CDI effectively in outbreak settings. For example, during the B1/NAP1/O27 outbreak, a hospital in Quebec, Canada, was successfully able to control CDI with a nonrestrictive antibiotic stewardship program involving guideline dissemination and reinforcement of guidelines through pharmacist telephone feedback to physicians.[67] Use of targeted antibiotics (second- and third-generation cephalosporins, ciprofloxacin, clindamycin, and macrolides) decreased by 54% followed by decrease in CDI incidence by 60%. Numerous other studies have demonstrated decreases in CDI incidence by reducing use of multiple antibiotic classes, including cephalosporins, clindamycin, and fluoroquinolones.[66–68] An academic tertiary care hospital was able to demonstrate that implementation of a strong antibiotic stewardship program could result in sustained benefits. They examined their institution over a 13-year period and found a 62.8% reduction in antibiotic use. This reduction resulted in decreasing CDI, MRSA infection, and quinolone-resistant *Pseudomonas aeruginosa* rates by 43%, 57%, and 72%, respectively.[69] A 2014 systematic review and meta-analysis of 16 quasi-experimental studies conducted in nonoutbreak settings also concluded that antibiotic stewardship programs had a significant protective effect on CDI incidence (pooled risk ratio: 0.48; 95% confidence interval: 0.38–0.62).[70] Restrictive policies were found to be more effective than persuasive policies. A more recent systematic review and meta-analysis also noted a 32% decrease in CDI incidence associated with antibiotic stewardship interventions.[71] In conclusion, efforts to reduce unnecessary antibiotic prescribing and decreased use of high-risk medications can have a substantial impact on *C difficile* prevention. A reduction of antibiotic use is achievable by implementation of effective antibiotic stewardship interventions.

Avoiding Gastric Acid Suppression

Two different meta-analyses have noted an association between PPI/histamine type 2 receptor antagonist use and increased risk of CDI.[45,72] In 2012, the US Food and Drug Administration published a safety notification that the likelihood of CDI increases after PPI administration. The report found an elevation in CDI risk by 1.4- to 2.75-fold in people using PPIs.[73] Despite this, a causal relationship between gastric acid suppression and CDI is unclear. Regardless, stewardship activities to limit unnecessary use are warranted.

Probiotics

Probiotics are live microorganisms that when administered can reach the intestines in sufficient numbers to confer health benefit to the host. Probiotics are thought to provide this benefit by several mechanisms including direct effects on the intestinal epithelium, altering the microbiota composition, competition with other microorganisms for nutrients and binding sites, and enhancement of mucosal immunity.[74] Systematic reviews of randomized trials have noted potential efficacy of probiotics for primary prevention of CDI.[75,76] A Cochrane review of 31 randomized controlled trials noted that use of probiotics reduced the risk of CDI by 60% in patients taking antibiotics, and the evidence supporting this finding was categorized to be of moderate certainty.[75] The risk of CDI was reduced regardless of the dose of probiotics used, whether they were administered in the inpatient versus outpatient setting, whether adults versus children were studied, and the type of probiotic used. However, it is to be noted that the largest trial (2941 patients) in the Cochrane review failed to show a significant benefit of a high dose preparation of *Lactobacilli* and *Bifidobacterium* in CDI prevention.[77] The baseline risk of CDI in the control group in this study was 1.2%. When the authors of the review conducted a subgroup analysis, studies with baseline CDI risk of 0% to 2% showed a nonsignificant CDI reduction of 23% (relative risk: 0.77, 95% CI: 0.45–1.32; $P = .34$), whereas studies with high baseline risk (>5%) demonstrated a significant risk reduction of 70% (RR: 0.30, 95% CI: 0.21–0.42; $P = .01$).[75] As the CDI risk in most health care settings is lower than 5%, the benefit of probiotics in this patient population is less clear. In addition, uncertainty exists with regards to the efficacy of various probiotic formulations and the duration of probiotic use. Owing to this, most major societies including SHEA and IDSA do not endorse routine use of probiotics for primary CDI prevention.[27] It is important to note that there is no role for probiotics in the management of acute CDI, and in fact, using probiotics in this setting can be harmful.[78,79]

Vaccination

An area of active research is *C difficile* vaccine development. Previous evidence demonstrated a function of naturally occurring toxin A antibodies in prevention of acute diarrhea and recurrence of CDI.[80,81] Higher concentration of antibodies to toxin B also correlate with protection from recurrent CDI, which is further strengthened by the fact that bezlotoxumab, a monoclonal antibody against toxin B, decreases rates of recurrent CDI.[82,83] These data suggest that active immunization with toxoid vaccines could be beneficial in disease prevention. Even though parenteral toxoid vaccines have been found to be immunogenic in phase 1/2 trials, one of the vaccines in phase 3 trial was withdrawn as data showed it failed to protect from CDI.[84–86] Results from another phase 3 trial of a toxoid vaccine in adults aged 50 years and older who are at risk of CDI are awaited (NCT03090191). Other studies have evaluated nonparenteral modes of vaccine delivery (such as oral and rectal) or nontoxin antigenic targets for vaccine development, but these are still in early stages of development.[87,88]

Diagnostic Stewardship

A significant proportion of hospitalized patients can be colonized with toxigenic *C difficile*.[6,7,63] Distinguishing *C difficile* colonization from infection can be a diagnostic challenge. Studies indicate that only about 60% of patients tested for *C difficile* have clinically significant diarrhea ($\geq$3 unformed stools in 24 hours).[89] In addition, about 19% of patients tested for *C difficile* had received laxatives in the past 48 hours.[89] Testing in patients who do not meet clinical criteria, especially with sensitive molecular assays, often leads to detection of asymptomatic carriers and falsely inflates a hospital's CDI rate and leads to unnecessary treatment. A study by Kelly and colleagues[90] noted that 15% of hospital-onset CDI cases were due to inappropriate testing and not representative of actual infection. In addition, a prospective cohort study indicated that up to 50% of hospitalized patients with a positive molecular test may not need treatment.[91]

Diagnostic stewardship aims to encourage rationale use of *C difficile* testing, improving the diagnosis of true CDI and reducing inappropriate testing and false-positive results.[92] Stewardship interventions have targeted various types of inappropriate testing including testing in the absence of clinically significant diarrhea, ordering repeat tests or tests of cure, testing formed stools, and testing in patients receiving laxatives.[93–95] Studies have also used various strategies to improve testing as part of diagnostic stewardship including provider education, use of computerized clinical decision support, real-time electronic tracking, and feedback and prior approval among others.[93–96] These interventions have resulted in a decrease in overall and inappropriate testing, and some have also noted decrease in hospital-onset CDI rates.[93–95] Despite the success of diagnostic stewardship interventions, concerns have been raised about adverse consequences related to underdiagnosis and delayed diagnosis of true CDI. Two studies noted that clinical outcomes were not significantly different between patients with tests that were determined to be inappropriate and were not ordered compared with patients with negative *C difficile* tests.[93,97] On the contrary, a study noted similar outcomes and illness severity among two groups of patients with CDI: those with and those without laxative use in the 48 hours before CDI diagnosis.[98] This latter observation indicates that the entire clinical picture needs to be considered when deciding to order *C difficile* testing and that the possibility of a CDI diagnosis cannot be discounted just because a patient is receiving laxatives.

SUMMARY

C.difficile remains a significant problem in the health care setting. Successful prevention efforts typically require a multifaceted bundled approach. A combination of hand hygiene, contact precautions, environmental decontamination, and antibiotic stewardship can result in significant reductions in CDI incidence. If CDI incidence remains higher than an institution's goal despite these measures, then CDI risk assessment should be performed. Based on the risk assessment findings, special approaches such as extended contact precautions, sporicidal disinfection (if not already instituted), no-touch disinfection technologies, and diagnostic stewardship can be considered.

CLINICS CARE POINTS

- Perform hand hygiene with soap and water instead of alcohol-based hand rub if hands are visibly soiled, during outbreaks or in setting of hyperendemic *C. difficile* infection (CDI).
- Contact precautions should be continued until 48 hours after diarrhea resolution. Start empiric contact precautions while waiting test results and continue contact precautions until discharge if facility CDI rates remain high.
- Use sporicidal agents for environmental decontamination during CDI outbreaks, hyperendemic CDI or when there is evidence of repeated cases of CDI in the same patient room.
- Before using no touch disinfection technology (Ultraviolet-C light or hydrogen peroxide systems), rooms should be cleaned of dirt and debris to increase their effectiveness.
- During CDI outbreak or hyperendemic settings, consider a restrictive policy to reduce use of high-risk antibiotics known to predispose to CDI.

DISCLOSURE

The authors have nothing to disclose.

REFERENCES

1. Bartlett JG. Clinical practice. Antibiotic-associated diarrhea. N Engl J Med 2002; 346(5):334–9.
2. Centers for Disease Control and Prevention. Antibiotic/Antimicrobial Resistance. 2019. Available at: https://www.cdc.gov/drugresistance/biggest-threats.html? CDC_AA_refVal=https%3A%2F%2Fwww.cdc.gov%2Fdrugresistance%2Fbiggest_threats.html. Accessed April 30, 2021.
3. Britton RA, Young VB. Interaction between the intestinal microbiota and host in Clostridium difficile colonization resistance. Trends Microbiol 2012;20(7):313–9.
4. Kuehne SA, Cartman ST, Minton NP. Both, toxin A and toxin B, are important in Clostridium difficile infection. Gut Microbes 2011;2(4):252–5.
5. Rao A, Jump RL, Pultz NJ, et al. In vitro killing of nosocomial pathogens by acid and acidified nitrite. Antimicrob Agents Chemother 2006;50(11):3901–4.

6. Kim KH, Fekety R, Batts DH, et al. Isolation of Clostridium difficile from the environment and contacts of patients with antibiotic-associated colitis. J Infect Dis 1981;143(1):42–50.

7. McFarland LV, Mulligan ME, Kwok RY, et al. Nosocomial acquisition of Clostridium difficile infection. N Engl J Med 1989;320(4):204–10.

8. Sethi AK, Al-Nassir WN, Nerandzic MM, et al. Persistence of skin contamination and environmental shedding of Clostridium difficile during and after treatment of C. difficile infection. Infect Control Hosp Epidemiol 2010;31(1):21–7.

9. Guh AY, Mu Y, Winston LG, et al. Trends in U.S. Burden of Clostridioides difficile Infection and Outcomes. N Engl J Med 2020;382(14):1320–30.

10. Chitnis AS, Holzbauer SM, Belflower RM, et al. Epidemiology of community-associated Clostridium difficile infection, 2009 through 2011. JAMA Intern Med 2013;173(14):1359–67.

11. Loo VG, Brassard P, Miller MA. Household Transmission of Clostridium difficile to Family Members and Domestic Pets. Infect Control Hosp Epidemiol 2016;37(11): 1342–8.

12. Knetsch CW, Connor TR, Mutreja A, et al. Whole genome sequencing reveals potential spread of Clostridium difficile between humans and farm animals in the Netherlands, 2002 to 2011. Euro Surveill 2014;19(45):20954.

13. McGlone SM, Bailey RR, Zimmer SM, et al. The economic burden of Clostridium difficile. Clin Microbiol Infect 2012;18(3):282–9.

14. Desai K, Gupta SB, Dubberke ER, et al. Epidemiological and economic burden of Clostridium difficile in the United States: estimates from a modeling approach. BMC Infect Dis 2016;16:303.

15. O'Connor JR, Johnson S, Gerding DN. Clostridium difficile infection caused by the epidemic BI/NAP1/027 strain. Gastroenterology 2009;136(6):1913–24.

16. Stevens V, Dumyati G, Fine LS, et al. Cumulative antibiotic exposures over time and the risk of Clostridium difficile infection. Clin Infect Dis 2011;53(1):42–8.

17. Privitera G, Scarpellini P, Ortisi G, et al. Prospective study of Clostridium difficile intestinal colonization and disease following single-dose antibiotic prophylaxis in surgery. Antimicrob Agents Chemother 1991;35(1):208–10.

18. Hensgens MP, Goorhuis A, Dekkers OM, et al. Time interval of increased risk for Clostridium difficile infection after exposure to antibiotics. J Antimicrob Chemother 2012;67(3):742–8.

19. Clabots CR, Johnson S, Olson MM, et al. Acquisition of Clostridium difficile by hospitalized patients: evidence for colonized new admissions as a source of infection. J Infect Dis 1992;166(3):561–7.

20. Guerrero DM, Nerandzic MM, Jury LA, et al. Acquisition of spores on gloved hands after contact with the skin of patients with Clostridium difficile infection and with environmental surfaces in their rooms. Am J Infect Control 2012;40(6): 556–8.

21. Pittet D, Mourouga P, Perneger TV. Compliance with handwashing in a teaching hospital. Infection Control Program. Ann Intern Med 1999;130(2):126–30.

22. Boyce JM. Using alcohol for hand antisepsis: dispelling old myths. Infect Control Hosp Epidemiol 2000;21(7):438–41.

23. Gordin FM, Schultz ME, Huber RA, et al. Reduction in nosocomial transmission of drug-resistant bacteria after introduction of an alcohol-based handrub. Infect Control Hosp Epidemiol 2005;26(7):650–3.

24. Clabots CR, Gerding SJ, Olson MM, et al. Detection of asymptomatic Clostridium difficile carriage by an alcohol shock procedure. J Clin Microbiol 1989;27(10): 2386–7.

25. Oughton MT, Loo VG, Dendukuri N, et al. Hand hygiene with soap and water is superior to alcohol rub and antiseptic wipes for removal of Clostridium difficile. Infect Control Hosp Epidemiol 2009;30(10):939–44.
26. Stone SP, Fuller C, Savage J, et al. Evaluation of the national Cleanyourhands campaign to reduce Staphylococcus aureus bacteraemia and Clostridium difficile infection in hospitals in England and Wales by improved hand hygiene: four year, prospective, ecological, interrupted time series study. BMJ 2012;344: e3005.
27. McDonald LC, Gerding DN, Johnson S, et al. Clinical Practice Guidelines for Clostridium difficile Infection in Adults and Children: 2017 Update by the Infectious Diseases Society of America (IDSA) and Society for Healthcare Epidemiology of America (SHEA). Clin Infect Dis 2018;66(7):e1–48.
28. Johnson S, Gerding DN, Olson MM, et al. Prospective, controlled study of vinyl glove use to interrupt Clostridium difficile nosocomial transmission. Am J Med 1990;88(2):137–40.
29. Perry C, Marshall R, Jones E. Bacterial contamination of uniforms. J Hosp Infect 2001;48(3):238–41.
30. Croft LD, Harris AD, Pineles L, et al. The Effect of Universal Glove and Gown Use on Adverse Events in Intensive Care Unit Patients. Clin Infect Dis 2015;61(4): 545–53.
31. Sunkesula VC, Kundrapu S, Jury LA, et al. Potential for transmission of spores by patients awaiting laboratory testing to confirm suspected Clostridium difficile infection. Infect Control Hosp Epidemiol 2013;34(3):306–8.
32. Teltsch DY, Hanley J, Loo V, et al. Infection acquisition following intensive care unit room privatization. Arch Intern Med 2011;171(1):32–8.
33. Islam J, Cheek E, Navani V, et al. Influence of cohorting patients with Clostridium difficile infection on risk of symptomatic recurrence. J Hosp Infect 2013;85(1): 17–21.
34. Brooks SE, Veal RO, Kramer M, et al. Reduction in the incidence of Clostridium difficile-associated diarrhea in an acute care hospital and a skilled nursing facility following replacement of electronic thermometers with single-use disposables. Infect Control Hosp Epidemiol 1992;13(2):98–103.
35. Jernigan JA, Siegman-Igra Y, Guerrant RC, et al. A randomized crossover study of disposable thermometers for prevention of Clostridium difficile and other nosocomial infections. Infect Control Hosp Epidemiol 1998;19(7):494–9.
36. Manian FA, Meyer L, Jenne J. Clostridium difficile contamination of blood pressure cuffs: a call for a closer look at gloving practices in the era of universal precautions. Infect Control Hosp Epidemiol 1996;17(3):180–2.
37. Vajravelu RK, Guerrero DM, Jury LA, et al. Evaluation of stethoscopes as vectors of Clostridium difficile and methicillin-resistant Staphylococcus aureus. Infect Control Hosp Epidemiol 2012;33(1):96–8.
38. Ye Z, Mukamel DB, Huang SS, et al. Healthcare-associated pathogens and nursing home policies and practices: results from a national survey. Infect Control Hosp Epidemiol 2015;36(7):759–66.
39. Shaughnessy MK, Micielli RL, DePestel DD, et al. Evaluation of hospital room assignment and acquisition of Clostridium difficile infection. Infect Control Hosp Epidemiol 2011;32(3):201–6.
40. Fawley WN, Underwood S, Freeman J, et al. Efficacy of hospital cleaning agents and germicides against epidemic Clostridium difficile strains. Infect Control Hosp Epidemiol 2007;28(8):920–5.

41. Marler LM, Siders JA, Wolters LC, et al. Comparison of five cultural procedures for isolation of Clostridium difficile from stools. J Clin Microbiol 1992;30(2):514–6.

42. McMullen KM, Zack J, Coopersmith CM, et al. Use of hypochlorite solution to decrease rates of Clostridium difficile-associated diarrhea. Infect Control Hosp Epidemiol 2007;28(2):205–7.

43. Mayfield JL, Leet T, Miller J, et al. Environmental control to reduce transmission of Clostridium difficile. Clin Infect Dis 2000;31(4):995–1000.

44. Vaughn VM, Greene MT, Ratz D, et al. Antibiotic stewardship teams and Clostridioides difficile practices in United States hospitals: A national survey in The Joint Commission antibiotic stewardship standard era. Infect Control Hosp Epidemiol 2020;41(2):143–8.

45. Janarthanan S, Ditah I, Adler DG, et al. Clostridium difficile-associated diarrhea and proton pump inhibitor therapy: a meta-analysis. Am J Gastroenterol 2012; 107(7):1001–10.

46. Rutala WA, Weber DJ. Uses of inorganic hypochlorite (bleach) in health-care facilities. Clin Microbiol Rev 1997;10(4):597–610.

47. Carling PC, Parry MM, Rupp ME, et al. Improving cleaning of the environment surrounding patients in 36 acute care hospitals. Infect Control Hosp Epidemiol 2008; 29(11):1035–41.

48. Boyce JM, Havill NL, Lipka A, et al. Variations in hospital daily cleaning practices. Infect Control Hosp Epidemiol 2010;31(1):99–101.

49. Sitzlar B, Deshpande A, Fertelli D, et al. An environmental disinfection odyssey: evaluation of sequential interventions to improve disinfection of Clostridium difficile isolation rooms. Infect Control Hosp Epidemiol 2013;34(5):459–65.

50. Jennings A, Sitzlar B, Jury L. A survey of environmental service workers' knowledge and opinions regarding environmental cleaning. Am J Infect Control 2013;41(2):177–9.

51. Carling PC, Parry MF, Bruno-Murtha LA, et al. Improving environmental hygiene in 27 intensive care units to decrease multidrug-resistant bacterial transmission. Crit Care Med 2010;38(4):1054–9.

52. Luick L, Thompson PA, Loock MH, et al. Diagnostic assessment of different environmental cleaning monitoring methods. Am J Infect Control 2013;41(8):751–2.

53. Ray AJ, Deshpande A, Fertelli D, et al. A Multicenter Randomized Trial to Determine the Effect of an Environmental Disinfection Intervention on the Incidence of Healthcare-Associated Clostridium difficile Infection. Infect Control Hosp Epidemiol 2017;38(7):777–83.

54. Smith A, Taggart LR, Lebovic G, et al. Clostridium difficile infection incidence: impact of audit and feedback programme to improve room cleaning. J Hosp Infect 2016;92(2):161–6.

55. Rutala WA, Weber DJ. Are room decontamination units needed to prevent transmission of environmental pathogens? Infect Control Hosp Epidemiol 2011;32(8): 743–7.

56. Rutala WA, Gergen MF, Weber DJ. Room decontamination with UV radiation. Infect Control Hosp Epidemiol 2010;31(10):1025–9.

57. Boyce JM, Havill NL, Otter JA, et al. Impact of hydrogen peroxide vapor room decontamination on Clostridium difficile environmental contamination and transmission in a healthcare setting. Infect Control Hosp Epidemiol 2008;29(8):723–9.

58. Anderson DJ, Chen LF, Weber DJ, et al. Enhanced terminal room disinfection and acquisition and infection caused by multidrug-resistant organisms and Clostridium difficile (the Benefits of Enhanced Terminal Room Disinfection study): a

cluster-randomised, multicentre, crossover study. Lancet 2017;389(10071): 805–14.

59. Anderson DJ, Moehring RW, Weber DJ, et al. Effectiveness of targeted enhanced terminal room disinfection on hospital-wide acquisition and infection with multidrug-resistant organisms and Clostridium difficile: a secondary analysis of a multicentre cluster randomised controlled trial with crossover design (BETR Disinfection). Lancet Infect Dis 2018;18(8):845–53.

60. Marra AR, Schweizer ML, Edmond MB. No-Touch Disinfection Methods to Decrease Multidrug-Resistant Organism Infections: A Systematic Review and Meta-analysis. Infect Control Hosp Epidemiol 2018;39(1):20–31.

61. Eyre DW, Cule ML, Wilson DJ, et al. Diverse sources of C. difficile infection identified on whole-genome sequencing. N Engl J Med 2013;369(13):1195–205.

62. Curry SR, Muto CA, Schlackman JL, et al. Use of multilocus variable number of tandem repeats analysis genotyping to determine the role of asymptomatic carriers in Clostridium difficile transmission. Clin Infect Dis 2013;57(8):1094–102.

63. Zacharioudakis IM, Zervou FN, Pliakos EE, et al. Colonization with toxinogenic C. difficile upon hospital admission, and risk of infection: a systematic review and meta-analysis. Am J Gastroenterol 2015;110(3):381–90 [quiz: 391].

64. Longtin Y, Paquet-Bolduc B, Gilca R, et al. Effect of Detecting and Isolating Clostridium difficile Carriers at Hospital Admission on the Incidence of C difficile Infections: A Quasi-Experimental Controlled Study. JAMA Intern Med 2016;176(6): 796–804.

65. Linsenmeyer K, O'Brien W, Brecher SM, et al. Clostridium difficile Screening for Colonization During an Outbreak Setting. Clin Infect Dis 2018;67(12):1912–4.

66. Pear SM, Williamson TH, Bettin KM, et al. Decrease in nosocomial Clostridium difficile-associated diarrhea by restricting clindamycin use. Ann Intern Med 1994;120(4):272–7.

67. Valiquette L, Cossette B, Garant MP, et al. Impact of a reduction in the use of high-risk antibiotics on the course of an epidemic of Clostridium difficile-associated disease caused by the hypervirulent NAP1/027 strain. Clin Infect Dis 2007;45(Suppl 2):S112–21.

68. Ludlam H, Brown N, Sule O, et al. An antibiotic policy associated with reduced risk of Clostridium difficile-associated diarrhoea. Age Ageing 1999;28(6):578–80.

69. Cook PP, Gooch M. Long-term effects of an antimicrobial stewardship programme at a tertiary-care teaching hospital. Int J Antimicrob Agents 2015; 45(3):262–7.

70. Feazel LM, Malhotra A, Perencevich EN, et al. Effect of antibiotic stewardship programmes on Clostridium difficile incidence: a systematic review and meta-analysis. J Antimicrob Chemother 2014;69(7):1748–54.

71. Baur D, Gladstone BP, Burkert F, et al. Effect of antibiotic stewardship on the incidence of infection and colonisation with antibiotic-resistant bacteria and Clostridium difficile infection: a systematic review and meta-analysis. Lancet Infect Dis 2017;17(9):990–1001.

72. Kwok CS, Arthur AK, Anibueze CI, et al. Risk of Clostridium difficile infection with acid suppressing drugs and antibiotics: meta-analysis. Am J Gastroenterol 2012; 107(7):1011–9.

73. FDA Drug Safety Communication: Clostridium difficile-associated diarrhea can be associated with stomach acid drugs known as proton pump inhibitors (PPIs). 2012. Available at: http://www.fda.gov/Drugs/DrugSafety/ucm290510. htm. Accessed April 30, 2021.

74. Ohland CL, Macnaughton WK. Probiotic bacteria and intestinal epithelial barrier function. Am J Physiol Gastrointest Liver Physiol 2010;298(6):G807–19.

75. Goldenberg JZ, Yap C, Lytvyn L, et al. Probiotics for the prevention of Clostridium difficile-associated diarrhea in adults and children. Cochrane Database Syst Rev 2017;12:CD006095.

76. Shen NT, Maw A, Tmanova LL, et al. Timely Use of Probiotics in Hospitalized Adults Prevents Clostridium difficile Infection: A Systematic Review With Meta-Regression Analysis. Gastroenterology 2017;152(8):1889–900.e9.

77. Allen SJ, Wareham K, Wang D, et al. Lactobacilli and bifidobacteria in the prevention of antibiotic-associated diarrhoea and Clostridium difficile diarrhoea in older inpatients (PLACIDE): a randomised, double-blind, placebo-controlled, multi-centre trial. Lancet 2013;382(9900):1249–57.

78. Su GL, Ko CW, Bercik P, et al. AGA Clinical Practice Guidelines on the Role of Probiotics in the Management of Gastrointestinal Disorders. Gastroenterology 2020;159(2):697–705.

79. Munoz P, Bouza E, Cuenca-Estrella M, et al. Saccharomyces cerevisiae fungemia: an emerging infectious disease. Clin Infect Dis 2005;40(11):1625–34.

80. Kyne L, Warny M, Qamar A, et al. Asymptomatic carriage of Clostridium difficile and serum levels of IgG antibody against toxin A. N Engl J Med 2000;342(6):390–7.

81. Kyne L, Warny M, Qamar A, et al. Association between antibody response to toxin A and protection against recurrent Clostridium difficile diarrhoea. Lancet 2001;357(9251):189–93.

82. Leav BA, Blair B, Leney M, et al. Serum anti-toxin B antibody correlates with protection from recurrent Clostridium difficile infection (CDI). Vaccine 2010;28(4):965–9.

83. Wilcox MH, Gerding DN, Poxton IR, et al. Bezlotoxumab for Prevention of Recurrent Clostridium difficile Infection. N Engl J Med 2017;376(4):305–17.

84. de Bruyn G, Saleh J, Workman D, et al. Defining the optimal formulation and schedule of a candidate toxoid vaccine against Clostridium difficile infection: A randomized Phase 2 clinical trial. Vaccine 2016;34(19):2170–8.

85. Sheldon E, Kitchin N, Peng Y, et al. A phase 1, placebo-controlled, randomized study of the safety, tolerability, and immunogenicity of a Clostridium difficile vaccine administered with or without aluminum hydroxide in healthy adults. Vaccine 2016;34(18):2082–91.

86. Sanofi. Sanofi Ends Development of Clostridium Difficile Vaccine. Available at: https://www.sanofi.com/en/media-room/press-releases/2017/2017-12-01-22-00-00. Accessed April 30, 2021.

87. Guo S, Yan W, McDonough SP, et al. The recombinant Lactococcus lactis oral vaccine induces protection against C. difficile spore challenge in a mouse model. Vaccine 2015;33(13):1586–95.

88. Bruxelle JF, Mizrahi A, Hoys S, et al. Immunogenic properties of the surface layer precursor of Clostridium difficile and vaccination assays in animal models. Anaerobe 2016;37:78–84.

89. Dubberke ER, Han Z, Bobo L, et al. Impact of clinical symptoms on interpretation of diagnostic assays for Clostridium difficile infections. J Clin Microbiol 2011;49(8):2887–93.

90. Kelly SG, Yarrington M, Zembower TR, et al. Inappropriate Clostridium difficile Testing and Consequent Overtreatment and Inaccurate Publicly Reported Metrics. Infect Control Hosp Epidemiol 2016;37(12):1395–400.

91. Polage CR, Gyorke CE, Kennedy MA, et al. Overdiagnosis of Clostridium difficile Infection in the Molecular Test Era. JAMA Intern Med 2015;175(11):1792–801.

92. Boly FJ, Reske KA, Kwon JH. The Role of Diagnostic Stewardship in Clostridioides difficile Testing: Challenges and Opportunities. Curr Infect Dis Rep 2020;22(3):7.

93. Truong CY, Gombar S, Wilson R, et al. Real-Time Electronic Tracking of Diarrheal Episodes and Laxative Therapy Enables Verification of Clostridium difficile Clinical Testing Criteria and Reduction of Clostridium difficile Infection Rates. J Clin Microbiol 2017;55(5):1276–84.

94. Howard-Anderson JR, Sexton ME, Robichaux C, et al. The impact of an electronic medical record nudge on reducing testing for hospital-onset Clostridioides difficile infection. Infect Control Hosp Epidemiol 2020;41(4):411–7.

95. Madden GR, German Mesner I, Cox HL, et al. Reduced Clostridium difficile Tests and Laboratory-Identified Events With a Computerized Clinical Decision Support Tool and Financial Incentive. Infect Control Hosp Epidemiol 2018;39(6):737–40.

96. Lin MY, Wiksten T, Tomich A, et al. 974. Impact of Mandatory Infectious Disease (ID) Specialist Approval on Hospital-Onset Clostridium difficile (HO-CDI) Testing and Infection Rates: Results of a Pilot Study. Open Forum Infect Dis 2018; 5(suppl_1):S38–9.

97. Madden GR, Enfield KB, Sifri CD. Patient Outcomes With Prevented vs Negative Clostridioides difficile Tests Using a Computerized Clinical Decision Support Tool. Open Forum Infect Dis 2020;7(4):ofaa094.

98. White NC, Mendo-Lopez R, Papamichael K, et al. Laxative Use Does Not Preclude Diagnosis or Reduce Disease Severity in Clostridiodes difficile Infection. Clin Infect Dis 2020;71(6):1472–8.

Prevention of *Mycobacterium tuberculosis* Transmission in Health Care Settings

Neeraja Swaminathan, MD[a], Sarah R. Perloff, DO[b,c],
Jerry M. Zuckerman, MD[d,e],*

KEYWORDS

- Tuberculosis • Health care setting • Infection control • Nosocomial spread
- *Mycobacterium tuberculosis*

KEY POINTS

- Controlling nosocomial transmission of tuberculosis (TB) is a key element in reducing disease incidence and achieving the goal of eventual TB eradication in the United States.
- The Centers for Disease Control and Prevention–recommended TB control plan relies on a trilevel hierarchy of controls—administrative, environmental, and respiratory protection.
- Administrative controls are the most important level of control and include protocols for prompt detection and isolation of suspect cases, timeliness of diagnostic tests, education, and implementation of a TB screening program for employees who may be exposed to TB.
- Environmental controls focus on preventing the spread and reducing the concentration of airborne particles containing *Mycobacterium tuberculosis*.
- Respiratory protective equipment is the final barrier to the spread of TB. Minimizing face-seal leakage is essential to optimize a respirator's protective ability.

EPIDEMIOLOGY
Worldwide

The World Health Organization (WHO) *Global Tuberculosis Report* of 2020 reports that worldwide, there were still 10 million incident cases of tuberculosis (TB) worldwide the prior year, accounting for 1.4 million deaths.[1] Drug-resistant TB also remains a threat,

[a] Department of Medicine, Einstein Medical Center, Klein Building, Suite 300, 5501 Old York Road, Philadelphia, PA 19141, USA; [b] Division of Infectious Disease, Department of Medicine, Einstein Medical Center, Klein Building, Suite 300, 5501 Old York Road, Philadelphia, PA 19141, USA; [c] Sidney Kimmel Medical College of Thomas Jefferson University, Philadelphia, PA, USA; [d] Department of Patient Safety and Quality, Hackensack Meridian Health, Edison, NJ, USA; [e] Hackensack Meridian School of Medicine, Nutley, NJ, USA
* Corresponding author. Department of Patient Safety and Quality, Hackensack Meridian Health, 343 Thornall Street, Edison, NJ 08837.
E-mail address: Jerry.zuckerman@hmhn.org

Infect Dis Clin N Am 35 (2021) 1013–1025
https://doi.org/10.1016/j.idc.2021.07.003
0891-5520/21/© 2021 Elsevier Inc. All rights reserved.

id.theclinics.com

with close to half a million people worldwide having rifampicin-resistant TB; a vast majority (78%) of these infections are due to isoniazid and rifampin-resistant TB (ie, multi-drug-resistant). Although WHO "End TB Strategy" adopted by the World Health Assembly of the United Nations in 2014 called for a reduction in TB deaths by 95% and in new cases by 90% between 2015 and 2035, the data presented in the *Global Tuberculosis Report* indicate it is unlikely that the 2020 milestone of a 20% reduction in TB cases and a 35% reduction in deaths will be attained. The cumulative reductions from 2015 to 2019 in cases and deaths were only 9% and 14%, respectively.

United States

Since 1992, the rate of TB cases in the United States continually decreased to a record low of 2.2 cases per 100,000 people in 2020 (7163 incident cases), with the rate among non–US-born persons accounting for 71% of reported cases according to the Centers for Disease Control and Prevention (CDC).[2] This case rate represents a 20% relative reduction from the prior year, when the case rate was 2.7 per 100,000 persons, although the proportion of cases among non–US born persons was unchanged. It is unclear whether this dramatic decrease in TB incidence is related to reduced transmission due to COVID mitigation measures or decreased detection during the COVID pandemic. Underreporting appears to not have played a significant role.[2]

Despite successes, the elimination of TB in the United States remains an elusive goal with pre-COVID pandemic reporting indicating a leveling off of annual case rates.[3] Although the annual incidence of TB has declined 62% since 2000, the rate of decline has slowed, averaging a 2.1% reduction per year from 2012 to 2019. Barriers to this goal include[3] (1) prevalence of TB among foreign-born persons residing in the United States, (2) delays in detecting and reporting cases of pulmonary TB, (3) varied public health responses in identifying close contacts of persons with infectious TB and surveillance for TB outbreaks, (4) persistence of a substantial population of persons living in the United States with either unidentified or untreated latent TB infection (LTBI) who are at risk for progression to TB disease; and (5) maintaining clinical and public health expertise in an era of declining TB incidence. The importance of treatment of LTBI is evident particularly in the CDC's TB data for the year 2020, when 32% of cases of TB in non–US-born persons occurred in patients who have been residing in the United States for at least 20 years.[2]

Preventing Nosocomial Spread of Tuberculosis: An Opportunity Not To Be Neglected

Between 1985 and 1992, there were several nosocomial outbreaks of TB, including multidrug-resistant strains, in health care facilities within the United States that resulted in TB transmission to other patients and health care workers (HCWs). These outbreaks occurred because of the failure to recognize and diagnose TB, resulting in delayed initiation of both effective antituberculous therapy and appropriate infection control measures, both of which were hampered further by reductions in funding for TB programs at the time. Many of these outbreaks also were associated with lapses in infection control procedures, particularly in congregate settings.[4] These nosocomial outbreaks were curtailed successfully by the widespread implementation of infection control measures recommended by the CDC.[4]

Nosocomial outbreaks still occur into the twenty-first century. In 2002, 5 cases of nosocomially acquired active TB (both in patients and in HCWs) were confirmed by genotype analysis of strains isolated from the index patient in a large community hospital in Washington, DC. In addition, 11.3% of staff members and 22.5% of patient contacts subsequently evaluated with tuberculin skin testing (TST) tested positive. Delayed recognition and isolation of the index patient were believed causative.[5]

In 2013, the Southern Nevada Health District reported 2 cases of active TB and 53 cases of health care-acquired LTBI from a Las Vegas hospital. The index patient was a young woman who delivered premature twins 2 months before her death in July 2013. She had been ill prior to and during her pregnancy. The twins remained in the neonatal intensive care unit (NICU) until their deaths (in June and August). Only after an autopsy on the mother revealed TB was the second baby diagnosed and treated for the same. Subsequently, 1 of the resulting active cases of TB was in an HCW who was exposed to the mother and the infants in the NICU.[6] These outbreaks highlight the importance of the continued vigilance HCWs must have to ensure the prevention of nosocomial spread of TB.

A meta-analysis by Uden and colleagues[7] included 21 studies, from 2007 through 2016, evaluating TB prevalence or incidence among HCWs and a control group. The studies originated from 16 different countries; 8 of them were classified by the WHO as high burden countries and none of them was from North America. The prevalence of LTBI among HCWs was 37%, and the mean incidence rate of active TB was 97/100,000 per year. Compared with the general population, the risk of LTBI was greater for HCWs (odds ratio 2.27; 95% CI, 1.61–3.20), and the incidence rate ratio for active TB was 2.94 (95% CI, 1.67–5.19).[7] A subgroup analysis demonstrated that the risk of LTBI or incidence of active TB was greater in high-TB burden countries compared with ones with a low TB burden. Although the number of cases were low, what prevented larger outbreaks in low burden areas was the lower incidence of TB rather than excellence in infection prevention and control practices.[8]

More recently, the impact of infectious disease resulting in workforce attrition during the COVID-19 pandemic has demonstrated the deleterious consequences to the functioning of the broader health care system. Although not of the same magnitude as COVID-19, TB acquisition by HCWs poses a risk to the effective functioning of poorly staffed health systems as well as to patient safety. HCWs are a limited resource, and occupational TB can lead to workforce attrition.[9]

TRANSMISSION OF TUBERCULOSIS

Transmission of TB occurs via airborne particles (droplet nuclei) containing *Mycobacterium tuberculosis* (MTB). Infectious droplet nuclei, 1 μm to 5 μm in size, are generated by individuals with pulmonary or laryngeal TB when they cough or talk. Although an increased frequency of coughing is associated with infectivity, several other aerosol-generating procedures, such as singing, sneezing, and talking, have been implicated in disease transmission.[10] Droplet nuclei remain airborne for prolonged periods of time and are small enough when inhaled to evade the mucociliary defenses in airways before being deposited in alveoli. The likelihood of TB being transmitted to another individual depends on the concentration of infectious droplet nuclei in the air and the duration of exposure. Patients with TB are more infectious if they have a cough, cavitation on chest radiograph, acid fast bacilli (AFB) detected on sputum smear, or laryngeal involvement. Transmission risk is increased further by cough-inducing or aerosol-generating procedures, endotracheal intubation, bronchoscopy, tuberculous abscess irrigation, and autopsy. Environmental factors that contribute to increased risk of transmission include exposure to TB in small, enclosed spaces, insufficient dilution and removal of infectious droplet nuclei from the air, and recirculation of contaminated air.[11–13]

COMPONENTS OF A TUBERCULOSIS INFECTION CONTROL PROGRAM

In 2005, the CDC published revised guidelines for preventing the spread of TB within health care settings.[14] These guidelines recommend that all health care settings have a TB infection control program to ensure prompt detection, isolation, and treatment of persons who have suspected or confirmed TB. The recommended TB control plan relies on a trilevel hierarchy of controls—administrative, environmental, and respiratory protection—and is based on an annual risk assessment performed for the setting. The salient features of these guidelines are summarized. For a more in-depth discussion, readers are advised to review the document available at http://www.cdc.gov/tb/publications/guidelines/infectioncontrol.htm. These recommendations, which were guided by scientific reasoning based on TB epidemiology, TB pathogenesis, and public health principles, were shown in a systematic review by Fox and colleagues[15] in 2020 to be associated with reduced transmission of MTB in health care settings.

ADMINISTRATIVE MEASURES

Administrative measures are the most important level of control to reduce the risk of exposure to persons who have suspected or confirmed TB. These measures include protocols to ensure the prompt detection and isolation of suspect cases, timeliness of diagnostic tests, education of HCWs, implementation of a screening program for employees who may be exposed to TB, and coordination of efforts with the local health department. Process measures, such as the time interval to initiation of airborne precautions and/or treatment in suspect or confirmed TB cases, duration of airborne infection isolation (AII), and compliance with discontinuation of airborne precautions criteria, should be used to assess the efficacy of the TB control plan.

Prompt Triage

The primary risk for health care–associated transmission is the unsuspected or undiagnosed patient with active pulmonary TB or laryngeal TB. A high index of suspicion and prompt initiation of airborne isolation are essential to minimize the exposure risk to HCWs and other patients. Patient characteristics that may increase a clinician's suspicion for TB infection should be identified at the time of triage. These features include identification of (1) a history of known TB exposure, latent infection, or prior disease; (2) signs or symptoms consistent with active pulmonary TB disease (ie, cough for >3 weeks duration, loss of appetite, unexplained weight loss, night sweats, fever, hemoptysis, hoarseness, fatigue, and chest pain); and (3) the presence of comorbidities or use of medications that increase susceptibility to TB infection or reactivation.[16]

In attempting to create a decision tool utilizing specific patient characteristics to aide in the triage of patients with pneumonia into a room with the appropriate isolation precautions, 1 study retrospectively identified and prospectively validated a decision instrument for predicting active TB infection in 11 university-affiliated US emergency departments. According to this study, patients unlikely to have TB are those without a history of active or latent TB, who are not immigrants or homeless, have not been recently incarcerated, who do not have any recent weight loss, and who do not have apical infiltrates or cavitary lesions on chest radiograph. This decision instrument exhibited a negative predictive value of 99.7% for TB.[17] A single-center retrospective case control study found that being non–US born and having a prior positive TB test predicted an 18.2% probability of pulmonary TB diagnosis when present, compared with 1.0% if both factors were not present.[18]

Isolation of Suspected Cases

The CDC and WHO each has specific criteria for appropriate patients to be in AII. For hospitalized individuals in whom TB disease is either confirmed or suspected, AII precautions should be maintained until TB is either no longer suspected or the patient is no longer considered infectious to others.

For suspected cases, the recommendations for discontinuation of isolation depend on the clinical scenario. When TB is considered less likely based on history, examination, and radiography, AII may be discontinued when an alternative diagnosis is established or when there are 3 consecutive negative sputum AFB smears. Alternatively, AII may be discontinued, if a patient has positive AFB smears and simultaneous negative sputum Xpert MTB/RIF (Cepheid, Sunnyvale, CA) tests and TB is considered unlikely.[19–21] In the latter scenario, a nontuberculous mycobacterial infection should be considered.

The decision to discontinue AII should not be based on negative sputum AFB smears or NAA tests alone. Before discontinuing AII, negative results must be interpreted in the context of the patient's clinical and radiographic presentation and the clinician's suspicion for MTB infection. If the clinical features are highly suggestive of MTB infection, the patient must be kept under AII until further work-up (eg, induced sputum or bronchoscopy) is done or a therapeutic trial of multidrug antituberculous therapy has resulted in clinical improvement. In highly suspect cases, negative smears alone are not considered tantamount to being noninfectious, as highlighted by 1 study performed in the Netherlands, which found that patients with smear-negative, culture-positive TB are responsible for 13% of TB transmission in the country.[22]

For confirmed cases, hospitalized patients must remain in AII until they have received at least 2 weeks of 4 drug anti-tuberculous therapy, demonstrated clinical improvement (eg, resolution of fever, decreased cough), and had 3 consecutive negative AFB sputum smears. Serial NAA tests should not be used to monitor response to treatment.[19] Medically stable patients can be discharged to home even if the sputum AFB smears remain positive as long as the following criteria are met: (1) follow-up care and directly observed therapy have been arranged, (2) there are no children younger than 4 years of age or immunocompromised persons of any age in the household, (3) all immunocompetent household members previously have been exposed to the patient prior to hospital admission, and (4) the patient is willing to remain on home quarantine pending conversion to negative sputum smears for AFB.[23] Although difficult to say with certainty due to the heterogeneity of studies included in 1 recent systematic review, there clearly was a trend toward reduced nosocomial TB transmission following the implementation of triage, isolation, and treatment of possible TB cases.[24]

Laboratory Diagnosis

Laboratories likewise must be proficient in infection control measures. Diagnostic testing for TB must occur in a designated biosafety level 2 or higher. The processing of TB specimens must be performed in a safe manner to minimize exposure risk of laboratory technicians. Personnel should be trained thoroughly in proper technique to minimize the production of aerosols. All specimens suspected or known to contain MTB must be handled in a class I or class II biological safety cabinet (BSC) with appropriate environmental and respiratory protection controls in place. Proper maintenance of the BSC and handling of clinical specimens are essential to minimize the risk of cross-contamination of specimens. The Association of Public Health Laboratories has developed a tool for mycobacteriology laboratories to self-assess the quality of their diagnostic TB practices and to identify areas that may be in need of improvement.[25] Systems also should be in place to ensure that laboratories report positive results from any specimen to clinicians within 24 hours.

False-positive culture results for MTB have been reported to occur in an estimated 1% to 2% of TB cases and may be secondary to laboratory cross-contamination, contaminated clinical equipment, or clerical errors.[26] Clinicians should consider this possibility when the clinical presentation is not consistent with TB disease. False-positive results also should be considered when there is a low percentage of culture-positive specimens from the same patient, there are low colony counts on solid media, or there is a prolonged incubation period before growth is detected in broth-based media. In addition, false-positive results should be considered when investigating potential outbreaks in the health care setting when specimens from multiple patients processed in the same laboratory on the same day are reported positive or isolates have unexpected and identical drug-resistance patterns, especially in a setting of atypical radiographic findings or inconsistent history for TB infection.[25–29] Mycobacteriology laboratories should have a plan for identification, review, and notification of possible false-positive culture results.

The rapidity of diagnostics has an impact on the duration of AII while admitted to the hospital for reasons discussed previously. Due to the importance of early recognition of TB infection, there has been increased interest in developing more rapid diagnostic tools. The use of nucleic acid amplification (NAA) can decrease the time to diagnosis from a mean of 3 weeks, when using a liquid broth culture, to 4 days.[30] The CDC recommends using an NAA test on at least 1 specimen, in addition to AFB smears, from all patients suspected of having TB to facilitate more rapid diagnosis and initiation of treatment,[12] thereby reducing the odds of transmission of infection. The WHO recommends NAA testing as the preferred initial diagnostic test for adults with signs and symptoms of or radiographic findings consistent with pulmonary TB.[31] Because NAA has a sensitivity of only 50% to 80% to detect TB on AFB smear-negative specimens (compared with >95% on AFB smear-positive specimens), culture remains the gold standard for diagnosis and exclusion, and is essential for susceptibility testing.

Although more costly than traditional organism identification methods, NAA testing decreases net expenditures by providing earlier diagnosis resulting in earlier removal from AII, shorter hospital length of stay, and decreased duration of unnecessary TB treatment.[32–34] A recent study concluded that, in individuals with suspicious clinical symptoms, computer-aided detection methods for interpreting digital chest radiographs is useful in identifying probable TB-infected patients who would more likely benefit from NAA testing. By specifically testing a screened population, the associated costs can be reduced.[35]

Adequate specimen collection is likewise vital. Various studies report that a single sputum AFB smear has a sensitivity of only 50% to 70%, and repeated testing increases this value. There is conflicting evidence regarding the difference in the diagnostic yield of 2 versus 3 sputum AFB smears, but a meta-analysis suggested a third sample is unnecessary because it adds little to the diagnostic yield; thus, the WHO advises that 2 specimens are sufficient. Specimens need not be collected 24 hours apart; 1 every 8 hours is adequate.[36,37] Lastly, the value of at least 1 early morning specimen cannot be overstated. In both WHO and CDC guidelines, 1 early morning specimen is specifically recommended in the diagnostic work-up as a result of several studies that demonstrated increased diagnostic yield. One observational cohort study done in Uganda found that among 2418 cases of suspected TB, 21 had confirmed disease. Random sputum smears combined with the use of mycobacterial growth indicator tubes (Becton, Dickinson and Company, Franklin Lakes, New Jersey) allowed detection of 57.1% of cases. Six patients were diagnosed by direct microscopy; the remainder were diagnosed by culture. Of those diagnosed by microscopy, only 42.9% were positive on random specimen but 100% were positive when an early morning specimen was used.[38]

Another useful tool is fluorescence microscopy. In Taiwan, a study comparing fluorescent to conventional microscopy found that sputum smear detection rate nearly doubled, resulting in more prompt initiation of AII.[39] The WHO also endorses the use of fluorescence rather than conventional microscopy if laboratory personnel receive adequate training and there is reliable external quality control.[31]

Contact Investigation

Health care facilities must have written policies detailing how to proceed when a patient or an employee is confirmed to have active TB. Investigation of the patients' family members and contacts in the community are conducted by public health officials, and contact investigation also must proceed within the health care facility if (1) there was a delay in institution of infection control measures for a patient with active TB or (2) an HCW in the facility is diagnosed with active TB.

Contact investigation[40] is conducted on all those exposed to the patient in a graduated approach, identifying high-priority and low-priority contacts, including HCWs and other patients in the facility. The process begins with performing either a TST or an interferon gamma release assay (IGRA) unless the individual is known to have tested positive previously. If the TST or IGRA is negative, then the test is repeated using the same modality initially employed 8 weeks to 10 weeks after the exposure. If an exposed patient or HCW has HIV infection; however, commencing treatment of LTBI is recommended regardless of the initial TST or IGRA results. If the second test performed 8 weeks to 10 weeks after exposure remains negative, LTBI treatment can be discontinued. If the result of the second test is positive and active TB disease then is ruled out, the contact is classified as recently infected and followed-up and treated appropriately. The contact investigation then should be expanded to include lower-priority contacts. Further details on contact investigation can be found in the CDC module, available at http://www.cdc.gov/tb/education/ssmodules/pdfs/Module8.pdf.

Although necessary, contact investigation of health care–associated TB exposure is a cost-intensive and labor-intensive endeavor for the health system. In a study retrospectively describing the experience of the labor resources needed to perform contact investigations following a health care TB exposure, a 3-hospital system in New York City with an average delay in time to AII of 3.3 days, a mean of 41 staff were exposed per patient and the estimated workload per index case was 38 person-hours.[41] This burden may be somewhat mitigated by utilizing data on access of the chart in the electronic medical record to identify potentially exposed patients and HCWs.[42]

Genotyping or restriction fragment length polymorphism analysis of TB isolates can facilitate the identification of TB outbreaks[27] by examining the genetic relatedness of isolates and thereby determining if cases in a health care setting are outbreak related or independent events.[43] Moreover, the CDC encourages universal genotyping, that is, at least one MTB isolate from every culture-positive TB case should be sent for genotyping, because it may uncover unrecognized outbreaks and clusters. In 2004, when the national TB genotyping services was initiated by the CDC, national genotyping laboratories located in Michigan and California were tasked with genotyping isolates at no cost to patients or health care providers. Laboratories ship MTB isolates for genotyping to these facilities. Genotyping has evolved over time and now can be performed as whole-genome sequencing (WGS). The CDC Division of Tuberculosis Elimination began universal WGS in 2018 with the intent of transitioning to WGS as the standard method for genotyping in 2021. The results of multilocus WGS typing are used to identify potential clusters/outbreaks.[43]

The TB Genotyping Information Management System (GIMS), a secure Web-based portal designed to improve access and dissemination of genotyping information nationwide, is another resource that can alert physicians to potential TB outbreaks in their jurisdictions and allows for the monitoring of TB transmission trends. Access to TB GIMS is limited to registered users and is coordinated by a designated TB GIMS administrator for each state TB control program. Health care providers desiring access should contact their TB GIMS administrator. Until the end of the transition period in 2021 when WGS becomes the standard modality for genotyping, WGS assessment of potential clusters will not be reported in TB GIMS.[43]

Screening of Health Care Workers

Given the declining incidence of TB infections in the United States and health care–associated transmission, the CDC updated guidelines for TB screening, testing, and treatment of HCWs.[44] An employee TB screening program is an essential component of the TB control plan. All HCWs should receive baseline TB screening on hire with an individual risk assessment (available at https://www.cdc.gov/tb/topic/infectioncontrol/pdf/healthCareSettings-assessment.pdf) and either a 2-step TST or a single IGRA. If an individual tests positive and their risk assessment determines they are low risk for TB, then a second TB test should be performed to confirm the result.[44]

During screening, if HCWs are detected to have LTBI, it also is important to offer treatment of the same to prevent progression to active TB.[14] Additionally TB screening for HCWs must pay special attention to confidential HIV testing and access to antiretroviral therapy as well because of the high risk of TB in HIV patients. In some countries/settings, the association of TB with HIV leads to stigma associated with the diagnosis leading to delays in diagnosis as well as treatment.[45]

Serial testing of all HCWs no longer is recommended unless there is a known exposure or ongoing TB transmission within a facility or department.[44] Annual TB screening can be considered for certain groups, identified by an annual facility risk assessment, who might be at increased risk for occupational exposures. In lieu of serial testing, all HCWs should receive TB education annually. Training includes information on TB risk factors, the signs and symptoms of TB disease and the organization's TB infection control policies and procedures. Additionally, HCWs with untreated LTBI should complete an annual TB symptom screen and assessed accordingly.

All HCWs exposed to an infectious TB case while not using appropriate personal protective equipment should undergo postexposure screening and testing.[44] Exposed individuals should complete a TB symptom screen and be evaluated accordingly if positive. If the individual had a negative TB test previously, they should be retested with either a TST or IGRA immediately and then again 8 weeks to 10 weeks after the last known exposure date. If either test is positive, then the HCW should be evaluated for active TB. Individuals with a documented history of a positive TB test do not need to be retested.

Individuals who newly test positive for TB should be evaluated further for symptoms and have a chest radiograph to assess for TB disease. If there is no evidence for active disease, then treatment of LTBI should be offered and strongly encouraged. HCWs who decline treatment should be monitored annually for symptoms; a yearly chest radiograph is not recommended unless they become symptomatic.[44]

ENVIRONMENTAL CONTROLS

After administrative controls, environmental controls form the second line of defense in TB control programs, and focus on preventing the spread and reducing the concentration of airborne particles containing MTB.

General ventilation systems dilute and remove contaminated air throughout the hospital and can be balanced to control airflow patterns in any room or clinical setting. In areas where infectious airborne droplet nuclei might be present (eg, AII rooms), a single-pass ventilation system with airflow circulation of at least 6 air changes per hour (12 air changes per hour for new construction) is preferred.[15] External exhaust of contaminated air is preferred but, if necessary, air may be recirculated through high-efficiency particulate absorbing (HEPA) filters or following UV germicidal irradiation.[14] All inpatient rooms are maintained at negative pressure to surrounding areas to prevent outflow of droplet nuclei to the outside environment. A pressure differential greater than or equal to 0.01 in of water is recommended, and monitoring of the negative pressure should be performed daily when the room is occupied by a patient with suspected or confirmed TB. Persons entering the room must wear appropriate respiratory protective equipment.

Other areas that should have negative pressure rooms include bronchoscopy and autopsy suites, sputum induction rooms, clinical laboratories, and other selected examination and treatment rooms in areas, such as the emergency department or outpatient offices. Routine preventative maintenance should be scheduled and regular quality control checks performed to ensure that environmental controls are functioning properly. Infection control preventionists should be notified of any malfunction of, or scheduled maintenance on, ventilation systems servicing care areas of patients with TB.

RESPIRATORY PROTECTION

Respiratory protective equipment is the last line of defense in a TB control plan, providing a final barrier to the spread of TB. Respirators used for TB protection must be certified to have 95% or greater filtration efficiency when challenged with 0.3-mm–sized particles (N95 masks). Because these masks filter air prior to inhalation, they are intended to be worn by any possible contacts and not by the patient. Respirators should be readily available for use prior to entering an AII room. All HCWs must have respirator fit testing and training in correct procedures for donning and doffing to ensure optimal protection during use.

Minimizing face-seal leakage of a respirator is essential to optimize the respirator's protective ability. The amount of face-seal leakage is determined by the fit characteristics of the respirator as well as the ability to properly don the respirator. A user-seal check should be performed before each use to ensure that the respirator is correctly positioned with minimal leakage. The use of respirators for TB in the United States is regulated by the Occupational Safety and Health Administration general industry standard for respiratory protection, which requires health care settings to perform respirator fit testing and annual training to ensure proper fit and use for all HCWs.[46] Those who fail the respirator fit testing must use a powered air purifying respirator, which consists of a facepiece and a blower to pass contaminated air through a HEPA filter removing contaminated air and supplying purified air to the user.

ROLE OF HEALTH CARE WORKERS

HCWs themselves are crucial to the goal of eradicating the spread of TB. They are specially equipped to be advocates for change by increasing awareness. In a systematic review that looked at barriers to implementation of TB control, one of the reasons for high rates of nosocomial transmission was an erroneous sense of safety—HCWs believing that they are not at risk either omit or incorrectly use their personal protective equipment. Thus, the attitude of HCWs also has an impact in their response to noso-comial TB transmission.[9]

SUMMARY

Patients with TB pose a risk to other patients and HCWs, and outbreaks in health care settings have occurred when the diagnosis is not suspected in a patient and/or appropriate infection control measures were not used. All health care facilities should have an operational TB infection control plan that emphasizes the use of a hierarchy of controls (administrative, environmental, and personal respiratory protection) to prevent the transmission of MTB.

CLINICS CARE POINTS

- Maintain a high degree of clinical suspicion for TB and isolate in airborne precautions while diagnostic evaluation is in progress.

- To expedite the diagnostic work-up for TB, send 3 sputum samples every 8 hours for both AFB smear and NAA testing. At least 1 of these samples should be a first morning sample because they have the highest yield in TB cases.

- Do not discontinue airborne isolation precautions based solely on negative test results. All test results should be interpreted in the context of a patient's clinical and radiographic presentation and the clinician's suspicion for MTB infection.

- In patients diagnosed with TB, discontinuation of AII precautions can be done safely when the patient has received at least 2 weeks of effective anti-TB therapy, has improved clinically, and has 3 consecutive negative AFB smears.

- Monitoring of negative pressure in AII rooms should be performed daily when the room is occupied by a patient with suspected or confirmed TB.

DISCLOSURE

The authors have nothing to disclose.

REFERENCES

1. Global tuberculosis report 2020. Geneva: World Health Organization; 2020. Licence: CC BY-NC-SA 3.0 IGO.
2. Deutsch-Feldman M, Pratt RH, Price SF, et al. Tuberculosis — United States, 2020. MMWR Morb Mortal Wkly Rep 2021;70:409–14.
3. Salinas JL, Mindra G, Haddad MB, et al. Leveling of Tuberculosis Incidence - United States, 2013-2015. MMWR Morb Mortal Wkly Rep 2016;65(11):273–8.
4. Cole B, Nilsen DM, Will L, et al. Essential components of a public health tuberculosis prevention, control, and elimination program: recommendations of the Advisory Council for the Elimination of Tuberculosis and the National Tuberculosis Controllers Association. MMWR Morb Mortal Wkly Rep 2020;69(No. RR-7):1–27.
5. Tuberculosis Outbreak in a Community Hospital — District of Columbia, 2002. MMWR Morb Mortal Wkly Rep 2004;53(10):214–6.
6. Southern Nevada health District Maternal TB investigation. Available at: https://www.southernnevadahealthdistrict.org/download/stats-reports/Maternal-TB-Investigation-Report-121615.pdf. Accessed April 17, 2021.

7. Uden L, Barber E, Ford N, et al. Risk of tuberculosis infection and disease for health care workers: an updated meta-analysis. Open Forum Infect Dis 2017; 4(3):ofx137.

8. Curran E. Outbreak column 21: Tuberculosis (TB): still a nosocomial threat. J Infect Prev 2017;19(3):144–50.

9. Nathavitharana R, Bond P, Dramowski A, et al. Agents of change: the role of healthcare workers in the prevention of nosocomial and occupational tuberculosis. Presse Med 2017;46(2):e53–62.

10. Patterson B, Morrow C, Singh V, et al. Detection of Mycobacterium tuberculosis bacilli in bio-aerosols from untreated TB patients. Gates Open Res 2018;1:11.

11. Centers for Disease Control and Prevention. Targeted tuberculin testing and treatment of latent tuberculosis infection. American Thoracic Society. MMWR Recomm Rep 2000;49(RR–6):1–51.

12. Lewinsohn DM, Leonard MK, LoBue PA, et al. Official American Thoracic Society/Infectious Diseases Society of America/Centers for Disease Control and Prevention clinical practice guidelines: diagnosis of tuberculosis in adults and children. Clin Infect Dis 2017;64(2):e1–33.

13. Nahid P, Dorman S, Alipanah N, et al. Official American Thoracic Society/Centers for Disease Control and Prevention/Infectious Diseases Society of America clinical practice guidelines: treatment of drug-susceptible tuberculosis. Clin Infect Dis 2016;63(7):e147–95.

14. Jensen PA, Lambert LA, Iademarco MF, et al. Guidelines for preventing the transmission of Mycobacterium tuberculosis in health-care settings, 2005. MMWR Recomm Rep 2005;54(RR–17):1–141.

15. Fox G, Redwood L, Chang V, et al. The effectiveness of individual and environmental infection control measures in reducing the transmission of mycobacterium tuberculosis: a systematic review. Clin Infect Dis 2020. https://doi.org/10.1093/cid/ciaa719.

16. Iwata K, Smith BA, Santos E, et al. Failure to implement respiratory isolation: why does it happen? Infect Control Hosp Epidemiol 2002;23(10):595–9.

17. Moran GJ, Barrett TW, Mower WR, et al. Decision instrument for the isolation of pneumonia patients with suspected pulmonary tuberculosis admitted through US Emergency Departments. Ann Emerg Med 2009;53(5):625–32.

18. England J, Byrne D, Harris B, et al. Use of airborne infection isolation in potential cases of pulmonary tuberculosis. Infect Control Hosp Epidemiol 2020;41(5): 505–9.

19. National Tuberculosis Controllers Association; Association of Public Health Laboratories. Consensus statement on the use of Cepheid Xpert MTB/RIF® assay in making decisions to discontinue airborne infection isolation in healthcare settings. Smyrna, GA: National Tuberculosis Controllers Association. Available at: http://www.tbcontrollers.org/resources/airborne-infection-isolation/#.W19aWdhKhmwexternal icon. Accessed April 5, 2021.

20. Chaisson LH, Duong D, Cattamanchi A, et al. Association of rapid molecular testing with duration of respiratory isolation for patients with possible tuberculosis in a US hospital. JAMA Intern Med 2018;178(10):1380–8.

21. Khan S, Nakasone A, Ghajar M, et al. Time to detection in culture supports prediction of low transmissibility of tuberculosis and discontinuation of isolation for low-risk patients with a single AFB-negative and NAAT-negative respiratory specimen. Infect Control Hosp Epidemiol 2018;39(5):619–21.

22. Tostmann A1, Kik SV, Kalisvaart NA, et al. Tuberculosis transmission by patients with smear-negative pulmonary tuberculosis in a large cohort in the Netherlands. Clin Infect Dis 2008;47(9):1135–42.

23. Sia IG, Wieland ML. Current concepts in the management of tuberculosis. Mayo Clin Proc 2011;86(4):348–61.

24. Karat A, Gregg M, Barton H, et al. Evidence for the use of triage, respiratory isolation, and effective treatment to reduce the transmission of mycobacterium tuberculosis in healthcare settings: a systematic review. Clin Infect Dis 2021;72(1): 155–72.

25. Association of Public Health Laboratories. Mycobacterium tuberculosis: assessing your laboratory. Available at: https://www.aphl.org/aboutAPHL/publications/Documents/ID-2019Apr-TB-Toolkit.pdf#search=tuberculosis. Accessed April 5, 2021.

26. Barac A, Karimzadeh-Esfahani H, Pourostadi M, et al. Laboratory cross-contamination of mycobacterium tuberculosis: a systematic review and meta-analysis. Lung 2019;197(5):651–61.

27. Guide to the application of genotyping to tuberculosis prevention and control. Available at: https://www.cdc.gov/tb/programs/genotyping/images/TBGenotyping Guide_June2004.pdf. Accessed April 11, 2021.

28. Burman WJ, Reves RR. Review of false-positive cultures for Mycobacterium tuberculosis and recommendations for avoiding unnecessary treatment. Clin Infect Dis 2000;31(6):1390–5.

29. Fitzpatrick L, Braden C, Cronin W, et al. Investigation of laboratory cross-contamination of Mycobacterium tuberculosis cultures. Clin Infect Dis 2004; 38(6):e52–4.

30. Moore DF, Guzman JA, Mikhail LT. Reduction in turnaround time for laboratory diagnosis of pulmonary tuberculosis by routine use of a nucleic acid amplification test. Diagn Microbiol Infect Dis 2005;52:247–54.

31. WHO consolidated guidelines on tuberculosis. Module 3: diagnosis – rapid diagnostics for tuberculosis detection. Geneva: World Health Organization; 2020.

32. Report of an expert consultation on the uses of nucelic acid amplification tests for the diagnosis of tuberculosis. CDC. Available at: https://www.cdc.gov/tb/publications/guidelines/amplification_tests/amplification_tests.pdf. Accessed April 15, 2021.

33. Chaisson LH, Duong D, Cattamanchi A, et al. Association of rapid molecular testing with duration of respiratory isolation for patients with possible tuberculosis in a US Hospital. JAMA Intern Med 2018;178(10):1380–8.

34. Poonawala H, Leekha S, Medina-Moreno S, et al. Use of a single xpert MTB/RIF assay to determine the duration of airborne isolation in hospitalized patients with suspected pulmonary tuberculosis. Infect Control Hosp Epidemiol 2018;39(5): 590–5.

35. Zaidi S, Habib S, Van Ginneken B, et al. Evaluation of the diagnostic accuracy of computer-aided detection of tuberculosis on chest radiography among private sector patients in Pakistan. Sci Rep 2018;8(1):12339.

36. Al Zahrani K, Al Jahdali H, Poirier L, et al. Yield of smear, culture and amplification tests from repeated sputum induction for the diagnosis of pulmonary tuberculosis. Int J Tuberc Lung Dis 2001;5(9):855–60.

37. Mase SR, Ramsay A, Ng V, et al. Yield of serial sputum specimen examinations in the diagnosis of pulmonary tuberculosis: a systematic review. Int J Tuberc Lung Dis 2007;11(5):485–95.

38. Ssengooba W, Kateete DP, Wajja A, et al. An early morning sputum sample is necessary for the diagnosis of pulmonary tuberculosis, even with more sensitive techniques: a prospective cohort study among adolescent TB-suspects in Uganda. Tuberculosis Res Treat 2012;2012:970203.
39. Sun HY, Wang JY, Chen YC, et al. Impact of introducing fluorescent microscopy on hospital tuberculosis control: a before-after study at a high caseload medical center in Taiwan. PLoS One 2020;15(4):e0230067.
40. Self-Study Module on Tuberculosis. Module 8 Contact Investigations for Tuberculosis. Available at: http://www.cdc.gov/tb/education/ssmodules/pdfs/Module8.pdf. Accessed April 5, 2021.
41. Kelly AM, D'Agostino JF, Andrada LV, et al. Delayed tuberculosis diagnosis and costs of contact investigations for hospital exposure: New York City, 2010-2014. Am J Infect Control 2017;45(5):483–6.
42. Usiak S, Romero F, Schwegman P, et al. Utilization of electronic health record events to conduct a tuberculosis contact investigation in a high-risk oncology unit. Infect Control Hosp Epidemiol 2017;38(10):1235–9.
43. Talarico S, Silk B, Shaw T, et al. Tuberculosis_WGS_Training_Module. Available at: https://www.cdc.gov/tb/programs/genotyping/Tuberculosis_WGS_Training_Module.pdf. Accessed April 5, 2021.
44. Sosa LE, Njie GJ, Lobato MN, et al. Tuberculosis screening, testing, and treatment of U.S. health care personnel: recommendations from the National Tuberculosis Controllers Association and CDC, 2019. MMWR Morb Mortal Wkly Rep 2019;68:439–43.
45. Flick R, Munthali A, Simon K, et al. Assessing infection control practices to protect health care workers and patients in Malawi from nosocomial transmission of Mycobacterium tuberculosis. PLoS One 2017;12(12):e0189140.
46. Occupational Safety and Health Administration. Respiratory Protection. -1910.134. Available at: https://www.osha.gov/pls/oshaweb/owadisp.show_document?p_table=STANDARDS&p_id=12716. Accessed April 5, 2021.

Nosocomial Fungal Infections
Epidemiology, Infection Control, and Prevention

Geehan Suleyman, MD, MLS (ASCP)[a], George J. Alangaden, MD[b],*

KEYWORDS

• Nosocomial • Fungal infection • *Candida* • *Aspergillus*

KEY POINTS

- Invasive candidiasis and mold infections are a common cause of hospital-acquired infections often related to the use of invasive lines, immunosuppression, and a contaminated environment.
- Traditional culture methodologies may be insensitive for the diagnosis of fungal infections and may require the use of more sensitive nonculture-based testing.
- The control and prevention of invasive fungal infections require a combination of traditional infection control practices, as well as the use of antifungal prophylaxis in high-risk individuals.
- There has been an increase in the rates of invasive fungal infection during the COVID-19 pandemic as a result of gaps in infection control practices and use of immunosuppression for treatment of COVID-19 infection.

IMPACT OF NOSOCOMIAL FUNGAL INFECTIONS

There has been an overall increase in fungal health care–associated infections (HAIs). The increase is partly due to the increased population of immunocompromised patients at risk for invasive fungal infection as a consequence of the wider use of treatment modalities, such as hematopoietic stem cell transplantation (HSCT), solid organ transplantation (SOT), and newer immunomodulatory agents (**Table 1**).[1–3] Moreover, the increasing use of invasive devices, especially central venous catheters (CVCs), has resulted in an increase in nosocomial central line-associated bloodstream infections (CLABSIs) due to *Candida* spp.[1,3,4] Exposure to airborne molds such as *Aspergillus* spp. within the hospital environment has caused outbreaks of nosocomial aspergillosis in severely immunocompromised patients such as allogeneic HSCT recipients and neutropenic patients with hematologic malignancies.[5]

---

[a] Infection Prevention and Control, Henry Ford Hospital, Wayne State University, 2799 West Grand Boulevard, CFP Suite 317, Detroit, MI 48202, USA; [b] Division of Infectious Diseases, Henry Ford Hospital, Wayne State University, 2799 West Grand Boulevard, CFP Suite 316, Detroit, MI 48202, USA
* Corresponding author.
E-mail address: GALANGA1@hfhs.org

Infect Dis Clin N Am 35 (2021) 1027–1053
https://doi.org/10.1016/j.idc.2021.08.002
0891-5520/21/© 2021 Elsevier Inc. All rights reserved.

id.theclinics.com

Table 1
Risk factors associated with invasive fungal infections

Candida	Aspergillus	Mucorales	Fusarium	Scedosporium
• Acute necrotizing pancreatitis	• Alemtuzumab	• CMV disease	• Corticosteroid	• Corticosteroid
• Abdominal surgery; anastomotic leak; or repeat laparotomies	• Allogeneic HSCT	• Corticosteroids	• Myeloma	• Neutropenia
• Broad-spectrum antibiotics	• Anastomotic complications in lung transplantation	• Diabetes mellitus	• Severe GVHD	• Severe GVHD
• Central venous catheters	• *Aspergillus* colonization	• Echinocandin use		
• Hemodialysis	• CMV disease	• Iron overload		
• HSCT	• Corticosteroids	• Malnutrition		
• Immunosuppression including corticosteroids, chemotherapy	• Infliximab	• Myelodysplasia		
• Malignancy	• Neutropenia	• Neutropenia		
• Mechanical ventilation >3 d	• Older age	• Older age		
• Multifocal candida colonization	• Prolonged ICU stay	• Renal failure		
• Neutropenia	• Renal failure requiring dialysis	• Severe GVHD		
• Prolonged ICU stay	• Retransplantation	• Voriconazole use		
• Prolonged hospitalization	• Severe GVHD			
• SOT (kidney and liver)	• T-cell depleting agents			
• Total parenteral nutrition				

Abbreviations: CMV, cytomegalovirus; GVHD, graft-versus-host disease; HSCT, hematopoietic stem cell transplantation; IA, intraabdominal; ICU, intensive care unit; SOT, solid organ transplantation.

Candida spp. are associated with serious HAIs, especially in patients in intensive care units (ICUs)[1,3,4,6] and are one of the most common causes of nosocomial bloodstream infections (BSIs) in US hospitals.[3,4] It is estimated that approximately 25,000 cases of invasive candidiasis (IC) occur in the United States each year.[7,8] The true incidence of candidemia is likely higher because of the poor sensitivity (approximately 50%) of blood cultures (BCs) for detection of Candida spp. Newer automated rapid nonculture-based test (NCT) molecular platforms have improved the diagnostic yield in patients with IC.[3] Candida auris, an emerging multidrug-resistant species that is difficult to identify, has been associated with nosocomial outbreaks and IC globally and in the United States.[7] The attributable mortality for IC, including candidemia, is significant, and the excess health care cost ranges from $35,000 to $68,000 for each episode of candidemia in the United States.[3,9]

The incidence rate of invasive aspergillosis (IA) per million persons rose from 32.8 in 2000 to 46.0 in 2013, especially in SOT recipients.[10] Aspergillosis accounted for 59% of all invasive fungal infections and was associated with a 6-week mortality rate of 22% in severely immunocompromised patients.[11,12]

Thus, the overall burden of disease caused by nosocomial fungal infections is substantial. Limitations of the current diagnostic tests, the emergence of resistant fungal pathogens, and significant mortality make the prevention of fungal HAIs increasingly important. The epidemiology, risk factors associated with nosocomial fungal infections, and control and prevention strategies are discussed in the following paragraphs.[13–15]

COMMON NOSOCOMIAL INFECTIONS CAUSED BY YEASTS
Candida spp.

Candida spp., especially Candida albicans, are part of the human microbial flora; hence, most candidal infections are endogenous in origin. IC, namely, candidemia, disseminated hematogenous infections, or deep-seated infections can occur in immunocompromised patients, such as those with neutropenia, and in critically ill patients. In patients with chemotherapy-induced neutropenia and mucositis, candidemia may originate from the gastrointestinal tract. However, in critically ill patients, the source of candidemia is most likely a CVC colonized by Candida spp. from the patient's endogenous microflora or acquired from the health care environment.[1,3] Candida spp. have been isolated from environmental cultures of the floor, countertops, and other inanimate surfaces in the hospital.[16,17] Patient acquisition and colonization with Candida spp. found in the hospital environment and food has been demonstrated.[8,16] The propensity of Candida spp., especially Candida parapsilosis, to cause CLABSIs is likely related to this pathogen's ability to form biofilms on catheters.[18]

Overall, Candida spp. accounted for 6.4% of 356,633 HAIs reported to the National Healthcare Safety Network (NHSN) at the Centers for Disease Control and Prevention (CDC) between 2015 and 2017.[4] Approximately, 11% of infections in North American ICUs were due to Candida spp.[19] Notably, Candida spp. were the most common cause of CLABSIs in the ICU and hospital wards, accounting for 25% and 16.7% of CLABSIs, respectively.[4] The increasing proportion of patients with candidemia in non-ICU settings is possibly due to the presence of long-term CVCs.[3] Additional risk factors for nosocomial candidemia are listed in **Table 1**. Candidemia-related hospitalization per 100,000 population rose by 52%, from 3.65 to 5.56 cases between 2000 and 2005.[20] However, from 2009 to 2017, the change in incidence of IC-related hospitalizations remained low at 1.3%.[21]

A study of IC from 203 centers in the United States between 2009 and 2017 identified *C albicans* (48%), *Candida glabrata* (24%), *C parapsilosis* (11%), and *C tropicalis* (7%) as the most common *Candida* pathogens.[21,22] The overall 90-day crude mortality rate associated with candidemia was 39%. Overall, there has been an increase in the proportion of infections caused by nonalbicans *Candida* spp.[22,23] In the United States, nonalbicans *Candida* spp. were reported to cause most candidemias.[22] Most of the nonalbicans species, particularly *C glabrata*, are reported from cancer centers in the United States.[22] In contrast, higher rates of *C parapsilosis* and *C tropicalis* are reported from Latin America.[24] Nonalbicans *Candida* spp. have an increased likelihood of resistance to fluconazole: 16% of *C glabrata*, 78% of *Candida krusei*, and 11% of *C guilliermondii*.[24]

Although most cases of IC are endogenous, exogenous transmission of *Candida* spp. may occur. Characteristics of specific *Candida* spp. may influence the risk for exogenous transmission and nosocomial infections in certain patient populations.

In molecular epidemiologic studies, *C albicans* has been implicated in nosocomial transmission among patients in burn units.[25] Person-to-person transmission has also been reported from geriatric short-stay units.[26]

C parapsilosis candidemia is common in the neonatal population[18,22] and transplant recipients.[18] *C parapsilosis* is commonly isolated from the hands of health care workers (HCWs), and a review of molecular epidemiologic studies of outbreaks suggests horizontal transmission from HCWs to neonates.[18] The ability of *C parapsilosis* to produce biofilms and its selective growth advantage in glucose-rich hyperalimentation solutions in total parenteral nutrition (TPN) may explain its propensity to cause outbreaks associated with CVCs.[18] Hence, the frequent isolation of *C parapsilosis* should prompt measures to enhance hand hygiene and appropriate care of CVCs.

Emerging *Candida* spp. that are relatively resistant to fluconazole such as *C auris*,[8] *C guilliermondii*,[27] and *Candida rugosa*[28] have also been associated with nosocomial outbreaks, some involving CVCs. *C auris* first isolated from the external ear canal of a hospitalized patient in Japan in 2009 has since been associated with nosocomial outbreaks in health care facilities globally.[8,29] Its ability to persistently colonize patients and survive on surfaces for months has contributed to outbreaks.[8,29–32]

The first *C auris* case in the United States was identified in New York in 2013.[30] As of March 19, 2021, there have been 1708 confirmed clinical cases in the United States, most of which have occurred in New York City, New Jersey, and Chicago, Illinois.[8] More recently, an outbreak was reported in patients with coronaviorus disease 2019 (COVID-19) who received care in a dedicated COVID-19 unit.[31] Infection and colonization have been detected mainly in critically ill patients with comorbidities and exposure to healthcare facility (HCF). Risk factors for *C auris* are similar as those for other *Candida* infections and include prolonged ICU stay, recent surgery, antibiotic and antifungal use, CVCs or indwelling urinary catheters, TPN, hematological malignancies, SOT, HSCT, and immunosuppression.[30,32]

C auris has been misidentified as *C haemulonii* when using conventional diagnostic methods.[8,29,30,32] It has been cultured from blood, urine, bile, wounds, and rectum.[8,30,32] Most of the reported *C auris* cases are BSIs, but pericarditis, otitis, and wound infections can occur.[30,32] *C auris* is often resistant to one or more classes of antifungal agents.[31–33] Of 35 isolates in the United States, 86% were resistant to fluconazole, 43% to amphotericin B, and 3% to echinocandins,[29] which is the drug of choice in clinical infections.[8,29] Despite geographic variability, overall mortality rates range from 35% to 72%.[32]

Other Yeasts

Malassezia spp. are lipophilic yeasts that are frequent skin colonizers and the cause of pityriasis. Outbreaks of *Malassezia* fungemia have been reported in premature neonates and immunocompromised patients.[34,35] Prolonged use of CVCs and TPN were important predisposing conditions.[34,35]

Trichosporon spp. fungemia has been reported in patients with hematologic malignancies and HSCT and SOT recipients.[36] Systemic disease has also been reported in premature neonates, diabetics, nonneutropenic ICU, and burn patients.[36,37] Common risk factors in cases of nosocomial trichosporonosis are the presence of a CVC and exposure to prior antibiotics.[37] Waterborne outbreaks have also been reported.[38] The reported mortality rate ranges from 42% to 83%.[36,37]

Most outbreaks of nosocomial IC and invasive infections with other yeasts have been associated with CVCs. Hence, infection control strategies targeted to improve adherence to hand hygiene recommendations, including avoidance of long nails and artificial nails, adherence to guidelines for insertion and care of CVCs, and prompt removal of unnecessary catheters are important in the prevention of these infections.[39]

NOSOCOMIAL INFECTIONS CAUSED BY MOLDS

Unlike IC, which can affect relatively immunocompetent patients, invasive disease caused by *Aspergillus* spp. and other molds generally involves severely immunocompromised patients. *Aspergillus* spp. account for most mold infections: 76% among HSCT recipients and 81% among SOT recipients.[1] Although several outbreaks of environmental airborne fungal infection within hospital settings have been reported,[5] most cases of IA are sporadic. At present, there is no uniform definition of what constitutes nosocomial aspergillosis. One of the primary reasons for the difficulty in defining hospital-acquired aspergillosis is that the incubation period of IA is unknown.[2] Moreover, the prolonged period of immunosuppression in high-risk patients such as HSCT recipients and frequent hospital admissions and discharges make it difficult to determine if exposure to *Aspergillus* spores occurred during hospitalization or within the community. Generally, invasive disease that occurs after 1 week of hospitalization is considered nosocomial.[2] Although most hospital outbreaks have been caused by *Aspergillus* spp.,[5] other airborne molds have also been implicated, including *Zygomycetes* spp.,[5,40] *Fusarium* spp.,[5] and *Scedosporium* spp.[5,41] The risks factors for mold infections and vehicles of transmission are summarized in **Table 1** and **Table 2**.

Table 2
Reported vehicles of transmission in invasive mold infections and associated types of infections

Mold	Reservoir or Source	Type of Infection
Aspergillus	Contaminated air, ventilation system, air filters, false ceilings and insulation material, water supply, plumbing, showers, food, ornamental plants, arm boards, dressing package	Invasive pulmonary and disseminated aspergillosis, cutaneous disease
Mucorales	Contaminated air, Elastoplast adhesive dressing, karaya ostomy bag, wooden tongue depressor, ventilation systems, water-damaged plaster, cornstarch, linens	Cutaneous infections, sinopulmonary disease, gastrointestinal mucormycosis
Fusarium	Contaminated air, contact lens solution, showers, sink drains and faucets, water tanks	Keratitis, disseminated fusariosis
Scedosporium	Contaminated air	Pulmonary and disseminated disease, cutaneous lesions

Aspergillus spp.

Aspergillus spp. are ubiquitous molds found widely in the environment. Exposure to airborne spores of Aspergillus occurs frequently in the environment, especially near decaying organic matter. Although these conidia (2.5–3.0 mm in diameter) are frequently inhaled, invasive pulmonary disease is rare in immunocompetent persons. Opportunistic IA occurs primarily in high-risk severely immunocompromised patients namely allogeneic HSCT and neutropenic patients with hematologic malignancies. Aspergillus fumigatus is most often associated with invasive disease, although Aspergillus flavus, Aspergillus niger, and Aspergillus terreus have also been isolated from patients.[1,42] Aspergillosis is an important cause of morbidity and mortality ranging from 65% to 92% in this high-risk population.[2,43]

SOT recipients,[2,44] patients with acquired immunodeficiency syndrome (AIDS), and those with chronic granulomatous disease are also at risk for IA.[2] There are increasing reports of IA in critically ill patients in the ICU, including patients with chronic obstructive pulmonary disease, severe influenza, COVID-19, liver cirrhosis, and those receiving corticosteroids.[2,45–47]

Aspergillus outbreaks

The information on the environmental exposures and the association with infection has been derived from investigations of outbreaks of aspergillosis in hospital settings. An extensive review of nosocomial aspergillosis identified 53 reported outbreaks involving 458 patients.[48] Of these, 33 outbreaks involving 299 patients (65%) occurred in HSCT recipients or patients with hematologic malignancies. Other patient populations involved in these outbreaks were SOT recipients (10%), predominately renal transplant recipients; patients without severe immunodeficiency (8%); and patients on high-dose steroids (3%).[48] Aspergillosis was associated with mortality greater than 50% in patients with hematologic malignancies, HSCT and SOT recipients, and patients with severe immunodeficiency. The lung was the most common site of infection, with 5% involving the surgical site or skin. A fumigatus and A flavus were the most identified species. Volumetric air sampling performed during epidemiologic investigations in 24 of the outbreaks noted spore counts ranging from 0 to 100 spores per cubic meter. Outbreaks were primarily attributed to airborne infections related to construction or renovation activities in about 50% of cases and to compromised air quality in 17%.[48] The various environmental vehicles implicated in the transmission of Aspergillus spp. and other molds have also been detailed in the CDC guidelines for environmental infection control in HCFs (see **Table 2**).[14]

The most frequent nosocomial source of Aspergillus infection is contaminated air, but Aspergillus has also been recovered from the hospital water supply and plumbing systems.[2,38] The highest airborne Aspergillus spore counts were detected in patient's bathrooms, suggesting possible aerosolization of Aspergillus spores from the shower facilities.[2] The clinical implications of this finding remain to be defined.

Although the association between construction and IA has often been reported, there is poor correlation of the Aspergillus spp. recovered from the hospital environment and species isolated from patients with aspergillosis.[2] One explanation for this discordance between hospital and patient strains of Aspergillus might relate to the lack of a clearly defined incubation period for aspergillosis and the relationship to exposure within the hospital environment and subsequent infection.[2] Other factors include the methods of air sampling used, the broad diversity of Aspergillus spp. in the environment, and the various methods used for typing of Aspergillus and other pathogenic molds.[49,50]

Zygomycetes

Zygomycetes are ubiquitous molds found in the soil and decaying organic matter in the environment. Infection often occurs via inhalation of fungal spores, resulting in sinopulmonary disease, but systemic infection can result from inoculation of the skin or gastrointestinal mucosa.[51] Although infection caused by Zygomycetes is uncommon, it is often a fatal disease. In a review of 929 patients with zygomycosis, mortality was 76% with pulmonary zygomycosis and 100% with disseminated and central nervous system diseases.[52]

Nosocomial infections caused by Zygomycetes have been recently reviewed.[40] Clusters of cutaneous infections have occurred in orthopedic and cardiothoracic patients, children with leukemia, and burn patients. These infections were associated with Elastoplast adhesive dressings possibly contaminated with Rhizopus and Absidia spp.[40] Outbreaks in patients with hematologic malignancies have resulted from airborne transmission associated with contamination of hospital ventilation systems.[5] Use of negative pressure rooms during construction has also been implicated in a cluster of invasive mucormycosis infection among SOT recipients during a 12-month period.[53] Water-damaged plaster has been associated with Rhizomucor pusillius outbreak in patients with leukemia.[40] Unusual routes of transmission have been traced to the use of contaminated wooden tongue depressors, nonsterile karaya (plant-derived adhesive) for securing ostomy bags, and wooden tongue depressors.[40] An outbreak of gastrointestinal zygomycosis caused by Rhizopus in 12 patients with hematologic malignances was traced to contaminated cornstarch used as an excipient in the manufacture of allopurinol and ready-to-eat foods.[54] Additionally, hospital linens have also been implicated in outbreaks.[55]

Fusarium spp.

Fusarium is a soil saprophyte and causes keratitis and onychomycosis in humans.[56] Outbreaks of keratitis caused by possible contamination of contact lens solutions have been described.[56,57] Invasive disease has been reported in patients with prolonged neutropenia, especially in HSCT recipients[56,58] and to a lesser extent in SOT recipients.[56] The incidence of fusariosis is estimated to be 4 to 5 cases per 1000 matched allogeneic HSCT recipients to as high as 20 cases per 1000 mismatched recipients.[59] Fusariosis in HSCT recipients has a bimodal distribution, with a peak before engraftment and later during the period of graft-versus-host disease (GVHD), and is associated with an actuarial survival of 13%.[58] Most infections are believed to be caused by airborne transmission; however, contamination of the water system in the hospital has been reported to result in dispersal of airborne conidia.[38]

Other Molds

Several other pathogenic molds have been associated with HAIs. Nosocomial outbreaks caused by Scedosporium spp. during hospital reconstruction have been reported.[60] Phialemonium spp. have been linked to outbreaks of intravascular infections in patients undergoing hemodialysis (HD), resulting from contamination of water distribution systems.[61] A multistate outbreak of fungal meningitis, parameningeal, and joint infections occurred in 753 patients who received injections of contaminated methylprednisone acetate solutions, resulting in 64 (8.5%) deaths across 20 states. The predominant pathogen detected in this outbreak was Exserophilum.[62]

Pneumocystis jiroveci

Opportunistic pneumonia caused by *Pneumocystis jirovecii* has been traditionally attributed to reactivation of latent infection during periods of severe T-cell–mediated immunosuppression, particularly in transplant recipients and patients with AIDS. However, recent data suggest possible person-to-person transmission or common environmental source as a potential mode of transmission.[63] Molecular evidence has also identified nosocomial person-to-person transmission of *Pneumocystis jiroveci* to be the likely cause of outbreaks of *Pneumocystis* pneumonia, particularly among renal transplant recipients.[63] In a meta-analysis of 30 outbreaks, more than 80% occurred among renal transplant recipients. None of the patients received appropriate antipneumocystis prophylaxis.

STRATEGIES FOR PREVENTION OF NOSOCOMIAL CANDIDIASIS
Prevention of Intravascular Catheter-Related Candidemia

Guidelines for the prevention of CLABSI have been published.[13] Although randomized clinical trials have shown that daily 2% chlorhexidine gluconate (CHG) bathing of patients in the ICU decreases the incidence of nosocomial multidrug-resistant bacterial BSIs, few studies have evaluated the impact on candidemia.[64,65] A meta-analysis of five randomized controlled trials evaluating the efficacy of CHG bathing in reducing BSIs showed that CHG had no effect on fungal BSIs.[65] However, a more recent meta-analysis of 26 randomized and nonrandomized studies demonstrated that CHG bathing was associated with a significant reduction in BSIs, including those due to *Candida* spp.[64] A multicenter, randomized, crossover study also found that the incidence of fungal CLABSIs was 90% lower during the CHG intervention period compared with the control period.[66] Despite the conflicting results, use of daily CHG bathing in patients in the ICU is a simple and effective strategy to decrease the overall rate of primary BSIs.

Additionally, the use of disinfection caps, which include alcohol or alcohol/CHG combinations, placed on needleless connectors or access ports has demonstrated decreased CLABSI rates.[67,68]

Unlike other *Candida* spp., *C auris* can spread rapidly in HCFs and lead to nosocomial outbreaks that can be difficult to contain. Patients can remain colonized even after a year, leading to environmental shedding where it can survive and persist on a wide range of surfaces.[32] A single case of *C auris* requires rapid implementation of infection control measures and investigation. When *C auris* is suspected or confirmed, the patient should be placed in a single room under contact precautions with reinforcement of hand hygiene practices. Additional infection prevention and control measures include daily and terminal cleaning and disinfection of patient care areas using an Environmental Protection Agency–registered hospital-grade disinfectant effective against *Clostridioides difficile* spores, contact tracing and testing, prospective laboratory surveillance to identify other potential cases for at least 1 month until there is no evidence of ongoing transmission, and interfacility communication during patient transfer.[8,29]

STRATEGIES FOR PREVENTION OF NOSOCOMIAL ASPERGILLOSIS AND MOLD INFECTIONS

Aspergillosis is primarily acquired by inhalation of fungal spores and subsequent invasive disease in immunocompromised patients. Hence, the primary infection control strategy is to minimize exposure to airborne environmental fungal spores within HCFs during the high-risk period. Exposure to fungal spores of *Aspergillus* spp. and other pathogenic molds after hospital discharge may occur in high-risk patients, such as allogeneic HSCT recipients with chronic GVHD who are administered corticosteroids. Patient education to minimize exposures to fungal spores and chemoprophylaxis with antifungal agents may be necessary. Guidelines for the use of antifungal agents for prophylaxis against IA have been previously published[15] and updated.[2]

The CDC and Healthcare Infection Control Practices Advisory Committee have published recommendations regarding environmental infection control measures to prevent nosocomial mold infections in HCFs.[14] These recommendations include infection control strategies and engineering controls directed primarily for the prevention of exposure of immunocompromised patients to environmental airborne fungal spores of *Aspergillus* and other molds.[14]

Because opportunistic *Aspergillus* and airborne mold infections occur primarily in severely immunocompromised patients such as HSCT recipients; one of the main components of these prevention strategies is the provision of a protected environment (PE) for these patients within the HCF.

Protected Environment

A PE is a specialized patient care environment in acute care hospitals for the care of allogeneic HSCT recipients.[13,14] The benefit of a PE for other immunocompromised patients such as autologous HSCT or SOT recipients remains undefined.[14,60] A PE is designed to minimize HSCT patient exposure to airborne environmental *Aspergillus* and other fungal spores. The essential features of a PE are shown in **Box 1**. Additional infection control measures for patients housed in a PE include (1) daily monitoring and maintenance of a positive pressure in PE areas, (2) minimizing exposures to activities that can cause aerosolization of fungal spores (eg, vacuuming), (3) minimizing the length of time that the patients are outside the PE for procedures, and (4) provision of high-efficiency respiratory protection (eg, N95 respirators) when outside the PE if there is ongoing construction activity in the HCF.[14] The effectiveness of respirators in the absence of construction or the use of surgical masks to prevent fungal infection has not been evaluated.

The other infection control strategies and engineering control recommendations that reduce exposure to environmental airborne *Aspergillus* and other fungal spores emphasize the provision of safe air during routine care and importantly during hospital construction.[14] These strategies are outlined in **Table 3**.

Box 1
Protective environment

Requirements of protective environment rooms
- Central or point-of-use high-efficiency particulate air (HEPA) filters with 99.97% efficiency for removing particles 0.3 mm or larger
- Directed airflow, air intake occurs at 1 side and air exhaust occurs at the opposite side of the room
- Positive air pressure differential between the room and corridor ($\geq$2.5 Pa)
- Maintenance of 12 or more air changes per hour
- Well-sealed patient rooms

Data from Sehulster L, Chinn RY. Guidelines for environmental infection control in health-care facilities. Recommendations of CDC and the Healthcare Infection Control Practices Advisory Committee (HICPAC). MMWR Recomm Rep 2003;52(RR–10):1–42.

Table 3
Environmental infection control measures in healthcare facilities to minimize exposure to fungal spores

Recommendations	Rating Category
Air handling systems	
Use the American Institute of Architects (AIA) guidelines or state regulations for design and construction of ventilations systems[164]	1C
Conduct ICRA and provide adequate number of PE rooms for the HSCT population	1A, 1C
Monitor ventilation systems for removal of particulates and excess moisture Proper location and maintenance of air intake and exhaust outlets, for example, removal of bird roosts from near air intake outlets to prevent entry of fungal spores Appropriate installation, maintenance, and disposal of HVAC filters Monitor PE areas for ACH, filtration, and pressure differentials	1B, 1C
Develop a contingency plan for backup capacity in case of a power failure	1C
Coordinate HVAC system shutdowns with infection control staff to allow for safe air handling to PE areas and to relocate immunocompromised patients if necessary	1C
Infection control measures during construction projects	
Set up a multidisciplinary team that includes infection control staff to coordinate proactive preventive measures to reduce exposure to fungal spores and monitor adherence	1B, 1C
Provide education to HCWs and the construction crew in immunocompromised patient care areas regarding airborne infections	1C
Perform an ICRA to assess potential exposure of high-risk patients to high ambient air fungal spore count	1B, 1C
Develop and implement measures to keep airborne spores from construction areas away from patient care units Dust control measures (eg, dust barriers, safe air handling, negative pressure in construction work zones) Water damage response plan to prevent fungal growth	1B, 1C
Maintain surveillance for cases of HCF-associated aspergillosis and mold infections in immunocompromised patients	1B
Undertake an epidemiologic investigation if a case of nosocomial *Aspergillus* or other mold infection is detected Surveillance for additional cases Determine appropriate air handling in the PE and in construction areas. Conduct environmental assessment to identify the source Take corrective action to improve deficiencies identified and to eliminate the source of fungal spores	1B
Environmental service recommendations to minimize exposure to fungal spores	
Avoid carpeting and upholstered furniture and furnishings in areas housing immunocompromised patients	1B

(continued on next page)

Table 3 (*continued*)	
Recommendations	**Rating Category**

Avoid cleaning methods that disperse dust
  Wet dust horizontal surfaces using EPA-registered hospital
    disinfectant
  Equip vacuums with HEPA filters
  Close the doors of rooms of immunocompromised patients when
    cleaning
  Dry carpeting immediately if wet to prevent growth of fungi,
    replace if wet after 72 h
	1B

Avoid fresh flowers and potted plants in areas housing immunocompromised patients	II

Abbreviations: ACH, air changes per hour; EPA, Environmental Protection Agency; HCW, health care worker; HSCT, hematopoeitic stem cell transplantation; HVAC, heating ventilation air conditioning; 1A, strongly recommended for all hospitals and supported by well-designed experimental or epidemiologic evidence; 1B, strongly recommended for all hospitals and viewed as effective by experts because of strong rationale and suggestive evidence; 1C, required by state or federal regulation or representing an established association standard; ICRA, infection control risk assessment; II, suggested for implementation in many hospitals, supported by suggestive clinical or epidemiologic studies with a strong theoretical rationale or definitive studies applicable to some but not all hospitals; PE, protected environment.

Data from Sehulster L, Chinn RY. Guidelines for environmental infection control in health-care facilities. Recommendations of CDC and the Healthcare Infection Control Practices Advisory Committee (HICPAC). MMWR Recomm Rep 2003;52(RR–10):1–42; and Tablan OC, Anderson LJ, Besser R, et al. Guidelines for preventing health-care–associated pneumonia, 2003: recommen- dations of CDC and the Healthcare Infection Control Practices Advisory Committee. MMWR Recomm Rep 2004;53(RR–3):1–36.

Infection Control Risk Assessment

Infection control risk assessment is a multistep process that determines the potential effect of construction within an HCF on the environment and exposure of at-risk patients to infectious agents, particularly fungal spores.[69] Implementation of recommended infection control strategies during hospital construction has been successful in the prevention of fungal contamination of air in patient care areas in prospective environmental surveillance studies using cultures and polymerase chain reaction (PCR) assays for detection of airborne fungi.[70,71] Newer mobile nonfiltration-based air treatment systems that use exposure to electric fields and electrostatic nanofiltration to destroy airborne organisms have also been effective in preventing fungal contamination during construction.[72,73] Additional recommendations for the prevention and control of nosocomial aspergillosis are included in **Table 4**.

STRATEGIES FOR PREVENTION OF FUNGAL INFECTION IN HEMATOPOIETIC STEM CELL TRANSPLANTATION RECIPIENTS

To implement strategies to prevent fungal infections in the severely immunocompromised population, it is important to define the high-risk periods. In the allogeneic HSCT recipient, the risk of infections is related to the time from transplant.[15] The post-HSCT period is generally divided into 3 phases:

- Phase I: the preengraftment period (<30 days after HSCT). Risk of infection is related to prolonged neutropenia and disruption of the mucocutaneous barriers

Table 4
Recommendations for prevention and control of healthcare–associated pulmonary aspergillosis

Recommendations	Rating Category
Staff education	
Educate HCWs about infection control procedures to reduce HCA-PA	II
Surveillance	
Conduct surveillance for HCA-PA in severely immunocompromised patients[a]	1A
Monitor for HCA-PA by surveillance and periodic review of microbiologic and histopathologic data	II
Do not perform routine surveillance cultures of patients or devices	1B
Monitor ventilation status of PE and maintain appropriate standards	1B
Specialized care units for high-risk patients	
Provide a PE for care of allogeneic HSCT recipients	1B
Do not routinely use LAF in the PE	1B
No recommendation for a PE for autologous HSCT and SOT recipients	UR
Minimize the time high-risk patients are outside the PE for procedures	II
High-risk patients to wear N95 respirators outside the PE during ongoing construction.	
No recommendation for type of mask outside the PE when no construction	
When case of aspergillosis occurs	
Assess if health care related or community acquired	
Determine if there is an increase in the number of cases of HCA-PA and IB length of hospital stay	1B
Determine if there is ventilation deficiency in the PE	1B
If not health care related, continue routine maintenance as mentioned earlier	
If health care related, conduct epidemiologic investigation to identify and eliminate source	1B
Use EPA-registered antifungal biocide for decontamination of structural materials	

Abbreviations: EPA, Environmental Protection Agency; HCA-PA, health care–associated pulmonary aspergillosis; HCW, health care worker; HSCT, hematopoeitic stem cell transplantation; 1B, strongly recommended for all hospitals and supported by well-designed experimental or epidemiologic evidence; 1b, strongly recommended for all hospitals and viewed as effective by experts because of strong rationale and suggestive evidence; II, suggested for implementation in many hospitals, supported by suggestive clinical or epidemiologic studies with a strong theoretical rationale or definitive studies applicable to some but not all hospitals; LAF, laminar airflow; PE, protective environment; SOT, solid organ transplantation; UR, unresolved, practices for which insufficient evidence or consensus regarding efficacy exists.

[a] Severely immunocompromised patients, those with absolute neutrophil counts less than 500/mm^3 × 2 wk or less than 100/mm^3 × 1 wk, for example, HSCT and SOT recipients and patients on prolonged high-dose steroids.

Data from Sehulster L, Chinn RY. Guidelines for environmental infection control in health-care facilities. Recommendations of CDC and the Healthcare Infection Control Practices Advisory Committee (HICPAC). MMWR Recomm Rep 2003;52(RR-10):1–42; and Tablan OC, Anderson LJ, Besser R, et al. Guidelines for preventing health-care–associated pneumonia, 2003: recom- mendations of CDC and the Healthcare Infection Control Practices Advisory Committee. MMWR Recomm Rep 2004;53(RR-3):1–36.

because of cytotoxic chemotherapy. Infections during this period are generally caused by bacteria, *Herpes simplex virus*, *Candida*, and *Aspergillus* spp.

- Phase II: the postengraftment phase (30–100 days after HSCT). Risk of infection is related to impaired cell-mediated immunity based on the severity of GVHD and the intensity of immunosuppressive therapy used for treatment. Infections during this period are caused by cytomegalovirus (CMV), *Aspergillus* spp, and *P jiroveci*.
- Phase III: the late phase (>100 days after HSCT). Risk of infection is dictated by chronic GVHD and its treatment. Pathogens are primarily CMV, varicella-zoster virus, encapsulated bacteria, and *Aspergillus* spp.

As a general measure, avoidance of certain foods has been recommended to reduce exposure to fungi, primarily during the high-risk period of neutropenia (such as during receipt of conditioning therapy).[15] These foods include unpasteurized dairy products, cheeses made from mold cultures, uncooked eggs, meat, fish, tofu, unwashed vegetables, and fruits.[15]

IA displays a bimodal distribution, with increasing number of cases of late-onset disease (>40 days after HSCT) that is associated with immunosuppression for chronic GVHD.[12] A similar pattern of late-onset disease has also been noted with invasive infection with Zygomycetes and Fusarium[58] spp. in HSCT recipients. Educating the patient in minimizing exposure to *Aspergillus* spp. and pathogenic molds outside the hospital is important. However, because the risk of exposure within the hospital and community settings cannot be eliminated, strategies such as the use of antifungal prophylaxis may be necessary.

Prevention of Invasive Candidiasis

Antifungal chemoprophylaxis during the preengraftment period of neutropenia and mucositis can prevent the dissemination of endogenous *Candida* spp. from the gastrointestinal tract of patients. The antifungals are outlined in **Table 5**.

Diagnosis of Invasive Candidiasis

Although BCs are positive in about 50% of patients with IC, they are considered the gold standard for the diagnosis of candidiasis.[3,74] Thus, the true incidence of nosocomial candidemia is often underestimated. This has resulted in the increasing use of fungal biomarkers for the detection of candidemia and IC. These assays are used in the clinical management of patients with suspected IC in situations where BCs may be negative. However, the use of these assays for routine surveillance of nosocomial IC is yet to be defined. 1,3 β-D-Glucan (BG) assays and PCR-based assays are some of these tests used to aid in the diagnosis of IC (**Table 6**).[3] Although β-D glucan has high false-positive rates and is not specific, it has been shown to have a high negative predictive value in the ICU setting.[3,75] In-house PCR assays are not validated or standardized.[3,74]

NCT molecular platforms, including fully automated multiplex T2 Magnetic Resonance (T2MR) and T2Candida Panel (T2 Biosystems, Lexington, Massachusetts),[74,75] have the potential to improve early diagnosis and management of IC in high-risk patients and outbreak settings. The Food and Drug Administration (FDA)-approved T2Candida Panel detects the five most common *Candida* spp. from whole blood by category: *C albicans* and/or *C tropicalis* (A/T); *C parapsilosis* (P); *C krusei*, and/or *C glabrata* (K/G).[75,76]

C auris, a nationally reportable pathogen, is difficult to identify and has been often misidentified as *C haemulonii*, *C famata, C sake, Rhodotorula glutinis, Rhodotorula mucilaginosa*, and *Saccharomyces* or less commonly as *C catenulate, Candida lusitaniae, C guilliermondii*, or *C parapsilosis* or only to the *Candida* spp. level when using

Table 5
List of antifungal agents used for the prevention and treatment of invasive fungal infections

Antifungal Agent	Spectrum of Activity	Expected Resistance	Adverse Events	Drug Interactions	Clinical Considerations
Polyenes					
Conventional and lipid-based formulations of amphotericin B	Most yeast Dimorphic fungi Molds: *Aspergillus fumigatus*, *Aspergillus lentulus*, *Mucor* spp., *Rhizopus* spp., *Fusarium* spp.	*Candida lusitaniae*, *C guillermondii*, *C rugosa*, non-*fumigatus* *Aspergillus* (*Aspergillus terreus*, *A. ustus*), *Trichosporon* spp., *Scedosporium apiospermum*, *Scedosporium prolificans*	Infusion reactions (hypoxia, fever, chills), phlebitis, nausea, vomiting, anemia, nephrotoxicity, elevated liver enzymes, hypersensitivity reaction	Increased risk of nephrotoxicity with other nephrotoxic agents and hypotension with blood pressure lowering agents	Lipid formulations are associated with less nephrotoxicity and infusion reactions
Triazoles					
Fluconazole[a]	Most yeast, including most *Candida* spp. Dimorphic fungi	*Candida krusei* Increasing resistance in *C glabrata* Molds Dematiaceous fungi	Nausea, vomiting, diarrhea, headaches, hepatitis, cholestasis and fulminant hepatitis, allergic reactions	Inhibits CYP1A2, CYP2C19 CYP2C9, and CYP3A4 and may increase the concentration of several classes of drugs, including, anticonvulsants, antiarrhythmics, steroids, QT-prolonging agents, immunosuppressant and antineoplastic agents, anticoagulants, ergot alkaloids, HMG-CoA reductase inhibitors (statins)	Dose adjustment required if GFR is < 50 mL/min Excellent oral bioavailability Highest penetration in CSF and vitreous among azoles High urine concentration and preferred for cystitis Step-down therapy in a critically ill patient who becomes stable Alternative initial therapy in noncritically ill patients

Drug	Spectrum	Adverse effects	Drug interactions	Comments
Isavuconazole	Yeast, including all *Candida* spp. Mold: most *Aspergillus* spp. and *Mucor* spp. Dimorphic fungi	Nausea, vomiting, diarrhea, abdominal pain, constipation, headache, rash, peripheral edema, dyspnea, cough, hepatotoxicity, hypokalemia, Dose-dependent QT shortening	Moderate inhibitor of CYP3A4 and inhibits the metabolism of sirolimus, tacrolimus, cyclosporine, mycophenolate mofetil, and other drugs metabolized by CYP3A4	Excellent oral bioavailability Large volume of distribution with long half-life Newly approved extended spectrum triazole for invasive aspergillosis and mucormycosis Use with caution in patients with severe hepatic impairment
Itraconazole[b]	Most yeast Dimorphic fungi Molds: most *Aspergillus* spp. Dematiaceous fungi	*Candida krusei*, *Aspergillus lentulus*, *Aspergillus terreus*, *Fusarium solani*, *Rhizopus* spp., *Mucor* spp., *S apiospermum*, *S prolificans*	Nausea, vomiting, diarrhea, abdominal discomfort, peripheral and pulmonary edema, CHF, hypertension, hypokalemia, hepatotoxicity	Potent CYP3A4 and P-glycoprotein inhibitor that increases the concentration of several classes of drugs, including calcium channel blockers, antiarrhythmics, immunosuppressant agents, anticoagulants, ergot alkaloids, HMG-CoA reductase inhibitors Contraindicated in patients with ventricular failure	No IV formulation available Not well studied for invasive candidiasis Primarily used in dimorphic fungi infections Therapeutic drug monitoring required Use with caution in patients with liver and renal failure
Posaconazole[a,b]	Yeast Dimorphic fungi Molds: *Aspergillus* spp., *F solani*, *Mucor* spp., *Rhizopus* spp. Dematiaceous fungi	*Scedosporium prolificans*, *S apiospermum*	Nausea, vomiting, diarrhea, fever, headache, coughing, hypokalemia, and liver enzyme elevation	Potent CYP3A4 inhibitor Concomitant use of drugs that are metabolized through CYP3A4 (sirolimus, ergot alkaloids, HMG-CoA reductase inhibitors) or CYP3A4 substrates that prolong the QT interval (pimozide, quinidine) is contraindicated	Indicated for oropharyngeal but not primary candidiasis Primarily used for invasive *Aspergillus* and *Candida* prophylaxis in high-risk patients Oral suspension has unpredictable bioavailability

(continued on next page)

Table 5
(continued)

Antifungal Agent	Spectrum of Activity	Expected Resistance	Adverse Events	Drug Interactions	Clinical Considerations
					IV formulation should be avoided if GFR <50 mL/min
Voriconazole	Yeast Dimorphic fungi molds: most *Aspergillus* spp. Dematiaceous fungi	*Aspergillus lentulus,* *Rhizopus* spp., *Mucor* spp.	Skin rash, photosensitivity, hepatic toxicity, transient visual disturbances, hallucinations, periostitis,	Inhibits CYP2C19, CYP2C9, and CYP3A4 and increases the concentration of several classes of drugs, including steroids, anticonvulsants, antiarrhythmics, QT- prolonging agents, immunosuppressant and antineoplastic agents, anticoagulants, ergot alkaloids, HMG-CoA reductase inhibitors	IV formulation: cyclodextrin vehicle can accumulate if GFR <50 mL/min Dose adjustment required in hepatic impairment Good CSF and vitreous penetration Therapeutic drug monitoring required First-line therapy for *Aspergillus* infections Step-down oral therapy for patients with fluconazole-resistant *Candida* spp.
Echinocandins					
Anidulafungin	*Candida* spp. *Aspergillus* spp. Dimorphic fungi	*Cryptococcus* spp. *Trichosporon* spp. *Aspergillus lentulus* *Fusarium* spp. *S prolificans* *Mucor* spp. Dematiaceous fungi	Nausea, vomiting, diarrhea, fever, rash, insomnia, infusion reaction, edema, elevated liver enzymes, hypokalemia, hypomagnesemia	No major drug interactions	Only available in IV formulation Does not penetrate the eye, CNS, or urine Fist-line therapy in invasive candidiasis

Drug	Active	Not active	Adverse effects	Drug interactions	Comments
Caspofungin	Candida spp. Aspergillus spp. Dimorphic fungi	Cryptococcus spp. Trichosporon spp. Aspergillus lentulus Fusarium spp. S prolificans Mucor spp. Dematiaceous fungi	Nausea, vomiting, diarrhea, headache edema, chills, rash, phlebitis, hypotension, hypokalemia, anemia, elevated liver enzymes	May decrease the serum concentration of tacrolimus Cyclosporine may increase and rifampin may decrease the concentration of caspofungin	Only available in IV formulation Does not penetrate the eye, CNS, or urine Dose adjustment in patients with moderate hepatic impairment Fist-line therapy in invasive candidiasis
Micafungin[a]	Candida spp. Aspergillus spp. Dimorphic fungi	Cryptococcus spp. Trichosporon spp. Aspergillus lentulus Fusarium spp. S prolificans Mucor spp. Dematiaceous fungi	Nausea, vomiting, diarrhea, abdominal pain, headache, insomnia, phlebitis, skin reactions, hepatotoxicity, hemolytic anemia, renal failure	Micafungin may increase the serum concentration of sirolimus	Only available in IV formulation Does not penetrate the eye, CNS, or urine Fist-line therapy in invasive candidiasis

[a] FDA-approved for candidiasis prophylaxis.
[b] FDA-approved for aspergillosis prophylaxis.

Table 6
Nonculture-based microbiologic tests for detection of invasive fungal infections

Assay	1,3 β-D-Glucan (BG)	Galactomannan (GM)	T2MR Assay
Method	Protease zymogen-based colorimetric assay	Anti-GM monoclonal antibody	Amplification and detection of Candida DNA by PCR and T2 magnetic resonance
Clinical application	Early detection of IFI	Early detection of invasive aspergillosis	Early detection of candidemia (C albicans, C glabrata, C krusei, C parapsilosis, C tropicalis
Specimen type	Serum	Serum, BAL	Whole blood
Result Interpretation	Negative < 60 pg/mL Intermediate 60–79 pg/mL Positive >80 pg/mL	Negative <0.50 Positive >0.50	Negative Positive Indeterminate
Sensitivity	67%–84%	BAL: 72%–92% Serum: 59%–83%	91.1%
Specificity	80%–90%	BAL: 78%–92% Serum: 92%–94%	99.4%
Cross-reactivity	Pneumocystis jiroveci, Coccidioides immitis, Histoplasma encapsulatum, Candida spp., Acremonium, Fusarium spp., Trichosporon spp., Aspergillus spp.	Aspergillus spp., Fusarium spp., Paecilomyces, Penicillium spp., Alternaria spp., Histoplasma encapsulatum, Blastomyces dermatitidis, Cryptococcus neoformans	Candida bracarensis, C metapsilosis, C orthopsilosis, Saccharomyces cerevisiae
False positives	Semisynthetic β-lactam antibiotics Hemodialysis with cellulose membranes, Bacteremia Transfusion given through cellulose membranes Gauze Intravenous imunoglobulins and albumin	Semisynthetic β-lactam antibiotics Mucositis or GI tract GVHD Multiple myeloma Plasmalyte used in BAL Cotton swabs	Cross-contamination

(continued on next page)

Table 6 (*continued*)			
Assay	**1,3 β-D-Glucan (BG)**	**Galactomannan (GM)**	**T2MR Assay**
False negatives	Concomitant use of antifungals	Concomitant use of antifungals	Insufficient blood volume, clotted blood sample, specimen not at room temperature, presence of inhibitors, technical error, infection caused by an organism not detected by the panel

standard laboratory methods.[8,29,32] If the aforementioned species are identified or species identity cannot be determined, the CDC recommends further characterization using alternative methodology, including matrix-assisted laser desorption/ionization time-of-flight or molecular-based methods. The GenMark ePlex BC Identification Fungal Pathogen Panel is the first FDA-approved multiplex molecular panel that detects 16 fungal targets, including *C auris*, from positive BC with a high sensitivity and specificity.[77] The T2Cauris Panel, available for research use, is able to directly detect several Candida spp. from skin, blood, and environmental samples.[78] Various other PCR methods have been developed for the detection of *C auris*.

The use of newer NCTs such as T2Candida could impact the reporting of CLABSIs to NHSN. A positive NCT result may meet the laboratory-confirmed BSI (LCBI) criteria regardless of the BC result. In response to concerns from reporting health care institutions, NHSN revised reporting criteria starting January 1, 2020: If an NCT is positive but the BC is negative 2 days before, the day of, or 1 day after for the same organism, the NCT result is disregarded. However, if no BC is collected within this timeframe, the NCT result is used for LCBI surveillance determination and will be reported as a CLABSI if criteria are met.[79]

Prevention of Aspergillosis

Given the prolonged duration of the risk for aspergillosis in HSCT recipients with chronic GVHD, guidelines recommend the use of an antimold prophylaxis (see **Table 5**).[2] The duration of prophylaxis is not clearly defined but is generally dictated by the severity of GVHD and the intensity of immunosuppression used to treat GVHD. Antimold prophylaxis has also been recommended for patients with acute myelogenous leukemia and myelodysplastic syndromes during periods of prolonged neutropenia.[2] Among patients receiving SOT, lung transplant recipients are at the greatest risk for IA. Current guidelines recommend prophylaxis with an antimold azole agent or inhaled amphotericin B product for 3 to 4 months after lung transplantation.[2] Reinitiation of prophylaxis is also recommended after intensification of immunosuppression for episodes of rejection.[2] Antimold prophylaxis may be considered in high-risk patients during institutional outbreaks of mold infection.[2]

Diagnosis of Invasive Aspergillosis

The true incidence of community-associated or nosocomial IA may be underestimated as BCs are almost always negative. Diagnosis of invasive pulmonary aspergillosis

(IPA) has traditionally relied on the isolation of fungi in culture in combination with compatible histopathologic or radiographic findings. Moreover, it is often difficult to perform invasive testing in the severely immunocompromised patients to obtain specimens for microbiological testing. This has led to the increasing use of fungal biomarkers for the detection of IA, including the BG and the galactomannan (GM) assay (see **Table 6**). These assays are increasingly used in the clinical management of patients with suspected IA. Serum and bronchoalveolar lavage (BAL) GM and BG are recommended for the diagnosis of IA in patients with hematologic malignancies and HSCT recipients. However, GM is not recommended in nonneutropenic patients given its low sensitivity, and BG is not specific for Aspergillus spp.[2] Historically, molecular assays such as PCR were excluded due to lack of standardization and validation. However, recent efforts have been directed at addressing these limitations and optimizing assay performance using various specimens.[80–82] The use of these NCTs for routine surveillance of nosocomial IA is undefined.

Prevention of Pneumocystis Pneumonia

Pneumocystis pneumonia prophylaxis is recommended for HSCT and SOT recipients during high-risk periods of immunosuppression, especially the first 100 days after transplantation.[15] Although there is potential for person-to-person transmission of *P jirovecii* leading to nosocomial outbreaks, current guidelines do not recommend specific isolation measures for the care of these hospitalized patients.[14] However, they do recommend avoiding cohorting infected patients with those who are immunocompromised.[14]

Diagnosis of Pneumocystis Pneumonia

P jirovecii cannot be cultured, and microscopic visualization of cysts and/or trophozoites in lower respiratory samples (LRSs) such as induced sputum and BAL fluids is the gold standard for diagnosis, despite the low sensitivity and specificity.[82] In recent decades, molecular diagnostics such as PCR are increasingly being used for detection of *P jirovecii* in clinical respiratory samples; although the sensitivity (91%–100%) is high, specificity is much lower (86%) and false-negative results can occur in LRSs.[81] Conversely, PCR of oropharyngeal wash fluid has a higher specificity (93%) compared with LRSs.[82] As such, quantitative PCR is preferred to qualitative PCR to establish probable disease. However, threshold for positivity has not been determined.[80]

Coronavirus Disease 2019–Associated Candidiasis

Candidemia is increasing reported in critically ill patients with COVID-19, a condition termed COVID-19–associated candidiasis (CAC).[83–86] No specific underlying COVID-19–associated immunologic defects that predispose to IC have been identified. The incidence of CAC ranges from 0.7% to 24% in case series reported from various geographic regions.[83–86] The median time from the hospital or ICU admission to diagnosis of CAC was 10 to 15 days, indicating that CAC is likely an HAI. The overall 30-day mortality in patients with CAC was 50% or higher.[83,85,86] Non-*C albicans* species including *C auris* were frequently isolated, and infection with non-*C albicans* spp. was associated with worse outcomes.[83] Potential risk factors included extended ICU stay, cardiovascular disease (CVD), diabetes mellitus (DM), mechanical ventilation (MV), HD and prolonged CVC dwell time, and use of tocilizumab.[83–86] Traditional risk factors such as cancer chemotherapy, neutropenia, or transplantation were uncommon.

These reports suggest that CAC predominately results from CVC infection, and the increased incidence may reflect the unique challenges of caring for critically ill patients in the ICU during a pandemic. It also highlights the importance of strict adherence to infection control measures in ICUs to prevent CLABSIs in critically ill patients with COVID-19.

CORONAVIRUS DISEASE 2019–ASSOCIATED PULMONARY ASPERGILLOSIS

Critically ill patients with influenza can develop secondary influenza-associated pulmonary aspergillosis.[46] Similarly, there have been increasing reports of pulmonary aspergillosis among critically ill patients with COVID-19, a condition termed COVID-19–associated pulmonary aspergillosis (CAPA).[47,87–92] It is believed that CAPA occurs as a consequence of direct damage to the airway epithelium, impaired immune function caused by Severe acute respiratory syndrome coronavirus 2 (SARS-CoV-2), and increased susceptibility to aspergillosis as a result of the use of immune modulatory therapies such as corticosteroids and IL-6 blockers.[92] The incidence of CAPA ranges from 4.8% to 33% in reports from various geographic locations, among ICU and non-ICU settings.[87–91] The wide range in incidence may be primarily due to the varying definitions used and the difficulty in establishing the diagnosis as sampling of the lower respiratory tract was limited due to the risk of aerosolization during bronchoscopy.[92] A recent study from 17 countries, done between March and August 2020, described 186 patients with CAPA defined using established standard criteria.[47] The incidence of CAPA among these patients with COVID-19 ranged from 0.1% to 9.7%, with increasing incidence of 1.0%–39.1% in patients in the ICU and 1.1%–47.4% in patients requiring MV.[47] In this study, the median time to diagnosis of CAPA was 10 days from diagnosis of COVID-19 (Interquartile range, IQR: 5–16 days) and 8 days from ICU admission (IQR: 3–14 days). The time to diagnosis of 7 or more days suggests that most of these cases of CAPA might be HAIs. CAPA was significantly associated with worse outcomes compared with patients with COVID-19 without CAPA.[88] The overall mortality has been in excess of 50% with worse outcomes in intubated patients,[47,88,89] with CAPA attributable mortality of 33%.[47] Treatment with voriconazole was associated with improved outcomes.[47,89] A fumigatus was the most commonly isolated species, followed by A flavus.[47,87–89] Unlike the traditional risk factors of prolonged neutropenia or transplantation reported with IPA, the underlying comorbidities associated with CAPA include COVID-19–associated acute respiratory distress syndrome, CVD, renal failure, DM, chronic lung disease and obesity, and use of cortocosteroids.[47,89] Similarly, the clinical and radiographic features differ from those previously described for IPA. The diagnosis was established using fungal cultures and NCTs, including BG, GM, aspergillus PCR, and lateral flow assays.[91] In order to standardize reporting, consensus criteria have been proposed for CAPA.[91] The diagnosis of CAPA requires entry criteria of laboratory-confirmed diagnosis of COVID-19 pneumonia in an ICU patient and then stratifies CAPA as proven, probable, or possible using a combination of histopathology, clinical features, imaging, and microbiology.

From an infection prevention perspective, the increasing incidence of CAPA in critically ill patients with COVID-19 emphasizes the need for surveillance for nosocomial aspergillosis in this population and strict adherence to standard measures for mitigating risk for nosocomial aspergillosis as previously described.

SUMMARY

Nosocomial fungal infections, especially IC, including candidemia and IA, can result in significant morbidity and mortality in critically ill and severely immunocompromised patients. Implementation of recommended infection control strategies can prevent catheter-related candidemia and minimize exposure of severely immunocompromised patients to airborne Aspergillus spores within the hospital environment. In select patient populations at high risk for invasive fungal infections, antifungal prophylaxis should be considered during the periods of intense immunosuppression. Newer nonculture-based methods have the potential to improve the diagnosis of nosocomial fungal infections.

CLINICS CARE POINTS

- Surveillance for new entities of COVID-19–associated invasive candidiasis and aspergillosis and emerging fungal pathogen *C auris* is important.

- Thoughtful application of newer nonculture-based fungal diagnostics can improve identification of nosocomial infections.

- Adherence to established infection prevention and control practices is essential to minimize risk of nosocomial fungal infections.

REFERENCES

1. Vazquez JA, Miceli MH, Alangaden G. Invasive fungal infections in transplant recipients. Ther Adv Infect Dis 2013;1(3):85–105.
2. Patterson TF, Thompson GR III, Denning DW, et al. Practice guidelines for the diagnosis and management of Aspergillosis: 2016 update by the Infectious Diseases Society of America. Clin Infect Dis 2016;63(4):e1–60.
3. Pappas PG, Kauffman CA, Andes DR. Clinical practice guideline for the management of candiadiasis; 2016 update by the Infectious Diseases Society of America. Clin Infect Dis 2016;62(4):e1–50.
4. Weiner-Lastinger L, Abner S, Edwards J, et al. Antimicrobial-resistant pathogens associated with adult healthcare-associated infections: summary of data reported to the National Healthcare Safety Network, 2015–2017. Infect Control Hosp Epidemiol 2020;41(1):1–18.
5. Kanamori H, Rutala WA, Sickbert-Bennett EE, et al. Review of fungal outbreaks and infection prevention in healthcare settings during construction and renovation. Clin Infect Dis 2015;61(3):433–44.
6. Yapar N. Epidemiology and risk factors for invasive candidiasis. Ther Clin Risk Manag 2014;10:95–105.
7. Tsay S, Williams S, Mu Y, et al. National burden of candidemia, United States. Open Forum Infect Dis 2018;5(Suppl 1):S142–3.
8. Available at: https://www.cdc.gov/fungal/diseases/candidiasis/invasive/statistics.html. Accessed May 27, 2021.
9. Ha YE, Peck KR, Joo EJ, et al. Impact of first-line antifungal agents on the outcomes and costs of candidemia. Antimicrobial Agents Chemother 2012;56(7):3950–6.
10. Vallabhaneni S, Benedict K, Derado G, et al. Trends in hospitalizations related to invasive aspergillosis and mucormycosis in the United States, 2000-2013. Open Forum Infect Dis 2017;4(1):ofw268.
11. Neofytos D, Horn D, Anaissie E, et al. Epidemiology and outcome of invasive fungal infection in adult hematopoietic stem cell transplant recipients: analysis of Multicenter Prospective Antifungal Therapy (PATH) Alliance registry. Clin Infect Dis 2009;48(3):265–73.
12. Upton A, Kirby KA, Carpenter P, et al. Invasive aspergillosis following hematopoietic cell transplantation: outcomes and prognostic factors associated with mortality. Clin Infect Dis 2007;44(4):531–40.

13. O'Grady NP, Alexander M, Burns LA, et al. Guidelines for the prevention of intra-vascular catheter-related infections, 2011. Centers for Disease Control and Prevention. Clin Infect Dis 2011;52(9):e162–93.
14. Siegel JD, Rhinehart E, Jackson M, et al. Guidelines for isolation precautions: preventing transmission of infectious agents in healthcare settings. 2007. Available at: http://www.cdc.gov/ncidod/dhqp/pdf/isolation2007.pdf. Accessed April 20, 2021.
15. Tomblyn M, Chiller T, Einsele H, et al. Guidelines for preventing infectious complications among hematopoietic cell transplantation recipients: a global perspective. Biol Blood Marrow Transplant 2009;15(10):1143–238.
16. Vazquez JA, Sanchez V, Dmuchowski C, et al. Nosocomial acquisition of *Candida albicans*: an epidemiologic study. J Infect Dis 1993;168(1):195–201.
17. Vazquez JA, Dembry LM, Sanchez V, et al. Nosocomial *Candida glabrata* colonization: an epidemiologic study. J Clin Microbiol 1998;36(2):421–6.
18. Trofa D, Gacser A, Nosanchuk JD. Candida parapsilosis, an emerging fungal pathogen. Clin Microbiol Rev 2008;21(4):606–25.
19. Vincent J, Sakr Y, Singer M, et al. Prevalence and outcomes of infection among patients in intensive care units in 2017. JAMA 2020;323(15):1478–87.
20. Zilberberg M, Shorr A, Kollef M. Secular trends in candidemia-related hospitalization in the United States, 2000–2005. Infect Control Hosp Epidemiol 2008;29:978–80.
21. Ricotta EE, Lai YL, Babiker A, et al. Invasive candidiasis species distribution and trends, United States, 2009-2017. J Infect Dis 2021;223(7):1295–302.
22. Pfaller M, Neofytos D, Diekema D, et al. Epidemiology and outcomes of candidemia in 3648 patients: data from the Prospective Antifungal Therapy (PATH Alliance®) registry, 2004–2008. Diagn Microbiol Infect Dis 2012;74(4):323–31.
23. Azie N, Neofytos D, Pfaller M, et al. The PATH (Prospective Antifungal Therapy) Alliance® registry and invasive fungal infections: update 2012. Diagn Microbiol Infect Dis 2012;73(4):293–300.
24. Pfaller MA, Diekema DJ, Gibbs DL, et al. Results from the ARTEMIS DISK Global Antifungal Surveillance Study, 1997 to 2007: a 10.5-year analysis of susceptibilities of *Candida* Species to fluconazole and voriconazole as determined by CLSI standardized disk diffusion. J Clin Microbiol 2010;48(4):1366–77.
25. Gupta N, Haque A, Lattif AA, et al. Epidemiology and molecular typing of *Candida* isolates from burn patients. Mycopathologia 2004;158(4):397–405.
26. Fanello S, Bouchara JP, Jousset N, et al. Nosocomial *Candida albicans* acquisition in a geriatric unit: epidemiology and evidence for person-to-person transmission. J Hosp Infect 2001;47(1):46–52.
27. Masala L, Luzzati R, Maccacaro L, et al. Nosocomial cluster of *Candida guillermondii* fungemia in surgical patients. Eur J Clin Microbiol Infect Dis 2003;22(11):686–8.
28. Minces LR, Ho KS, Veldkamp PJ, et al. *Candida rugosa*: a distinctive emerging cause of candidaemia. A case report and review of the literature. Scand J Infect Dis 2009;41(11–12):892–7.
29. Tsay S, Kallen A, Jackson BR, et al. Approach to the investigation and management of patients with *Candida auris*, an emerging multidrug-resistant yeast. Clin Infect Dis 2018;66(2):306–11.
30. Vallabhaneni S, Kallen A, Tsay S, et al. Investigation of the first seven reported cases of *Candida auris*, a globally emerging invasive, multidrug-resistant fungus — United States, May 2013–August 2016. MMWR Morb Mortal Wkly Rep 2016;65:1234–7.

31. Prestel C, Anderson E, Forsberg K, et al. *Candida auris* outbreak in a COVID-19 specialty care unit — Florida, July–August 2020. MMWR Morb Mortal Wkly Rep 2021;70:56–7.

32. Jeffery-Smith A, Taori SK, Schelenz S, et al. *Candida auris*: a review of the literature. Clin Microbiol Rev 2017;31(1). e00029-17.

33. Ostrowsky B, Greenko J, Adams E, et al. *Candida auris* isolates resistant to three classes of antifungal medications — New York, 2019. MMWR Morb Mortal Wkly Rep 2020;69:6–9.

34. Rhimi W, Theelen B, Boekhout T, et al. *Malassezia* spp. Yeasts of emerging concern in fungemia. Front Cell Infect Microbiol 2020;10:370.

35. Iatta R, Cafarchia C, Cuna T, et al. Bloodstream infections by Malassezia and Candida species in critical care patients. Med Mycol 2014;52(3):264–9.

36. Liao Y, Lu X, Yang S, et al. Epidemiology and outcome of trichosporon fungemia: a review of 185 reported cases from 1975 to 2014. Open Forum Infect Dis 2015; 2(4):ofv141.

37. Ruan SY, Chien JY, Hsueh PR. Invasive trichosporonosis caused by *Trichosporon asahii* and other unusual *Trichosporon* species at a medical center in Taiwan. Clin Infect Dis 2009;49(1):e11–7.

38. Kanamori H, Weber DJ, Rutala WA. Healthcare Outbreaks associated with a water reservoir and infection prevention strategies. Clin Infect Dis 2016;62(11): 1423–35.

39. Available at: https://www.cdc.gov/infectioncontrol/guidelines/bsi/index.html. Accessed April 1, 2021.

40. Antoniadou A. Outbreaks of zygomycosis in hospitals. Clin Microbiol Infect 2009; 15(Suppl 5):55–9.

41. Guerrero A, Torres P, Duran MT, et al. Airborne outbreak of nosocomial *Scedosporium prolificans* infection. Lancet 2001;357(9264):1267–8.

42. Krishnan S, Manavathu EK, Chandrasekar PH. *Aspergillus flavus*: an emerging non-fumigatus *Aspergillus* species of significance. Mycoses 2009;52(3):206–22.

43. Barnes PD, Marr KA. Risks, diagnosis and outcomes of invasive fungal infections in haematopoietic stem cell transplant recipients. Br J Haematol 2007; 139(4):519–31.

44. Singh N, Husain S. Invasive aspergillosis in solid organ transplant recipients. Am J Transplant 2009;9(Suppl 4):S180–91.

45. Meersseman W, Lagrou K, Maertens J, et al. Invasive aspergillosis in the intensive care unit. Clin Infect Dis 2007;45(2):205–16.

46. Schauwvlieghe AFAD, Rijnders BJA, Philips N, et al, Dutch-Belgian Mycosis study group. Invasive aspergillosis in patients admitted to the intensive care unit with severe influenza: a retrospective cohort study. Lancet Respir Med 2018;6(10):782–92.

47. Salmanton-García J, Sprute R, Stemler J, et al, FungiScope European Confederation of Medical Mycology/The International Society for Human and Animal Mycology Working Group. COVID-19-Associated Pulmonary Aspergillosis, March-August 2020. Emerg Infect Dis 2021;27(4):1077–86.

48. Vonberg RP, Gastmeier P. Nosocomial aspergillosis in outbreak settings. J Hosp Infect 2006;63(3):246–54.

49. Kidd SE, Ling LM, Meyer W, et al. Molecular epidemiology of invasive aspergillosis: lessons learned from an outbreak investigation in an Australian hematology unit. Infect Control Hosp Epidemiol 2009;30(12):1223–6.

50. Balajee SA, Borman AM, Brandt ME, et al. Sequence-based identification of *Aspergillus, Fusarium,* and *Mucorales* species in the clinical mycology labora-

tory: where are we and where should we go from here? J Clin Microbiol 2009; 47(4):877–84.

51. Hamdi T, Karthikeyan V, Alangaden GJ. Mucormycosis in a renal transplant recipient. case report and comprehensive review of literature. Int J Nephrol 2014;2014: 950643.

52. Roden MM, Zaoutis TE, Buchanan WL, et al. Epidemiology and outcome of zygomycosis: a review of 929 reported cases. Clin Infect Dis 2005;41(5):634–53.

53. Novosad SA, Vasquez AM, Nambiar A, et al. Notes from the field. Probable Mucormycosis among adult solid organ transplant recipients at an acute care hospital — Pennsylvania, 2014–2015. MMWR Morb Mortal Wkly Rep 2016;65:481–2.

54. Cheng VCC, Chan JFW, Ngan AHY, et al. Outbreak of intestinal infection due to *Rhizopus microsporus*. J Clin Microbiol 2009;47(9):2834–43.

55. Duffy J, Harris J, Gade L, et al. Mucormycosis outbreak associated with hospital linens. Pediatr Infect Dis J 2014;33(5):472–6.

56. Batista BG, Chaves MA, Reginatto P, et al. Human fusariosis: An emerging infection that is difficult to treat. Rev Soc Bras Med Trop 2020;53:e20200013.

57. Chang DC, Grant GB, O'Donnell K, et al. Multistate outbreak of *Fusarium* keratitis associated with use of a contact lens solution. JAMA 2006;296(8):953–63.

58. Nucci M, Marr KA, Queiroz-Telles F, et al. *Fusarium* infection in hematopoietic stem cell transplant recipients. Clin Infect Dis 2004;38(9):1237–42.

59. O'Donnell K, Sutton DA, Rinaldi MG, et al. Genetic diversity of human pathogenic members of the *Fusarium oxysporum* complex inferred from multilocus DNA sequence data and amplified fragment length polymorphism analyses: evidence for the recent dispersion of a geographically widespread clonal lineage and nosocomial origin. J Clin Microbiol 2004;42(11):5109–20.

60. Ramirez-Garcia A, Pellon A, Rementeria A, et al. Scedosporium and Lomentospora: an updated overview of underrated opportunists. Med Mycol 2018; 56(suppl_1):102–25.

61. Rao CY, Pachucki C, Cali S, et al. Contaminated product water as the source of Phialemonium curvatum bloodstream infection among patients undergoing hemodialysis. Infect Control Hosp Epidemiol 2009;30(9):840–7.

62. McCotter OZ, Smith RM, Westercamp M, et al. Update on multistate outbreak of fungal infections associated with contaminated methylprednisolone injections, 2012–2014. MMWR Morb Mortal Wkly Rep 2015;64(42):1200–1.

63. Yiannakis EP, Boswell TC. Systematic review of outbreaks of Pneumocystis jirovecii pneumonia: evidence that P. jirovecii is a transmissible organism and the implications for healthcare infection control. J Hosp Infect 2016;93(1):1–8.

64. Musuuza JS, Guru PK, O'Horo JC, et al. The impact of chlorhexidine bathing on hospital-acquired bloodstream infections: a systematic review and meta-analysis. BMC Infect Dis 2019;19(1):416.

65. Choi EY, Park DA, Kim HJ, et al. Efficacy of chlorhexidine bathing for reducing healthcare associated bloodstream infections: a meta-analysis. Ann Intensive Care 2015;5(1):31.

66. Climo MW, Yokoe DS, Warren DK, et al. Effect of daily chlorhexidine bathing on hospital-acquired infection. N Engl J Med 2013;368(6):533–42.

67. Voor In 't Holt AF, Helder OK, Vos MC, et al. Antiseptic barrier cap effective in reducing central line-associated bloodstream infections: a systematic review and meta-analysis. Int J Nurs Stud 2017;69:34–40.

68. Kamboj M, Blair R, Bell N, et al. Use of disinfection cap to reduce central-line-associated bloodstream infection and blood culture contamination among

hematology-oncology patients. Infect Control Hosp Epidemiol 2015;36(12): 1401–8.

69. Guidelines for design and construction of hospital and health care facilities. Washington (DC): American Institute of Architects Facility Guidelines Institute AAoAfH, US Dept of Health & Human Services; 2006.

70. Goebes MD, Baron EJ, Mathews KL, et al. Effect of building construction on *Aspergillus* concentrations in a hospital. Infect Control Hosp Epidemiol 2008; 29(5):462–4.

71. Hansen D, Blahout B, Benner D, et al. Environmental sampling of particulate matter and fungal spores during demolition of a building on a hospital area. J Hosp Infect 2008;70(3):259–64.

72. Sautour M, Sixt N, Dalle F, et al. Prospective survey of indoor fungal contamination in hospital during a period of building construction. J Hosp Infect 2007;67(4): 367–73.

73. Sixt N, Dalle F, Lafon I, et al. Reduced fungal contamination of the indoor environment with the Plasmair (TM) system (Airinspace). J Hosp Infect 2007;65(2): 156–62.

74. Kullberg BJ, Arendrup MC. Invasive candidiasis. N Engl J Med 2015;373(15): 1445–56.

75. Pfaller MA, Wolk DM, Lowery TJ. T2MR and T2Candida: novel technology for the rapid diagnosis of candidemia and invasive candidiasis. Future Microbiol 2016; 11(1):103–17.

76. Monday LM, Parraga Acosta T, Alangaden G. T2Candida for the diagnosis and management of invasive candida infections. J Fungi (Basel) 2021;7(3):178.

77. Available at: https://genmarkdx.com/panels/eplex-panels/bcid-panels/. Accessed May 27, 2021.

78. T2 biosystems, products & technology international: product pipeline-T2Cauris panel RUO. Available at: https://www.t2biosystems.com/products-technology-ous/pipeline-ous/t2candida-auris-panel-ruo-ous/. Accessed May 27, 2021.

79. National Healthcare Safety Network (NHSN). Patient safety component manual. 2021. Available at: https://www.cdc.gov/nhsn/pdfs/pscmanual/pcsmanual_current.pdf. Accessed January 16, 2021.

80. Donnelly JP, Chen SC, Kauffman CA, et al. Revision and update of the consensus definitions of invasive fungal disease from the European Organization for Research and Treatment of Cancer and the Mycoses Study Group Education and Research Consortium. Clin Infect Dis 2020;71(6):1367–76.

81. White PL, Wingard JR, Bretagne S, et al. Aspergillus polymerase chain reaction: systematic review of evidence for clinical use in comparison with antigen testing. Clin Infect Dis 2015;61(8):1293–303.

82. Otašević S, Momčilović S, Stojanović NM, et al. Non-culture based assays for the detection of fungal pathogens. J Mycol Med 2018;28(2):236–48.

83. Arastehfar A, Carvalho A, Nguyen MH. COVID-19-Associated Candidiasis (CAC): an underestimated complication in the absence of immunological predispositions? J Fungi (Basel) 2020;6(4):211.

84. Nucci M, Barreiros G, Guimarães LF, et al. Increased incidence of candidemia in a tertiary care hospital with the COVID-19 pandemic. Mycoses 2021;64(2):152–6.

85. Mastrangelo A, Germinario BN, Ferrante M, et al, COVID-BioB Study Group. Candidemia in COVID-19 patients: incidence and characteristics in a prospective cohort compared to historical non-COVID-19 controls. Clin Infect Dis 2020. ciaa1594.

86. Macauley P, Epelbaum O. Epidemiology and Mycology of Candidaemia in non-oncological medical intensive care unit patients in a tertiary center in the United States: overall analysis and comparison between non-COVID-19 and COVID-19 cases. Mycoses 2021.
87. van Arkel ALE, Rijpstra TA, Belderbos HNA, et al. COVID-19 associated pulmonary aspergillosis. Am J Respir Crit Care Med 2020;202:132–5.
88. Bartoletti M, Pascale R, Cricca M, et al. Epidemiology of invasive pulmonary aspergillosis among COVID-19 intubated patients: a prospective study. Clin Infect Dis 2020. ciaa1065.
89. White PL, Dhillon R, Cordey A, et al. A national strategy to diagnose COVID-19 associated invasive fungal disease in the ICU. Clin Infect Dis 2020. ciaa1298.
90. Fekkar A, Lampros A, Mayaux J, et al. Occurrence of invasive pulmonary fungal infections in patients with severe COVID-19 admitted to the ICU. Am J Respir Crit Care Med 2021;203(3):307–17.
91. Koehler P, Bassetti M, Chakrabarti A, et al. Defining and managing COVID-19-associated pulmonary aspergillosis: the 2020 ECMM/ISHAM consensus criteria for research and clinical guidance. Lancet Infect Dis 2021;21(6):e149–62.
92. Hoenigl M. Invasive fungal disease complicating COVID-19: when it rains it pours. Clin Infect Dis 2020;ciaa1342. https://doi.org/10.1093/cid/ciaa1342.

Health Care–Acquired Viral Respiratory Diseases

Joshua G. Petrie, PhD[a], Thomas R. Talbot, MD, MPH, FSHCA, FIDSA[b],*

KEYWORDS

- Influenza • SARS-CoV-2 • COVID-19 • Coronavirus • Respiratory virus
- Infection prevention • Nosocomial infection • Health care–acquired infection

KEY POINTS

- Health care–acquired viral respiratory infections are common, with increased patient morbidity and mortality.
- Multicomponent infection control measures consisting of education, hand washing, isolation, consistent use of personal protective equipment, cohorting patients, and cohort nursing reduces transmission of respiratory infections.
- Health care worker influenza vaccination is recommended, with mandatory vaccination policies becoming more common.

INTRODUCTION

Although the threat of viral respiratory infection has been underscored by the current coronavirus disease 2019 (COVID-19) pandemic, respiratory viruses have a significant impact in health care settings even under normal circumstances. It is estimated that approximately 19,000 nosocomial respiratory virus infections occur in US hospitals each year, resulting in increased patient morbidity, mortality, and health care costs.[1] Approximately 20% of patients with health care–associated pneumonia have viral respiratory infections, with an incidence that typically reflects the level of virus activity within the community.[2,3] Respiratory viruses can be transmitted through multiple pathways, including contact, droplet, and airborne routes, with the relative contributions of each route depending on the viral species and environmental factors. Controlled laboratory studies to determine which transmission routes are possible and epidemiologic studies to determine which routes most contribute to real-world transmission are both needed to inform prevention and control. This article describes the current

This work was funded in whole or in part with federal funds by the National Institute of Allergy and Infectious Diseases (Grant No. K01 AI141579 to J.G.P.).

[a] Department of Epidemiology, University of Michigan School of Public Health, 1415 Washington Heights, Ann Arbor, MI 48109, USA; [b] Division of Infectious Diseases, Department of Medicine, Vanderbilt University School of Medicine, 1161 21st Avenue South, A-2200 MCN, Nashville, TN 37232, USA

* Corresponding author.

E-mail address: tom.talbot@vumc.org

understanding of the epidemiology, transmission, and control of health care–associated respiratory viral infections.

SEVERE ACUTE RESPIRATORY SYNDROME CORONAVIRUS-2 AND OTHER HUMAN CORONAVIRUSES
Epidemiology

Among the human coronaviruses (HCoVs), there are 4 seasonal viruses (229E, OC43, NL63, and HKU1) that cause annual epidemics of primarily mild respiratory infections. In addition, several novel coronaviruses have emerged from zoonotic reservoirs in recent decades causing severe lower respiratory disease, most notably the severe acute respiratory syndrome coronavirus-2 (SARS-CoV-2) virus responsible for the recent COVID-19 pandemic.

As of March 1, 2021, the COVID-19 pandemic caused by SARS-CoV-2 resulted in 113,467,303 confirmed cases and 2,520,550 deaths worldwide, with the United States accounting for approximately 25% of the cases and 20% of the deaths.[4,5] A large study performed in the United States and United Kingdom found that health care personnel (HCP) were more than 3 times more likely to be infected with SARS-CoV-2 compared with the general community after adjusting for likelihood of testing.[6] These infections strained health care capacity and put patient safety at risk. Characterizations of nosocomial outbreaks early in the pandemic noted that mortality among patients with health care–acquired COVID-19 was much higher than in the general population, potentially reflecting older age and poorer health.[7–9] Residents of long-term care facilities have accounted for more than a quarter of all US COVID-19 deaths as of mid-February 2021.[10]

Although the COVID-19 pandemic is the first documented pandemic caused by an HCoV, there are other recent examples of novel HCoV emergence causing epidemics. In 2002 to 2003, the novel SARS-CoV caused an epidemic of severe respiratory illness (coined severe acute respiratory syndrome [SARS]) resulting in 8096 cases globally and 774 deaths (9.6% case fatality ratio) with notable nosocomial outbreaks in Singapore and Toronto.[11,12] Middle East Respiratory Syndrome Coronavirus (MERS-CoV) was identified in the Arabian Peninsula in 2012.[13] As of January 2021, 2566 cases in 27 countries have been reported, with 882 deaths (34.4% case fatality ratio).[14,15] Although direct contact with dromedary camels has remained a major risk factor for MERS, there have been multiple MERS nosocomial outbreaks and 13% to 70% of nosocomial MERS infections were among HCP.[15–19]

Nosocomial infection with seasonal coronaviruses has also been described,[1,20,21] including large outbreaks among patients and HCP in pediatric and neonatal intensive care units.[22]

Transmission

The median incubation period of SARS-CoV-2 is 4 to 5 days, with symptoms developing within 12 days in 95% of symptomatic infections.[23,24] Between 1 in 3 and 1 in 6 SARS-CoV-2 infections remain asymptomatic.[25,26] Asymptomatic patients may have viral loads higher or comparable with symptomatic patients, but shorter durations of shedding.[27,28] Among symptomatic individuals, viral shedding peaks on or just before the day of symptom onset.[28] In uncomplicated infections, shedding of virus capable of replication lasts less than 10 days,[28] but individuals with severe COVID-19[29] or who are immunocompromised[30] may be infectious for much longer. Taken together, the long incubation period, high proportion of asymptomatic infections, presymptomatic shedding, and long duration of shedding contribute to a high proportion of unobserved transmission.

SARS-CoV-2 is predominantly transmitted through close contact via the large droplet and direct contact routes.[31,32] However, there is evidence that SARS-CoV-2 may be transmitted over longer distances and periods of time via smaller droplets or aerosols in certain circumstances.[32–34] Aerosol transmission may be of particular concern in health care settings where procedures are performed that can generate infectious respiratory droplets and aerosols (aerosol-generating procedures) such as endotracheal intubation and extubation, nebulizer administration, and airway suctioning.[35] Studies have also shown frequent contamination of surfaces, with prolonged infectivity up to 96 hours on nonporous surfaces and up to 72 hours on cardboard.[34,36] However, instances of indirect fomite transmission have not been conclusively documented.

In contrast with SARS-CoV-2, MERS-CoV has low human-to-human transmission potential. However, inadequate or inconsistent infection control measures have been cited as factors in MERS-CoV transmission during nosocomial outbreaks.[16,17] MERS-CoV may transmit by large droplets, contact, and aerosols following aerosol-generating procedures.[37]

The seasonal HCoVs, unlike their higher-severity counterparts, seem to be largely spread by droplet transmission.[38] Performing aerosol-generating procedures and contact with pediatric patients have been identified as risk factors for HCP infection with seasonal HCoV.[39]

Prevention and Control

Patients with suspected or confirmed SARS-CoV-2 infection, or those who would otherwise be required to quarantine, should be placed in single rooms with a closed door and dedicated bathroom.[40] Patients undergoing aerosol-generating procedures should be placed in airborne infection isolation rooms if possible. Limiting patients with SARS-CoV-2 to specific units should be considered, and their movement should be limited. In addition to standard precautions, HCP entering the rooms of patients with SARS-CoV-2 should use an N-95-equivalent or higher-level respirator, eye protection, gloves, and a gown. These best practices have not always been feasible given limited personal protective equipment (PPE) resources, and the US Centers for Disease Control and Prevention (CDC) has outlined contingencies and strategies to preserve PPE.[41] The World Health Organization (WHO) and several US state health departments have issued more lenient guidance permitting use of medical masks rather than respirators in the absence of aerosol-generating procedures.[42] Although the SARS-CoV-2 research base has developed in an extraordinarily short time, these differing recommendations highlight remaining gaps in the knowledge of SARS-CoV-2 epidemiology, transmission, and infection control best practices.[43]

CDC has also recommended general measures to reduce health care–associated transmission.[40] These measures have been extremely effective for reducing risk of health care–associated SARS-CoV-2 infection and could be considered for use during nonpandemic respiratory virus seasons.[44,45]

- Telehealth strategies should be used to reduce in-person medical visits where possible.
- Visitors to the health care facility should be limited, especially during times of high community transmission.
- All patients, visitors, and HCP should be screened for symptoms of COVID-19 or contact with a suspected or confirmed case in the past 14 days.
- Patients, visitors, and HCP should wear a well-fitting cloth mask,[46] surgical mask, or respirator at all times as a method of universal source control.

- Physical distancing should be encouraged to maintain at least 2 m (6 feet) between individuals when possible.

Both the Infectious Diseases Society of America (IDSA) and CDC recommend nucleic acid amplification testing for all individuals, hospitalized or in the community, with either symptoms of COVID-19 or who have been exposed to a suspected or confirmed patient with SARS-CoV-2 infection.[47,48] Negative results in symptomatic hospitalized patients should be treated with suspicion with repeated testing, including specimens from the lower respiratory tract if possible. Testing of asymptomatic patients on hospital admission is also recommended by IDSA and CDC during periods of high community transmission.[40,48] Periodic testing of asymptomatic HCP without known exposure is recommended for those working in long-term care facilities, and may be considered in hospital settings if resources are available.[49]

As of March 2021, 3 vaccines for the prevention of COVID-19 have received emergency use authorizations from the US Food and Drug Administration (FDA), and all have shown substantial efficacy, particularly against severe disease.[50–52] Frontline HCP are among those designated as highest priority for vaccination by the CDC's Advisory Committee for Immunization Practices (ACIP).[53,54] High HCP vaccination coverage is critical to protecting both HCP and patients. It remains to be seen whether requirements for HCP COVID vaccination will emerge as has occurred with influenza vaccination. As the experience and comfort with these new vaccines increases and full FDA approval is issued, such requirements may be justified, especially if an impact on transmission is confirmed.

Hospitalized patients with MERS-CoV should be placed in contact and airborne precautions with the use of eye protection.[55]

Although seasonal HCoV are not specifically mentioned in CDC infection prevention guidelines, droplet and contact precautions may be considered based on likely routes of transmission.[38]

SEASONAL INFLUENZA
Epidemiology

Influenza infects approximately 2% to 10% of the US population annually, resulting in 140,000 to 810,000 hospitalizations and 12,000 to 61,000 deaths.[56,57] Transmission of influenza has been reported in a variety of health care settings, and HCP are often implicated as index cases for nosocomial outbreaks.[58] A recent study found that nearly 90% of influenza-infected HCP were asymptomatic or mildly symptomatic with no fever or cough.[59] Although asymptomatic and mildly symptomatic individuals shed less virus for shorter duration than those who are symptomatic,[60] there is still potential for transmitting infection to patients or other HCP. Even when symptomatic, HCP often work while acutely ill for a variety of reasons.[61,62] High levels of patient and HCP infection can also disrupt hospital operations during seasonal influenza epidemics.[63,64]

Transmission

The average incubation period for influenza is approximately 3 days, but can range from 1 to 4 days.[65] Viral shedding begins before the appearance of symptoms and within the first 24 hours following infection, peaks on the second day following infection, and usually declines rapidly thereafter.[65,66] Virus is typically no longer detectable after 6 to 10 days after inoculation. Prolonged viral shedding has been documented in children,[67] those hospitalized for severe influenza,[68] and immunocompromised adults.[69]

The possibility for influenza transmission to occur through direct contact,[70,71] indirect contact with fomites,[72,73] large droplet,[74,75] and aerosol[76,77] routes has been shown in both laboratory and field studies. However, in both the community and health care settings, large droplet and direct contact transmission predominates.[78] Although possible, indirect fomite transmission and aerosol transmission across long distances and time periods have not been conclusively shown and are unlikely. Consistent with this, several randomized controlled trials have found that no significant advantage of N95 respirators compared with surgical masks has been shown for standard clinical care.[79–81] The exception may be for aerosol-generating procedures, which can increase risk of transmission to health care workers involved in or in close proximity to the procedure.[82,83]

Prevention and Control

In addition to standard precautions, the CDC recommends implementation of droplet precautions to prevent health care–associated influenza (**Tables 1** and **2**).[3,84,85] Droplet precautions should continue for 7 days after illness onset or until 24 hours after the resolution of fever and respiratory symptoms, whichever is longer, but may be extended for immunocompromised or other patients who may have prolonged viral shedding. HCP should wear respiratory protection equivalent to a fitted N95 filtering respirator mask if patients with influenza undergo aerosol-generating procedures.[85]

Annual influenza vaccination is recommended for HCP by the ACIP.[86] Although influenza vaccine effectiveness can vary annually, it is the best available tool for the prevention of influenza infection (**Fig. 1**).[87] Vaccinated HCP are less likely to miss work because of respiratory illness and miss fewer days when they are ill.[88,89] Improved HCP vaccination coverage has also been linked with decreased health care–associated influenza among patients and personnel,[90,91] and reduced mortality among nursing home patients.[92–96] Since 2013, multiple professional societies and safety advocacy organizations have endorsed policies for mandatory influenza vaccination for HCP (**Box 1**). As a result, the proportion of hospitals with mandatory influenza vaccination programs increased from 37% in 2013 to 61% in 2017.[97] During the 2019 to 2020 influenza season, HCP vaccination coverage was 81% overall; 52% in settings where vaccines were not required, promoted, or offered on site; and 94% where vaccination was required.[98]

Data from observational studies and controlled trials support recommendations to provide antiviral chemoprophylaxis to residents in long-term care facilities, regardless of vaccination status, during an institutional influenza outbreak.[99,100] In this setting, chemoprophylaxis should be continued for 14 days or for at least 7 days after the onset of symptoms in the last person infected, whichever is longer.[99,100] Effectiveness of employee chemoprophylaxis in the acute care setting is unclear, but may be considered for unvaccinated or high-risk HCP during an institutional outbreak.[99,100]

In addition to vaccination and antiviral chemoprophylaxis, interventions to prevent health care–associated influenza include source control (ie, wearing a mask), cohort nursing, exclusion of ill HCP and visitors through comprehensive sick leave policies and entry screening, and early diagnostic testing of symptomatic patients.[85,99] Influenza testing is recommended on admission for all hospitalized patients with acute respiratory illness during the influenza season.[99]

NOVEL PANDEMIC INFLUENZA

Over the past century, there have been 4 major influenza pandemics caused by novel viruses resulting from reassortment of human influenza genes with those of avian or swine strains: 1918 to 1919 A (H1N1), 1957 to 1958 A (H2N2), 1968 to 1969 A (H3N2), and 2009 A (H1N1). Several zoonotic influenza viruses are currently being monitored for pandemic potential, including avian H5 and H7 viruses.

Table 1
Precautions for preventing transmission of respiratory infections

Precautions	Component	Recommendation
Standard	Hand hygiene	Wash hands with soap and water or use an alcohol-based hand rub: • Before and after contact with a patient • After contact with respiratory secretions, and • After contact with potentially contaminated items in the patient's vicinity, including equipment and environmental surfaces
	Respiratory hygiene	Instruct staff and visitors with signs and symptoms of a respiratory infection to: • Cover the mouth and nose when sneezing or coughing • Perform hand hygiene after soiling hands with respiratory secretions • Wear masks when tolerated, and • Maintain spatial separation from others (>1 m [3 feet]) when in common waiting areas, if possible
	Gloves	Wear when contact with respiratory secretions could occur
	Gowns	Wear during procedures and activities when contact of clothing or exposed skin with respiratory secretions is anticipated
	Masks and eye protection	Wear during procedures and activities likely to generate splashes or sprays of respiratory secretions
Contact[a]	Patient placement	Place patient in a single-patient room, if possible, or cohort with other patients infected with the same organism Limit patient movement to medically necessary purposes
	Gloves and gowns	Wear on room entry whenever contact is likely with the patient, patient's respiratory secretions, or potentially contaminated items in the patient's vicinity, including equipment and environmental surfaces
	Masks and eye protection	As per standard precautions
Droplet[a]	Patient placement	Place patient in a single-patient room, if possible, or cohort with other patients infected with the same organism Limit patient movement to medically necessary purposes, and patients should wear a mask and follow respiratory hygiene during transport
	Gloves, gowns, and eye protection	As per standard precautions
	Masks	Wear a surgical mask on room entry if close contact (eg, <1 m [3 feet]) with the patient is anticipated

(continued on next page)

Table 1 (*continued*)		
Precautions	**Component**	**Recommendation**
Airborne[a]	Patient placement	Place infected patients in a single-patient airborne infection isolation room[b]
		Limit patient movement to medically necessary purposes, and patients should wear a mask and follow respiratory hygiene during transport
	Gloves, gowns, and eye protection	As per standard precautions
	Masks	Wear a fit-tested N95 respirator before room entry

[a] Contact, droplet, and airborne precautions include hand hygiene and respiratory hygiene as per standard precautions.
[b] Airborne infection isolation room consists of negative pressure relative to the surrounding area, 6 to 12 air changes per hour, and air is exhausted directly to the outside or recirculated through high-efficiency particulate air (HEPA) filtration before return.
From Siegel JD, Rhinehart E, Jackson M, et al; Health Care Infection Control Practices Advisory C. 2007 Guideline for isolation precautions: preventing transmission of infectious agents in health care settings. Am J Infect Control 2007;35:S65–164; with permission.

Highly pathogenic avian influenza A (H5N1) virus was first reported to cause human infections in 1997 in China; however, no other human infections were reported until the virus reemerged in Hong Kong in 2003.[101] Since that time, it has caused 862 infections worldwide, of whom 455 patients have died (case fatality ratio: 53%), although only 1 case was identified in 2020.[102] Human infection with avian influenza A (H7N9) was first reported 2013 in China, subsequently causing seasonal outbreaks of severe respiratory illness accounting for a total of 616 deaths from a total of 1568 cases (case fatality ratio: 39%).[103] However, only 4 human cases have been identified following mass immunization of Chinese poultry with a bivalent influenza A (H7N9) and A (H5N1) vaccine beginning in September 2017.[103,104]

The CDC has issued interim guidelines for infection control for patients with suspected novel influenza A infection associated with severe disease, including H5N1, H7N9, and other emerging strains. Avian influenza should be suspected in patients presenting with a severe respiratory illness with recent contact with potentially infected birds or with travel to a country with avian influenza activity in the past 10 days.[105] Contact and airborne precautions should be used for patients with suspected novel influenza (see **Tables 1** and **2**). In addition, all HCP should wear eye protection when entering the patient's room. Transmission-based precautions for novel influenza should be continued throughout the duration of the patient's stay. Antiviral chemoprophylaxis for 5 days should also be considered for HCP with unprotected exposures if the exposure was not ongoing, or for 10 days if the exposure was ongoing.[106]

RESPIRATORY SYNCYTIAL VIRUS
Epidemiology

Respiratory syncytial virus (RSV) is the most common cause of pneumonia and bronchiolitis in infants[107] and a common cause of hospitalization in older and high-risk adults.[108] Rates of respiratory hospitalizations secondary to RSV infection are highest among infants, although older patients ($\geq$75 years) have similar rates to children aged 1 to 4 years.[109] Outbreaks of RSV have occurred in a variety of health care settings.[110–113] Secondary infection risks between 19% and 45% among patients, and

Table 2
Infection prevention recommendations for viral respiratory pathogens

Common Measures for Reducing Transmission in the Health Care Setting

Hand hygiene

Respiratory hygiene/cough etiquette

Standard precautions

Restrict ill visitors[a]

Restrict ill personnel (prevent so-called presenteeism)

Cohort nursing

Prompt diagnosis of respiratory infections among patients by diagnostic tests[b]

Restrict elective admissions of patients during outbreaks in the community and/or facility

Surveillance for an increase in activity of viral infections within the community

Universal source control with well-fitting masks

Measures for Reducing Transmission of Specific Pathogens in the Health Care Setting

Intervention	RSV	Adenovirus	Parainfluenza Virus/HMPV	Rhinovirus	Influenza Seasonal	Influenza Novel	Novel Coronavirus
Precautions	—	—	—	—	—	—	—
Contact	●	●	●	—	—	●	●
Droplet	—	●	—	●	●		●
Airborne	—	—	—	—	●[c]	●	○[d]
Eye protection	—	—	—	—	—	●	●
Vaccination of personnel	—	—	—	—	●	—	—
Chemoprophylaxis	○[e]	—	—	—	○[f]	○	—

Closed circles (●) denote recommended measures. Open circles (○) denote measures recommended in certain circumstances.

Abbreviations: HMPV, human metapneumovirus; RSV, respiratory syncytial virus.

[a] Institutions may restrict only young children and/or screen all visitors for illness by using a trained health care worker to assess for signs and symptoms or by using an educational patient information list to advise ill visitors.

[b] To control outbreaks, institutions may perform preadmission screening of patients for infection.

[c] The Centers for Disease Control and Prevention recommends an N95 respirator for HCP performing aerosol-generating procedures.

[d] The Centers for Disease Control and Prevention recommends use of a fit-tested N95 respirator. The WHO and some US state health departments recommend medical masks.

[e] In addition to other infection control measures, palivizumab prophylaxis of high-risk infants has been used to control outbreaks in the neonatal intensive care unit.

[f] During a facility outbreak of influenza, administer antiviral chemoprophylaxis to all patients in the involved unit, regardless of vaccination status, and to unvaccinated HCP working in the involved unit. If feasible, administer facility-wide chemoprophylaxis for all residents in long-term care facilities. Chemoprophylaxis may also be administered to personnel when the outbreak strain is not well matched by the vaccine.

between 34% and 56% among HCP, on infant wards have been reported when limited or no infection control measures are implemented.[110,114,115] Most infected HCP are symptomatic, but asymptomatic shedding of RSV occurs in 15% to 20%.[116] As with other viruses, symptomatic HCP who work while ill are a concern, and this is reported to occur with a high frequency (51%–75%) in some populations.[117,118]

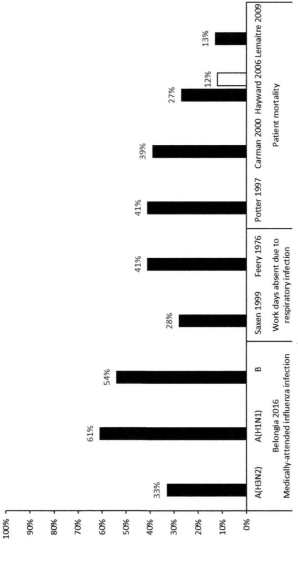

Fig. 1. Percentage reduction in noted outcomes in HCP receiving influenza vaccination. (*Data from* Refs.[58,94,95])

Box 1
Professional societies and safety advocacy organisms that recommend mandatory health care personnel influenza immunization

American Academy of Family Physicians (AAFP)

American Academy of Pediatrics (AAP)

American College of Physicians (ACP)

American Hospital Association (AHA)

American Medical Directors Association (AMDA)

American Nurses Association (ANA)

American Pharmacists Association

American Public Health Association (APHA)

Association for Professionals in Infection Control and Epidemiology (APIC)

IDSA

National Association of County and City Health Officials (NACCHO)

National Business Group on Health

National Patient Safety Foundation (NPSF)

Society for Healthcare Epidemiology of America (SHEA)

Veterans Health Administration (VHA) Department of Veterans Affairs

---

Transmission

Transmission of RSV occurs primarily through direct contact or by self-inoculation after touching contaminated fomites[119,120]; inoculation is most efficient via the eyes and nose.[121] RSV has been recovered on countertops for up to 6 hours, on rubber gloves for up to 2 hours, and on cloth gowns and hands for 15 to 60 minutes after contamination with infected nasal secretions.[122] The duration of viral shedding among hospitalized infants averages 6.7 days but can be as long as 21 days[123]; in a large Kenyan household cohort, shedding averaged 11 days, with approximately 13% shedding for more than 21 days.[124] Similar durations of viral shedding have also been shown for older adults.[125] Younger children, infants with lower respiratory disease, and those with a compromised immune status have more prolonged shedding and shed greater quantities of virus.[123,124]

Prevention and Control

Although several RSV vaccines are in development,[126] there is no licensed vaccine or specific treatment readily available for RSV. Therefore, effective infection control measures are paramount for minimizing transmission. In addition to standard precautions, the CDC recommends contact precautions to prevent health care–associated RSV (see **Tables 1** and **2**).[84] These precautions should continue for the duration of illness but may be extended for immunocompromised patients because of prolonged viral shedding. Some studies have suggested that eye protection may further reduce transmission given the importance of the eye as a portal of entry.[127,128]

Palivizumab is a humanized mouse immunoglobulin G monoclonal antibody that is effective in preventing hospitalizations caused by RSV infections,[129] and the use of palivizumab as prophylaxis for susceptible infants to control outbreaks in neonatal intensive care units has been described.[111,130] The American Academy of Pediatrics recommends that palivizumab be administered to the following groups of patients[131,132]:

- Infants younger than 12 months of age and born before 29 weeks' gestation at the beginning of RSV season
- Preterm infants with chronic lung disease of prematurity who are born before 32 weeks' gestation during the first year of life
- Infants younger than 12 months of age with hemodynamically significant heart disease

OTHER RESPIRATORY VIRUSES

Adenovirus

Health care–associated outbreaks of adenovirus have been reported from various settings with high secondary infection risks among patients (15%–56%).[133–135] Adenoviruses can result in severe or fatal disseminated disease among severely immunocompromised patients.[136] Adenoviruses are transmitted through large respiratory droplets but are also notable for their ability to survive on nonporous surfaces for up to 49 days.[137] As a result, transmission also occurs via self-inoculation after contact with contaminated fomites. In addition to standard precautions, the CDC recommends contact and droplet precautions to prevent health care–associated adenovirus infection (see **Tables 1** and **2**).[3,84]

Parainfluenza Virus

Transmission of parainfluenza has been documented in pediatric wards,[138] neonatal nurseries,[139] and adult transplant units.[140] Transmission of parainfluenza primarily occurs by direct person-to-person contact. Parainfluenza can survive up to 4 hours on porous surfaces and up to 10 hours on nonporous surfaces.[141] However, viral recovery from hands declines rapidly, with only 5% detected after 10 minutes.[142] The CDC recommends contact precautions for the prevention of health care–associated parainfluenza infection (see **Tables 1** and **2**).[3,84]

Rhinovirus

Among studies with broad molecular respiratory virus identification, rhinoviruses are typically the most common health care–associated respiratory viral infection among both children and adults.[1,20,21] Nosocomial rhinovirus infections have been linked with increased need for respiratory support and longer lengths of stay in high-risk neonates[143] and deaths in long-term care facilities.[144] However, the clinical significance of rhinovirus infections is debated because this virus is frequently detected in asymptomatic children.[145] The CDC recommends droplet precautions for the prevention of health care–associated rhinovirus infection (see **Tables 1** and **2**).[84]

Human Metapneumovirus

Nosocomial outbreaks of human metapneumovirus have been described in various settings with secondary infection risks ranging from 36% to 56%.[146–149] Human metapneumovirus survival on nonporous surfaces has been shown for up to 8 hours, but for much shorter durations on porous surfaces.[150] The CDC recommends contact precautions for the prevention of health care–associated human metapneumovirus infection (see **Tables 1** and **2**).[151]

EMPIRIC CLINICAL GUIDANCE FOR PATIENTS WITH SUSPECTED RESPIRATORY VIRAL INFECTIONS

For suspected respiratory virus infections, CDC recommends empiric contact plus droplet precautions until viruses specifically requiring droplet precautions can be ruled out.[3,84] Empiric treatment with influenza antiviral medications is also recommended for any patient with suspected or confirmed influenza infection who is hospitalized, has severe illness, or is at high risk of complications.[100]

Diagnostic Testing

In many cases, diagnosing a respiratory virus infection can inform clinical management, improve infection prevention,[152,153] and may improve antibiotic stewardship.[154] In addition to virus-specific guidance previously discussed for SARS-CoV-2 and influenza, IDSA recommends respiratory virus panel testing of immunocompromised patients who are hospitalized with respiratory symptoms, and advises that panel testing can be used more broadly in hospitalized patients if it might influence clinical care or infection prevention.[99] The diagnostic landscape continues to rapidly evolve and more research is needed regarding best practices, clinical interpretation, and cost-effectiveness of respiratory virus testing.[155]

SUMMARY

Transmission of respiratory viruses occurs in a variety of health care settings, resulting in increased patient morbidity and health care costs. Different viruses have different modes of transmission, and prevention of transmission requires early recognition of symptomatic patients and prompt institution of appropriate transmission-based precautions, in addition to adherence to basic infection control practices such as hand hygiene. In addition to virus-specific infection control measures, vaccination of HCP is a priority for prevention of health care–associated SARS-CoV-2 and influenza infection.

CLINICS CARE POINTS

- Vaccination of health care personnel is a priority for the prevention of healthcare acquired influenza and SARS-CoV-2 infection.
- Recommended precautions preventing healthcare acquired viral respiratory diseases vary by viral species.
- droplet precautions until viruses specifically requiring droplet precautions can be ruled out.
- In many cases, diagnosing a respiratory virus infection can inform clinical management, improve infection prevention, and may improve antibiotic stewardship.

DISCLOSURE

J.G. Petrie and T.R. Talbot have no disclosures.

REFERENCES

1. Chow EJ, Mermel LA. Hospital-Acquired Respiratory Viral Infections: Incidence, Morbidity, and Mortality in Pediatric and Adult Patients. Open Forum Infect Dis 2017;4(1). https://doi.org/10.1093/ofid/ofx006.
2. Hall CB. Nosocomial viral respiratory infections: Perennial weeds on pediatric wards. Am J Med 1981;70(3):670–6.
3. Tablan OC, Anderson LJ, Besser R, et al. Guidelines for preventing health-care-associated pneumonia, 2003: recommendations of CDC and the Healthcare Infection Control Practices Advisory Committee. MMWR Recomm Rep Morb Mortal Wkly Rep Recomm Rep Cent Dis Control 2004;53(RR-3):1–36.

4. Weekly operational update on COVID-19 - 1 March 2021. Available at: https://www. who.int/publications/m/item/weekly-operational-update-on-covid-19—1-march-2021. Accessed March 1, 2021.

5. Centers for Disease Control and Prevention. COVID Data Tracker weekly review. Centers for Disease Control and Prevention; 2021. Available at: https://www.cdc. gov/coronavirus/2019-ncov/covid-data/covidview/index.html. Accessed March 1, 2021.

6. Nguyen LH, Drew DA, Graham MS, et al. Risk of COVID-19 among front-line health-care workers and the general community: a prospective cohort study. Lancet Public Health 2020;5(9):e475–83.

7. Rickman HM, Rampling T, Shaw K, et al. Nosocomial Transmission of Coronavirus Disease 2019: A Retrospective Study of 66 Hospital-acquired Cases in a London Teaching Hospital. Clin Infect Dis 2021;72(4):690–3.

8. Van Praet JT, Claeys B, Coene A-S, et al. Prevention of nosocomial COVID-19: Another challenge of the pandemic. Infect Control Hosp Epidemiol 2020;41(11): 1355–6.

9. McMichael TM, Currie DW, Clark S, et al. Epidemiology of Covid-19 in a Long-Term Care Facility in King County, Washington. N Engl J Med 2020;382(21): 2005–11.

10. National Healthcare Safety Network (NHSN). COVID-19 Nursing Home Data. 2021. Available at: https://data.cms.gov/stories/s/COVID-19-Nursing-Home-Data/bkwz-xpvg/. Accessed March 2, 2021.

11. Goh K-T, Cutter J, Heng B-H, et al. Epidemiology and control of SARS in Singapore. Ann Acad Med Singap 2006;35(5):301–16.

12. Varia M, Wilson S, Sarwal S, et al. Investigation of a nosocomial outbreak of severe acute respiratory syndrome (SARS) in Toronto, Canada. CMAJ Can Med Assoc J 2003;169(4):285–92.

13. Zaki AM, van Boheemen S, Bestebroer TM, et al. Isolation of a novel coronavirus from a man with pneumonia in Saudi Arabia. N Engl J Med 2012;367(19): 1814–20.

14. WHO EMRO | MERS outbreaks | MERS-CoV | Health topics. Available at: http:// www.emro.who.int/health-topics/mers-cov/mers-outbreaks.html.   Accessed February 23, 2021.

15. Hui DS, Azhar EI, Kim Y-J, et al. Middle East respiratory syndrome coronavirus: risk factors and determinants of primary, household, and nosocomial transmission. Lancet Infect Dis 2018;18(8):e217–27.

16. Assiri A, McGeer A, Perl TM, et al. Hospital outbreak of Middle East respiratory syndrome coronavirus. N Engl J Med 2013;369(5):407–16.

17. Balkhy HH, Alenazi TH, Alshamrani MM, et al. Notes from the Field: Nosocomial Outbreak of Middle East Respiratory Syndrome in a Large Tertiary Care Hospital–Riyadh, Saudi Arabia, 2015. MMWR Morb Mortal Wkly Rep 2016;65(6): 163–4.

18. Hunter JC, Nguyen D, Aden B, et al. Transmission of Middle East Respiratory Syndrome Coronavirus Infections in Healthcare Settings, Abu Dhabi. Emerg Infect Dis 2016;22(4):647–56.

19. Chowell G, Abdirizak F, Lee S, et al. Transmission characteristics of MERS and SARS in the healthcare setting: a comparative study. BMC Med 2015;13:210.

20. Choi H-S, Kim M-N, Sung H, et al. Laboratory-based surveillance of hospital-acquired respiratory virus infection in a tertiary care hospital. Am J Infect Control 2017;45(5):e45–7.

21. Petrie JG, Lauring AS, Martin ET, et al. Hospital Associated Respiratory Virus Infection in Children and Adults: It Does Not Just Occur During Cold and Flu Season. Open Forum Infect Dis 2020;7(6). https://doi.org/10.1093/ofid/ofaa200.

22. Gagneur A, Vallet S, Talbot PJ, et al. Outbreaks of human coronavirus in a pediatric and neonatal intensive care unit. Eur J Pediatr 2008;167(12):1427–34.

23. Li Q, Guan X, Wu P, et al. Early Transmission Dynamics in Wuhan, China, of Novel Coronavirus-Infected Pneumonia. N Engl J Med 2020. https://doi.org/10.1056/NEJMoa2001316.

24. Lauer SA, Grantz KH, Bi Q, et al. The Incubation Period of Coronavirus Disease 2019 (COVID-19) From Publicly Reported Confirmed Cases: Estimation and Application. Ann Intern Med 2020. https://doi.org/10.7326/M20-0504.

25. Oran DP, Topol EJ. The Proportion of SARS-CoV-2 Infections That Are Asymptomatic. Ann Intern Med 2021. https://doi.org/10.7326/M20-6976.

26. Buitrago-Garcia D, Egli-Gany D, Counotte MJ, et al. Occurrence and transmission potential of asymptomatic and presymptomatic SARS-CoV-2 infections: A living systematic review and meta-analysis. PLOS Med 2020;17(9):e1003346.

27. Hasanoglu I, Korukluoglu G, Asilturk D, et al. Higher viral loads in asymptomatic COVID-19 patients might be the invisible part of the iceberg. Infection 2020;1–10. https://doi.org/10.1007/s15010-020-01548-8.

28. Cevik M, Tate M, Lloyd O, et al. SARS-CoV-2, SARS-CoV, and MERS-CoV viral load dynamics, duration of viral shedding, and infectiousness: a systematic review and meta-analysis. Lancet Microbe 2021;2(1):e13–22.

29. van Kampen JJA, van de Vijver DAMC, Fraaij PLA, et al. Duration and key determinants of infectious virus shedding in hospitalized patients with coronavirus disease-2019 (COVID-19). Nat Commun 2021;12(1):267.

30. Tarhini H, Recoing A, Bridier-Nahmias A, et al. Long term SARS-CoV-2 infectiousness among three immunocompromised patients: from prolonged viral shedding to SARS-CoV-2 superinfection. J Infect Dis 2021. https://doi.org/10.1093/infdis/jiab075.

31. World Health Organization (WHO). Transmission of SARS-CoV-2: implications for infection prevention precautions. Available at: https://www.who.int/newsroom/commentaries/detail/transmission-of-sars-cov-2-implications-for-infection-prevention-precautions. Accessed March 22, 2021.

32. Centers for Disease Control and Prevention. Science Brief: SARS-CoV-2 and Potential Airborne Transmission. 2020. Available at: https://www.cdc.gov/coronavirus/2019-ncov/more/scientific-brief-sars-cov-2.html. Accessed March 22, 2021.

33. Morawska L, Milton DK. It Is Time to Address Airborne Transmission of Coronavirus Disease 2019 (COVID-19). Clin Infect Dis 2020;71(9):2311–3.

34. van Doremalen N, Bushmaker T, Morris DH, et al. Aerosol and Surface Stability of SARS-CoV-2 as Compared with SARS-CoV-1. N Engl J Med 2020;382(16):1564–7.

35. Pasnick S, Carlos WG, Dela Cruz CS, et al. SARS-CoV-2 Transmission and the Risk of Aerosol-Generating Procedures. Am J Respir Crit Care Med 2020;202(4):P13–4.

36. Chia PY, Coleman KK, Tan YK, et al. Detection of air and surface contamination by SARS-CoV-2 in hospital rooms of infected patients. Nat Commun 2020;11(1):2800.

37. Otter JA, Donskey C, Yezli S, et al. Transmission of SARS and MERS coronaviruses and influenza virus in healthcare settings: the possible role of dry surface contamination. J Hosp Infect 2016;92(3):235–50.

38. Committee on Infectious Diseases; American Academy of Pediatrics, Kimberlin DW, Brady MT, Jackson MA, et al. Red Book® 2018 | red Book online 2018. Available at: https://redbook.solutions.aap.org/book.aspx?bookid=2205. Accessed March 25, 2021.
39. Cummings DAT, Radonovich LJ, Gorse GJ, et al. Risk Factors for Healthcare Personnel Infection with Endemic Coronaviruses (HKU1, OC43, NL63, 229E): Results from the Respiratory Protection Effectiveness Clinical Trial (ResPECT). Clin Infect Dis 2020. https://doi.org/10.1093/cid/ciaa900.
40. Centers for Disease Control and Prevention (CDC). Interim infection prevention and control recommendations for healthcare personnel during the coronavirus disease 2019 (COVID-19) pandemic 2020. Available at: https://www.cdc.gov/coronavirus/2019-ncov/hcp/infection-control-recommendations.html. Accessed March 2, 2021.
41. Centers for Disease Control and Prevention. Strategies for Optimizing the Supply of Facemasks. 2020. Available at: https://www.cdc.gov/coronavirus/2019-ncov/hcp/ppe-strategy/face-masks.html. Accessed March 2, 2021.
42. World Health Organization (WHO). Advice on the use of masks in the community, during home care and in healthcare settings in the context of the novel coronavirus (COVID-19) outbreak. Available at: https://www.who.int/publications/i/item/advice-on-the-use-of-masks-in-the-community-during-home-care-and-in-healthcare-settings-in-the-context-of-the-novel-coronavirus-(2019-ncov)-outbreak. Accessed March 17, 2021.
43. Mody L, Akinboyo IC, Babcock HM, et al. COVID-19 Research Agenda for Healthcare Epidemiology. Infect Control Hosp Epidemiol. 2021:1-81. doi:10.1017/ice.2021.25
44. Richterman A, Meyerowitz EA, Cevik M. Hospital-Acquired SARS-CoV-2 Infection: Lessons for Public Health. JAMA 2020. https://doi.org/10.1001/jama.2020.21399.
45. Wang X, Ferro EG, Zhou G, et al. Association Between Universal Masking in a Health Care System and SARS-CoV-2 Positivity Among Health Care Workers. JAMA 2020. https://doi.org/10.1001/jama.2020.12897.
46. Centers for Disease Control and Prevention. Your Guide to Masks. Available at: https://www.cdc.gov/coronavirus/2019-ncov/prevent-getting-sick/about-face-coverings.html. Accessed March 17, 2021.
47. Centers for Disease Control and Prevention. Overview of Testing for SARS-CoV-2 (COVID-19). 2020. Available at: https://www.cdc.gov/coronavirus/2019-ncov/hcp/testing-overview.html. Accessed March 5, 2021.
48. Hanson KE, Caliendo AM, Arias CA, et al. The Infectious Diseases Society of America Guidelines on the Diagnosis of COVID-19: Molecular Diagnostic Testing. Clin Infect Dis 2021. https://doi.org/10.1093/cid/ciab048. ciab048.
49. Centers for Disease Control and Prevention. Interim guidance on testing healthcare personnel for SARS-CoV-2 2020. Available at: https://www.cdc.gov/coronavirus/2019-ncov/hcp/testing-healthcare-personnel.html. Accessed March 5, 2021.
50. Food and Drug Administration. FACT SHEET FOR HEALTHCARE PROVIDERS ADMINISTERING VACCINE (VACCINATION PROVIDERS) EMERGENCY USE AUTHORIZATION (EUA) OF THE PFIZER-BIONTECH COVID-19 VACCINE TO PREVENT CORONAVIRUS DISEASE 2019 (COVID-19). 2021. Available at: https://www.fda.gov/media/144413/download. Accessed March 5, 2021.
51. Food and Drug Administration. FACT SHEET FOR HEALTHCARE PROVIDERS ADMINISTERING VACCINE (VACCINATION PROVIDERS) EMERGENCY USE AUTHORIZATION (EUA) OF THE MODERNA COVID-19 VACCINE TO PREVENT CORONAVIRUS DISEASE 2019 (COVID-19). 2020. Available at: https://www.fda.gov/media/144637/download. Accessed March 5, 2021.

52. Food and Drug Administration. FACT SHEET FOR HEALTHCARE PROVIDERS ADMINISTERING VACCINE (VACCINATION PROVIDERS) EMERGENCY USE AUTHORIZATION (EUA) OF THE JANSSEN COVID-19 VACCINE TO PREVENT CORONAVIRUS DISEASE 2019 (COVID-19). 2021. Available at: https://www.fda.gov/media/144413/download. Accessed March 5, 2021.

53. Dooling K. The Advisory Committee on Immunization Practices' Updated Interim Recommendation for Allocation of COVID-19 Vaccine — United States, December 2020. MMWR Morb Mortal Wkly Rep 2021;69. https://doi.org/10.15585/mmwr.mm695152e2.

54. Oliver SE. The Advisory Committee on Immunization Practices' Interim Recommendation for Use of Janssen COVID-19 Vaccine — United States, February 2021. MMWR Morb Mortal Wkly Rep 2021;70. https://doi.org/10.15585/mmwr.mm7009e4.

55. Centers for Disease Control and Prevention. MERS-CoV: Prevention and Control for Hospitalized Patients. Available at: https://www.cdc.gov/coronavirus/mers/infection-prevention-control.html. Accessed March 22, 2021.

56. Rolfes MA, Foppa IM, Garg S, et al. Annual estimates of the burden of seasonal influenza in the United States: A tool for strengthening influenza surveillance and preparedness. Influenza Other Respir Viruses 2018;12(1):132–7.

57. Centers for Disease Control and Prevention. Past seasons estimated influenza disease Burden 2020. Available at: https://www.cdc.gov/flu/about/burden/past-seasons.html. Accessed March 8, 2021.

58. Talbot TR, Bradley SF, Cosgrove SE, et al. Influenza Vaccination of Healthcare Workers and Vaccine Allocation for Healthcare Workers During Vaccine Shortages. Infect Control Hosp Epidemiol 2005;26(11):882–90.

59. Bénet T, Amour S, Valette M, et al. Incidence of asymptomatic and symptomatic influenza among healthcare workers: a multicenter prospective cohort study. Clin Infect Dis 2020. https://doi.org/10.1093/cid/ciaa1109.

60. Ip DKM, Lau LLH, Leung NHL, et al. Viral Shedding and Transmission Potential of Asymptomatic and Paucisymptomatic Influenza Virus Infections in the Community. Clin Infect Dis 2017;64(6):736–42.

61. Chow EJ, Mermel LA. More Than a Cold: Hospital-Acquired Respiratory Viral Infections, Sick Leave Policy, and A Need for Culture Change. Infect Control Hosp Epidemiol 2018;39(7):861–2.

62. Jiang L, McGeer A, McNeil S, et al. Which healthcare workers work with acute respiratory illness? Evidence from Canadian acute-care hospitals during 4 influenza seasons: 2010-2011 to 2013-2014. Infect Control Hosp Epidemiol 2019;40(8):889–96.

63. Shearer MP, Meyer D, Divya Hosangadi M, et al. Operational stresses on New York City Health+Hospitals Health System frontline hospitals during the 2017-18 influenza season. Am J Disaster Med 2020;15(2):99–111.

64. Poland GA, Tosh P, Jacobson RM. Requiring influenza vaccination for health care workers: seven truths we must accept. Vaccine 2005;23(17):2251–5.

65. Ip DKM, Lau LLH, Chan K-H, et al. The Dynamic Relationship Between Clinical Symptomatology and Viral Shedding in Naturally Acquired Seasonal and Pandemic Influenza Virus Infections. Clin Infect Dis 2016;62(4):431–7.

66. Murphy BR, Chalhub EG, Nusinoff SR, et al. Temperature-Sensitive Mutants of Influenza Virus. III. Further Characterization of the ts-1[E] Influenza A Recombinant (H3N2) Virus in Man. J Infect Dis 1973;128(4):479–87.

67. Hall CB, Douglas RG. Nosocomial Influenza Infection as a Cause of Intercurrent Fevers in Infants. Pediatrics 1975;55(5):673–7.

68. Lee N, Chan PKS, Hui DSC, et al. Viral loads and duration of viral shedding in adult patients hospitalized with influenza. J Infect Dis 2009;200(4):492–500.
69. Englund JA, Champlin RE, Wyde PR, et al. Common emergence of amantadine- and rimantadine-resistant influenza A viruses in symptomatic immunocompromised adults. Clin Infect Dis 1998;26(6):1418–24.
70. Grayson ML, Melvani S, Druce J, et al. Efficacy of soap and water and alcohol-based hand-rub preparations against live H1N1 influenza virus on the hands of human volunteers. Clin Infect Dis 2009;48(3):285–91.
71. Thomas Y, Boquete-Suter P, Koch D, et al. Survival of influenza virus on human fingers. Clin Microbiol Infect 2014;20(1):O58–64.
72. Bean B, Moore BM, Sterner B, et al. Survival of influenza viruses on environmental surfaces. J Infect Dis 1982;146(1):47–51.
73. Boone SA, Gerba CP. The occurrence of influenza A virus on household and day care center fomites. J Infect 2005;51(2):103–9.
74. Klontz KC, Hynes NA, Gunn RA, et al. An outbreak of influenza A/Taiwan/1/86 (H1N1) infections at a naval base and its association with airplane travel. Am J Epidemiol 1989;129(2):341–8.
75. Morens DM, Rash VM. Lessons from a nursing home outbreak of influenza A. Infect Control Hosp Epidemiol 1995;16(5):275–80.
76. Moser MR, Bender TR, Margolis HS, et al. An outbreak of influenza aboard a commercial airliner. Am J Epidemiol 1979;110(1):1–6.
77. Milton DK, Fabian MP, Cowling BJ, et al. Influenza virus aerosols in human exhaled breath: particle size, culturability, and effect of surgical masks. PLoS Pathog 2013;9(3):e1003205.
78. Brankston G, Gitterman L, Hirji Z, et al. Transmission of influenza A in human beings. Lancet Infect Dis 2007;7(4):257–65.
79. Radonovich LJ, Simberkoff MS, Bessesen MT, et al. N95 Respirators vs Medical Masks for Preventing Influenza Among Health Care Personnel: A Randomized Clinical Trial. JAMA 2019;322(9):824–33.
80. Loeb M, Dafoe N, Mahony J, et al. Surgical mask vs N95 respirator for preventing influenza among health care workers: a randomized trial. JAMA 2009; 302(17):1865–71.
81. MacIntyre CR, Wang Q, Cauchemez S, et al. A cluster randomized clinical trial comparing fit-tested and non-fit-tested N95 respirators to medical masks to prevent respiratory virus infection in health care workers. Influenza Other Respir Viruses 2011;5(3):170–9.
82. Kuster SP, Coleman BL, Raboud J, et al. Risk factors for influenza among health care workers during 2009 pandemic, Toronto, Ontario, Canada. Emerg Infect Dis 2013;19(4):606–15.
83. Tellier R. Aerosol transmission of influenza A virus: a review of new studies. J R Soc Interf 2009;6(suppl_6):S783–90.
84. Siegel JD, Rhinehart E, Jackson M, et al. 2007 Guideline for Isolation Precautions: Preventing Transmission of Infectious Agents in Health Care Settings. Am J Infect Control 2007;35(10, Supplement 2):S65–164.
85. Centers for Disease Control and Prevention (CDC). Prevention Strategies for Seasonal Influenza in Healthcare Settings. Available at: https://www.cdc.gov/flu/professionals/infectioncontrol/healthcaresettings.htm. Accessed March 15, 2021.
86. Advisory Committee on Immunization Practices, Centers for Disease Control and Prevention (CDC). Immunization of health-care personnel:

recommendations of the Advisory Committee on Immunization Practices (ACIP). MMWR Recomm Rep Morb Mortal Wkly Rep Recomm Rep 2011;60(RR-7):1–45.

87. Belongia EA, Simpson MD, King JP, et al. Variable influenza vaccine effectiveness by subtype: a systematic review and meta-analysis of test-negative design studies. Lancet Infect Dis 2016;16(8):942–51.

88. Murti M, Otterstatter M, Orth A, et al. Measuring the impact of influenza vaccination on healthcare worker absenteeism in the context of a province-wide mandatory vaccinate-or-mask policy. Vaccine 2019;37(30):4001–7.

89. Frederick J, Brown AC, Cummings DA, et al. Protecting Healthcare Personnel in Outpatient Settings: The Influence of Mandatory Versus Nonmandatory Influenza Vaccination Policies on Workplace Absenteeism During Multiple Respiratory Virus Seasons. Infect Control Hosp Epidemiol 2018;39(4):452–61.

90. Saxén H, Virtanen M. Randomized, placebo-controlled double blind study on the efficacy of influenza immunization on absenteeism of health care workers. Pediatr Infect Dis J 1999;18(9):779–83.

91. Feery BJ, Evered MG, Morrison EI. Different Protection Rates in Various Groups of Volunteers Given Subunit Influenza Virus Vaccine in 1976. J Infect Dis 1979; 139(2):237–41.

92. Carman WF, Elder AG, Wallace LA, et al. Effects of influenza vaccination of health-care workers on mortality of elderly people in long-term care: a randomised controlled trial. Lancet 2000;355(9198):93–7.

93. Potter J, Stott DJ, Roberts MA, et al. Influenza Vaccination of Health Care Workers in Long-Term-Care Hospitals Reduces the Mortality of Elderly Patients. J Infect Dis 1997;175(1):1–6.

94. Hayward AC, Harling R, Wetten S, et al. Effectiveness of an influenza vaccine programme for care home staff to prevent death, morbidity, and health service use among residents: cluster randomised controlled trial. BMJ 2006;333(7581): 1241.

95. Lemaitre M, Meret T, Rothan-Tondeur M, et al. Effect of Influenza Vaccination of Nursing Home Staff on Mortality of Residents: A Cluster-Randomized Trial. J Am Geriatr Soc 2009;57(9):1580–6.

96. Ahmed F, Lindley MC, Allred N, et al. Effect of influenza vaccination of health-care personnel on morbidity and mortality among patients: systematic review and grading of evidence. Clin Infect Dis 2014;58(1):50–7.

97. Greene MT, Fowler KE, Ratz D, et al. Changes in Influenza Vaccination Requirements for Health Care Personnel in US Hospitals. JAMA Netw Open 2018;1(2): e180143.

98. Centers for Disease Control and Prevention. Influenza Vaccination Information for Health Care Workers. Available at: https://www.cdc.gov/flu/professionals/ healthcareworkers.htm. Accessed March 16, 2021.

99. Uyeki TM, Bernstein HH, Bradley JS, et al. Clinical Practice Guidelines by the Infectious Diseases Society of America: 2018 Update on Diagnosis, Treatment, Chemoprophylaxis, and Institutional Outbreak Management of Seasonal Influenza. Clin Infect Dis 2019;68(6):e1–47.

100. Centers for Disease Control and Prevention. Influenza Antiviral Medications: Clinician Summary. 2021. Available at: https://www.cdc.gov/flu/professionals/ antivirals/summary-clinicians.htm. Accessed March 16, 2021.

101. World Health Organization (WHO). H5N1 highly pathogenic avian influenza: Timeline of major events. 2014. Available at: https://www.who.int/influenza/human_ animal_interface/H5N1_avian_influenza_update20140317.pdf. Accessed March 17, 2021.

102. World Health Organization (WHO). Cumulative number of confirmed human cases of avian influenza A(H5N1) reported to WHO. Available at: http://www.who.int/influenza/human_animal_interface/H5N1_cumulative_table_archives/en/. Accessed March 17, 2021.

103. Food and Agriculture Organization of the United Nations (FAO). H7N9 situation update. 2021. Available at: http://www.fao.org/ag/againfo/programmes/en/empres/H7N9/situation_update.html. Accessed March 17, 2021.

104. Wu J, Ke C, Lau EHY, et al. Influenza H5/H7 Virus Vaccination in Poultry and Reduction of Zoonotic Infections, Guangdong Province, China, 2017–18. Emerg Infect Dis 2019;25(1). https://doi.org/10.3201/eid2501.181259.

105. Centers for Disease Control and Prevention. Interim Guidance on Case Definitions for Investigations of Human Infection with Highly Pathogenic Avian Influenza A H5 Viruses in the United States. Available at: https://www.cdc.gov/flu/avianflu/hpai/case-definitions.htm. Accessed March 17, 2021..

106. Centers for Disease Control and Prevention. Interim Guidance on Follow-up of Close Contacts of Persons Infected with Novel Influenza A Viruses Associated with Severe Human Disease and on the Use of Antiviral Medications for Chemoprophylaxis. Available at: https://www.cdc.gov/flu/avianflu/novel-av-chemoprophylaxis-guidance.htm. Accessed March 17, 2021.

107. Shay DK, Holman RC, Newman RD, et al. Bronchiolitis-associated hospitalizations among US children, 1980-1996. J Am Med Assoc 1999;282(15):1440–6.

108. Falsey AR, Hennessey PA, Formica MA, et al. Respiratory syncytial virus infection in elderly and high-risk adults. N Engl J Med 2005;352(17):1749–59.

109. Goldstein E, Greene SK, Olson DR, et al. Estimating the hospitalization burden associated with influenza and respiratory syncytial virus in New York City, 2003–2011. Influenza Other Respir Viruses 2015;9(5):225–33.

110. Hall CB, Douglas RG, Geiman JM, et al. Nosocomial Respiratory Syncytial Virus Infections. N Engl J Med 1975;293(26):1343–6.

111. Halasa NB, Williams JV, Wilson GJ, et al. Medical and Economic Impact of a Respiratory Syncytial Virus Outbreak in a Neonatal Intensive Care Unit. Pediatr Infect Dis J 2005;24(12):1040–4.

112. Englund JA, Anderson LJ, Rhame FS. Nosocomial transmission of respiratory syncytial virus in immunocompromised adults. J Clin Microbiol 1991;29(1):115–9.

113. Mathur U, Bentley DW, Hall CB. Concurrent Respiratory Syncytial Virus and Influenza A Infections in the Institutionalized Elderly and Chronically Ill. Ann Intern Med 1980;93(1_Part_1):49–52.

114. Hall BC, Geiman JM, Douglas RG Jr, et al. Control of nosocomial respiratory syncytial viral infections. Pediatrics 1978;62(5):728–32.

115. Hall CB, Kopelman AE, Douglas RG Jr, et al. Neonatal Respiratory Syncytial Virus Infection. N Engl J Med 1979;300(8):393–6.

116. Weinstein RA, Hall CB. Nosocomial Respiratory Syncytial Virus Infections: The "Cold War" Has Not Ended. Clin Infect Dis 2000;31(2):590–6.

117. Jena AB, Baldwin DC, Daugherty SR, et al. Presenteeism among resident physicians. JAMA 2010;304(11):1166–8.

118. Jena AB, Meltzer DO, Press VG, et al. Why physicians work when sick. Arch Intern Med 2012;172(14):1107–8.

119. Hall CB, Douglas RG. Modes of transmission of respiratory syncytial virus. J Pediatr 1981;99(1):100–3.

120. Leclair JM, Freeman J, Sullivan BF, et al. Prevention of nosocomial respiratory syncytial virus infections through compliance with glove and gown isolation precautions. N Engl J Med 1987;317(6):329–34.

121. Hall CB, Douglas RG, Schnabel KC, et al. Infectivity of respiratory syncytial virus by various routes of inoculation. Infect Immun 1981;33(3):779–83.

122. Hall CB, Douglas RG Jr, Geiman JM. Possible Transmission by Fomites of Respiratory Syncytial Virus. J Infect Dis 1980;141(1):98–102.

123. Hall CB, Douglas RG, Geiman JM. Respiratory syncytial virus infections in infants: Quantitation and duration of shedding. J Pediatr 1976;89(1):11–5.

124. Munywoki PK, Koech DC, Agoti CN, et al. Influence of age, severity of infection, and co-infection on the duration of respiratory syncytial virus (RSV) shedding. Epidemiol Infect 2015;143(4):804–12.

125. Walsh EE, Peterson DR, Kalkanoglu AE, et al. Viral Shedding and Immune Responses to Respiratory Syncytial Virus Infection in Older Adults. J Infect Dis 2013;207(9):1424–32.

126. PATH. RSV Vaccine and mAb Snapshot. Available at: https://www.path.org/resources/rsv-vaccine-and-mab-snapshot/. Accessed March 18, 2021.

127. Gala CL, Hall CB, Schnabel KC, et al. The use of eye-nose goggles to control nosocomial respiratory syncytial virus infection. JAMA 1986;256(19):2706–8.

128. Agah R, Cherry JD, Garakian AJ, et al. Respiratory syncytial virus (RSV) infection rate in personnel caring for children with RSV infections. Routine isolation procedure vs routine procedure supplemented by use of masks and goggles. Am J Dis Child 1987;141(6):695–7.

129. Feltes TF, Cabalka AK, Meissner HC, et al. Palivizumab prophylaxis reduces hospitalization due to respiratory syncytial virus in young children with hemodynamically significant congenital heart disease. J Pediatr 2003;143(4):532–40.

130. Kurz H, Herbich K, Janata O, et al. Experience with the use of palivizumab together with infection control measures to prevent respiratory syncytial virus outbreaks in neonatal intensive care units. J Hosp Infect 2008;70(3):246–52.

131. American Academy of Pediatrics Committee on Infectious Diseases; American Academy of Pediatrics Bronchiolitis Guidelines Committee. Updated Guidance for Palivizumab Prophylaxis Among Infants and Young Children at Increased Risk of Hospitalization for Respiratory Syncytial Virus Infection. Pediatrics 2014;134(2):e620–38.

132. Pediatrics AA of. AAP Publications Reaffirmed. Pediatrics 2019;144(2). https://doi.org/10.1542/peds.2019-1767.

133. Brummitt CF, Cherrington JM, Katzenstein DA, et al. Nosocomial Adenovirus Infections: Molecular Epidemiology of an Outbreak Due to Adenovirus 3a. J Infect Dis 1988;158(2):423–32.

134. James L, Vernon MO, Jones RC, et al. Outbreak of Human Adenovirus Type 3 Infection in a Pediatric Long-Term Care Facility—Illinois, 2005. Clin Infect Dis 2007;45(4):416–20.

135. Lessa FC, Gould PL, Pascoe N, et al. Health Care Transmission of a Newly Emergent Adenovirus Serotype in Health Care Personnel at a Military Hospital in Texas, 2007. J Infect Dis 2009;200(11):1759–65.

136. Ison MG. Adenovirus Infections in Transplant Recipients. Clin Infect Dis 2006;43(3):331–9.

137. Gordon YJ, Gordon RY, Romanowski E, et al. Prolonged recovery of desiccated adenoviral serotypes 5, 8, and 19 from plastic and metal surfaces in vitro. Ophthalmology 1993;100(12):1835–9 [discussion: 1839–40].

138. Karron RA, O'Brien KL, Froehlich JL, et al. Molecular epidemiology of a parainfluenza type 3 virus outbreak on a pediatric ward. J Infect Dis 1993;167(6): 1441–5.
139. Meissner HC, Murray SA, Kiernan MA, et al. A simultaneous outbreak of respiratory syncytial virus and parainfluenza virus type 3 in a newborn nursery. J Pediatr 1984;104(5):680–4.
140. Zambon M, Bull T, Sadler CJ, et al. Molecular Epidemiology of Two Consecutive Outbreaks of Parainfluenza 3 in a Bone Marrow Transplant Unit. J Clin Microbiol 1998;36(8):2289–93.
141. Brady MT, Evans J, Cuartas J. Survival and disinfection of parainfluenza viruses on environmental surfaces. Am J Infect Control 1990;18(1):18–23.
142. Ansari SA, Springthorpe VS, Sattar SA, et al. Potential role of hands in the spread of respiratory viral infections: studies with human parainfluenza virus 3 and rhinovirus 14. J Clin Microbiol 1991;29(10):2115–9.
143. Zinna S, Lakshmanan A, Tan S, et al. Outcomes of Nosocomial Viral Respiratory Infections in High-Risk Neonates. Pediatrics 2016;138(5):e20161675.
144. Louie JK, Yagi S, Nelson FA, et al. Rhinovirus outbreak in a long term care facility for elderly persons associated with unusually high mortality. Clin Infect Dis 2005; 41(2):262–5.
145. Rhedin S, Lindstrand A, Rotzén-Östlund M, et al. Clinical utility of PCR for common viruses in acute respiratory illness. Pediatrics 2014;133(3):e538–45.
146. Liao RS, Appelgate DM, Pelz RK. An outbreak of severe respiratory tract infection due to human metapneumovirus in a long-term care facility for the elderly in Oregon. J Clin Virol 2012;53(2):171–3.
147. Lee N, Chan PKS, Yu IT, et al. Co-circulation of human metapneumovirus and SARS-associated coronavirus during a major nosocomial SARS outbreak in Hong Kong. J Clin Virol 2007;40(4):333–7.
148. Cheng VCC, Wu AKL, Cheung CHY, et al. Outbreak of human metapneumovirus infection in psychiatric inpatients: implications for directly observed use of alcohol hand rub in prevention of nosocomial outbreaks. J Hosp Infect 2007;67(4):336–43.
149. Kim S, Sung H, Im HJ, et al. Molecular epidemiological investigation of a nosocomial outbreak of human metapneumovirus infection in a pediatric hematooncology patient population. J Clin Microbiol 2009;47(4):1221–4.
150. Kutter JS, Spronken MI, Fraaij PL, et al. Transmission routes of respiratory viruses among humans. Curr Opin Virol 2018;28:142–51.
151. Tollefson SJ, Cox RG, Williams JV. Studies of culture conditions and environmental stability of human metapneumovirus. Virus Res 2010;151(1):54–9.
152. van Rijn AL, Nijhuis RHT, Bekker V, et al. Clinical implications of rapid ePlex® Respiratory Pathogen Panel testing compared to laboratory-developed real-time PCR. Eur J Clin Microbiol Infect Dis 2018;37(3):571–7.
153. Youngs J, Marshall B, Farragher M, et al. Implementation of influenza point-of-care testing and patient cohorting during a high-incidence season: a retrospective analysis of impact on infection prevention and control and clinical outcomes. J Hosp Infect 2019;101(3):276–84.
154. Barlam TF, Cosgrove SE, Abbo LM, et al. Implementing an Antibiotic Stewardship Program: Guidelines by the Infectious Diseases Society of America and the Society for Healthcare Epidemiology of America. Clin Infect Dis 2016;62(10):e51–77.
155. Hanson KE. America (IDSA) for the DC of the IDS of, Azar MM, et al. Molecular Testing for Acute Respiratory Tract Infections: Clinical and Diagnostic Recommendations From the IDSA's Diagnostics Committee. Clin Infect Dis 2020; 71(10):2744–51.

Pandemic Preparedness

Casey E. Godshall, MD, David B. Banach, MD, MPH, MS*

KEYWORDS

- Pandemic • Occupational health and safety • Incident management • Ethics
- Wellness

KEY POINTS

- Pandemic preparedness is an essential function of any health care facility. An Emergency Management Program can guide a facility through a pandemic response, and the Hospital Incident Command System can centralize communication and coordination to rapidly respond to a crisis.
- Plans for staffing and utilization of space to prepare for the continued provision of routine inpatient and outpatient care, as well as the surge of pandemic-related patients, must be developed and be reviewed and revised routinely.
- Consideration should be given to the ethical challenges inherent to a pandemic in which there may be a scarcity of resources.
- The maintenance of psychological health and well-being of health care workers making difficult treatment decisions under highly stressful conditions and potentially putting their own health at risk should be incorporated into pandemic preparedness planning.

INTRODUCTION

The coronavirus disease 2019 (COVID-19) pandemic has illustrated the ways in which many health care facilities and health systems were not adequately prepared for the crisis conditions caused by a rapidly emerging respiratory virus. Major challenges faced early on during the pandemic included shortages of personal protective equipment (PPE), health care personnel frequently being exposed to or infected with severe acute respiratory syndrome coronavirus 2 (SARS-CoV-2), and insufficient preparations for the surge of patients.[1] Although a discussion of all aspects of pandemic preparedness is beyond the scope of this review, we address several aspects of pandemic preparedness focused on health care facilities to provide clinicians and facility administrators guiding principles in preparation for future pandemics.

The authors have no disclosures relevant to this article.
Department of Medicine, University of Connecticut School of Medicine, Farmington, CT, USA
* Corresponding author. University of Connecticut School of Medicine, 263 Farmington Avenue, Farmington, CT 06030.
E-mail address: dbanach@uchc.edu

INCIDENT MANAGEMENT DURING A PANDEMIC

Previously published guidance for outbreak management and response has recommended the incorporation of an Emergency Management Program (EMP) to provide guidance through the 4 phases of incident management: preparedness, mitigation, response, and recovery.[2] The use of an all-hazards self-assessment can help facility leadership prepare in fulfilling its core mission of patient care during a pandemic. The National Incident Management System provides guidance to government, nongovernmental organizations, and the private sector to work together to prevent, protect against, mitigate, and respond to incidents, including infectious diseases pandemics.[3] The Hospital Incident Command System (HICS) is a structure within the EMP that coordinates the hospital command functions that have been identified during incident management and describes how responsibility is distributed within the management team in a facility (**Fig. 1**). This group may operate out of a single Incident

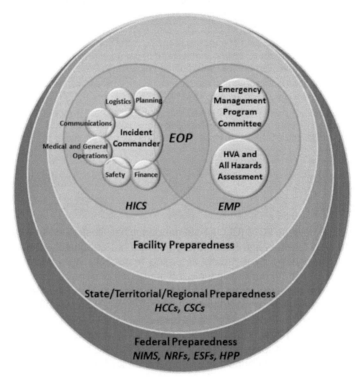

Fig. 1. Diagram of incident management preparedness structures and frameworks. This diagram was created by the authors of the Society of Healthcare Epidemiology of America Outbreak Response Training Program expert guidance document to illustrate how US preparedness structures and frameworks relate, starting at the federal level and moving to the facility level. CSC, Crisis Standards of Care; EMP, Emergency Management Program; EOP, Emergency Operations Plan; ESF, Emergency Support Function; HCC, Health Care Coalition; HICS, Hospital Incident Command System; HPP, Hospital Preparedness Program, NIMS, National Incident Management System; HVA, hazard vulnerability analysis; NRF, National Response Framework. (*From* Banach DB, Johnston BL, Al-Zubeidi D, et al. Outbreak response and incident management: SHEA guidance and resources for healthcare epidemiologists in United States acute-care hospitals. Infect Control Hosp Epidemiol. 2017;38(12):1393-419. https://doi.org/10.1017/ice.2017.212; with permission.)

Command Center (ICC) in a physical location at the facility, or through teleconference or video communication systems, as necessary. Depending on the nature of the pandemic event and the associated operations required to respond, a facility may need to activate either the entire HICS system or various components. Familiarity with the facility's HICS is required for rapid, effective, and sustained function of the system, which requires training team members and the deployment of exercises that use the system to identify any gaps or challenges. Institutional experiences during the initial COVID-19 crisis have further delineated specific roles of key administrative leadership in the incident management response, and they have reported effective strategies for coordinating members of the incident management team within a facility.[4–6]

In pandemic preparedness planning activities, the membership of the ICC should be frequently revisited and updated as new individuals join the organization's pandemic response team and as roles change within the structure of the HICS. One of the key roles of the HICS is to identify the key internal and external stakeholders required in pandemic response.[1] Internal stakeholders can be divided into 4 categories: direct care providers, administrative leadership, patient care support services, and facility services. External stakeholders may include a broader group, depending on the nature and impact of the outbreak/pandemic. This group would likely include local, regional, or national public health agencies; regional health care facilities and collaborative networks; and local municipalities. Understanding the local and regional infrastructures for emergency response and establishing a system to rapidly communicate and coordinate with the key stakeholders is a critical component of pandemic preparedness.

HEALTH CARE PERSONNEL PROTECTION AND SAFETY

Occupational health and safety among the health care workforce is a central priority in pandemic preparedness. The prevention of infection among those working in health care and other essential industries provides the ability to sustain the delivery of medical care and other essential services to the population during a pandemic. The understanding of infection transmission for the organism of concern coupled with the hierarchy of infection controls provides the basis for designing appropriate infection prevention strategies in health care settings.

Previous experiences with SARS, and most recently the COVID-19 pandemic, have highlighted the disproportionate impact of high-consequence respiratory viruses on health care personnel. During the early phases of the SARS epidemic in Toronto, Canada, health care personnel represented a large proportion of total infected individuals, more than 30% in a high infection incidence setting.[7] Most infections occurred in situations in which infection control precautions had not been initiated or were not implemented successfully.[8] During the COVID-19 pandemic, health care personnel were infected at a higher rate than the general population,[9] particularly in the early phases of the pandemic.[10] Health care personnel have also been infected at disproportionately higher rates in the setting of the recent Ebola and Marburg virus disease outbreaks over the past decade, generally in the setting of inadequate infection prevention measures and caring for patients with unsuspected infection.[11]

In the setting of a pandemic the optimal strategy for preventing infections among health care personnel depends on the organism of concern and its characteristics, particularly the route and mechanism of infection transmission. A strategy using the hierarchy of controls, frequently used in occupational medicine, has been used as a means of determining how to implement feasible and effective control solutions. This approach can guide pandemic preparedness programs, in developing strategies to protect health care personnel in the event of an infectious disease pandemic[12] (**Fig. 2**). The hierarchy of controls includes 3 components: engineering controls, administrative controls, and behavioral controls, each of which can be implemented in the context of infectious diseases pandemic response.

Engineering controls involve separating the health hazard (the patient with suspected or confirmed infection) from the health care worker, and when not possible, reduce the amount of contact between an infected patient and the organism of concern and the potentially infected health care worker. In the setting of an infectious disease pandemic, this may include specific wards or areas dedicated to patients with suspected or confirmed infection and creating a patient care environment that reduces transmission. Creating such an environment may include improving ventilation, use of negative pressure airborne isolation rooms and the use of high-efficiency particulate air (HEPA) filtration.[13] During the COVID-19 pandemic, indoor transmission in poorly ventilated environments was an important factor that facilitated transmission. Although most hospital facilities are generally well-ventilated, when nontraditional health care environments are involved in the care of infectious patients, as occurred during the COVID-19 pandemic, ensuring adequate ventilation is an important engineering control to address in pandemic preparation. HEPA filtration is highly effective in preventing the spread of organisms of 0.3 μm diameter or higher,[14] thus ensuring access to these devices may be warranted in pandemic planning. A layered approach to engineering controls in the prevention of SARS-CoV-2 transmission is

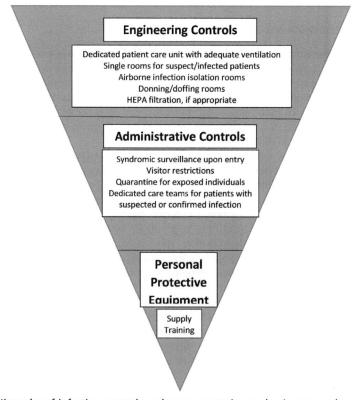

Fig. 2. Hierarchy of infection controls and components in pandemic preparedness.

recommended by Centers for Disease Control and Prevention (CDC) and can be supported for future pandemics in which airborne or droplet transmission occurs.[15]

Administrative controls, policies and procedures, and accompanying education are critical in preventing the spread of infectious diseases during pandemics. As part of the development of a pandemic preparedness plan, health care facility leadership should ensure that policies and protocols are designed to ensure rapid identification and isolation of potentially infectious patients and diagnostic testing and clinical management occurs in a setting that reduces the potential for exposure of others in the health care facility. This process includes detailed descriptions of movement within the facility and cleaning and disinfection of potentially contaminated surfaces. Although the details of these processes may need to be adjusted based on the organism of concern, pandemic preparation plans should identify locations and routes of patient movement that minimize spread of infection to health care personnel and others in the health care setting. These administrative controls may also include syndromic surveillance of all individuals entering the facility, visitor restrictions, and quarantining exposed personnel, all of which have been recommended in the COVID-19 pandemic response.[16] Importantly, health care personnel should be educated on these plans and easy, real-time access to the planning documents, when needed, should be ensured.

PPE, a barrier to protect individuals from exposure to the infectious agent, is an important part of the prevention strategy but remains the most prone to failure because it does not eliminate the hazard but rather reduces the risk of infection. Depending on the route of infection for a given pathogen, PPE will need to be adjusted. For many respiratory infections, PPE has focused primarily on the use of facemasks, and in some cases, higher-level filtration respiratory protection. The COVID-19 pandemic highlighted the role of eye protection in preventing infection.[17] Nonetheless, ensuring access to PPE, including a variety of sizes to accommodate all health care personnel, and education on how to properly don, doff, and wear PPE is a critical component of pandemic preparedness.

SUPPORTING INPATIENT CLINICAL ACTIVITIES DURING A PANDEMIC

The provision of inpatient clinical care and the associated supportive health care activities during a pandemic poses unique challenges. Guided by the emergency management plan, facility leadership within the incident command structure needs to continually evaluate the delivery of clinical services to patients and how this can be done in a safe and effective manner. The diversion of resources to provide care for infected patients may significantly impair the ability to provide care to those not infected by the organism of concern, resulting in deferral of care, particularly preventive and elective care.[18]

Surge capacity refers to the ability to evaluate and care for a markedly increased volume of patients that challenges or exceeds normal operating capacity, and there are public health principles that guide medical surge capacity and capability outlined by the United States Department of Health and Human Services.[19] Given the uncertainty surrounding the rate at which this increase can occur, preparations to respond to varying level of medical surge can guide decisions regarding resource allocation. Although most surge planning centers on ensuring sufficient hospital beds, personnel, pharmaceuticals, supplies, and equipment to provide care to patients, it is important to realize that flexibility will be needed to address the specific organism and disease epidemiology of concern. For instance, in the SARS-CoV-2 pandemic based on the frequency of critical illness,[20] expansion of critical care beds into areas of facilities such as operating rooms and perioperative areas was needed.[21] With these transitions, staff that are not typically responsible for the clinical management of critically ill patients need additional education and specialized training on how to safely provide standardized care to critically ill patients.

Beyond ensuring available space for patients, maintaining sufficient qualified health care personnel to provide care can be a primary challenge during a pandemic. During a pandemic, care services can be streamlined into focusing on the expanded numbers of patients who are impacted by the organism of concern and the deferral of elective care. Staffing will need to be rapidly expanded to adequately provide care to the increased number of patients in the facility. Thus, staffing modeling for the pandemics will need to be rapidly adjusted to accommodate this increase in clinical care needs, likely requiring frequent, potentially daily review by facility leadership. An additional challenge lies in the direct impact of the pandemic on the health care workforce,[22] including health care personnel who become infected and ill from exposure at work and in the community and those who are required to quarantine due to exposure to the infectious agent, as occurred during the COVID-19 pandemic. Thus, HICS leadership needs to work closely with nursing and human resource leaders to identify opportunities to adjust staffing scheduling and potentially expand the pool of available, adequately trained staff that can be rapidly deployed to provide clinical services. This process may involve measures such as rapidly hiring new staff and activating staff that may have training in clinical care but may not be engaged in direct care responsibilities. Expansion of the health care workforce at a regional level and the associated measures to address staffing needs during the COVID-19 pandemic have been described.[23] Notably, specialized expertise in certain areas, such as infectious diseases, emergency medicine, or critical care, may be limited. Thus, in pandemic preparedness, planning for the ability to mobilize clinical and technical expertise and coordinate collaboration with facility expertise in education and communication to provide real-time education and training to others to support these efforts is needed.

ROLE OF AMBULATORY CARE IN A PANDEMIC

In a pandemic due to a rapidly spreading contagious pathogen, health care focus naturally shifts to ensuring the ability to care for a surge of patients requiring hospitalization. However, health systems need to prepare for continued ambulatory care of patients with chronic illnesses, as well as care for those with mild to moderate pandemic-related infections who do not require hospitalization. The consequences of deferred care of chronic illnesses, as well as missed opportunities for preventive health care, create significant challenges for the health care system and increase overall costs.[24] In addition, ambulatory care services can be used to offload emergency department (ED) and urgent care settings by providing treatment to mild to moderately infected patients.

Telehealth is critical to providing continued routine care, and this technology can be leveraged to deliver a variety of services. Routine follow-ups and urgent visits for noninfectious complaints can temporarily be done via telehealth. During the COVID-19 pandemic, institutions that had little to no experience with telehealth were able to successfully convert to majority telehealth services and conduct thousands of billable visits using this platform.[25,26] Beyond these standard virtual visits, providers may choose to perform proactive population care, such as compiling registries of patients with certain poorly controlled health problems or conditions that place them at high risk for morbidity and mortality and reaching out to these vulnerable populations regularly to both ensure that chronic issues are being addressed and monitor for exposures to, or symptoms of, the emerging contagion.[27]

Telehealth tools, such as mobile device applications and interactive Web sites, can also be used for outpatients with mild to moderate infections. Apps or Web sites allowing patients to enter symptoms and self-triage can allow for streamlined outpatient care, offload some visits or calls to EDs and urgent care, and provide patients with education and guidance regarding treatment and quarantine.[28–30] Continued outpatient monitoring through interactive technology can permit care providers to track sick patients while they quarantine and guide them to higher levels of care as needed.[31]

During the COVID-19 pandemic, many outpatient offices were able to increase their capacity to offer acute care visits, screening, and diagnostic testing by performing these services in a walk-up or drive-through setting. An outdoor setting allows for additional distancing, as well as an open-air atmosphere that ensures additional safety for patients and staff by preventing transmission of a respiratory virus, especially during specimen collection for testing.[32]

As part of the effort to offload EDs during a pandemic surge, staff who typically work in an outpatient setting can be deployed to the ED to see noninfectious emergencies within their field. Physicians within surgical subspecialties, including obstetrics and gynecology, will likely not be performing elective procedures during this time and can potentially be deployed to assist in this fashion.[33]

Telehealth, outdoor screenings, and redeployment efforts are key ways to deliver care during a pandemic; however, ambulatory offices must also have plans for providing safe in-person care once it is deemed possible. The COVID-19 pandemic demonstrated the lack of preparedness that most ambulatory offices have to safely provide care during a pandemic with a respiratory pathogen. Most offices are not designed to have separate entrances and exits for patients, enough space for physical distancing in waiting rooms and lines, or proper ventilation systems or other engineering infection control measures.[34] It is critical that outpatient offices give thought to these renovations and system modifications to prepare for the next pandemic.

COMMUNICATION STRATEGIES

Given the rapidly changing conditions of a pandemic, a health care facility and its staff will need effective and efficient methods of internal and external communication to internal and external stakeholders. Keeping health care workers fully informed is a key component of providing adequate support to staff during a crisis to enable continued confidence in job performance. The CDC provides training for methods of communication during an emergency through their Crisis and Emergency Risk Communication (CERC) tool (**Table 1**). The most important principles outlined in this training are be first, be right, be credible, express empathy, promote action, and show respect. Members of the ICC should train themselves in CERC methods of communication for both internal and external messages sent during a pandemic.[35]

In terms of modes of communication, many options exist and using a variety of formats will increase impact and effectiveness of communication activities. Daily e-mails with important updates to all internal stakeholders, including health care personnel, can be an effective way to provide updated information on the pandemic response activities. Creating a living document or Web page that is frequently updated with protocols and procedures for staff to use as a daily resource is a way to have all important information that health care workers will reference in a centralized location.[32] Other options for daily updates and managing questions from staff include a text group or online chat board monitored by a content expert.[4] Hospitals can consider taking advantage of newer formats and platforms to keep staff updated, like creating a mobile phone app or starting a weekly or daily podcast on which

Table 1
Crisis and emergency risk communication

The Six Principles of CERC	The Five Pitfalls to Avoid
1. Be first: In a time-sensitive crisis, communicating early and quickly is crucial. The first source of information often becomes the preferred source	1. Mixed messages from multiple experts
2. Be right: Accuracy establishes credibility Information can include what is known, what is unknown, and what is being done to fill the gaps	2. Information released late
3. Be credible: Do not compromise honesty and truthfulness, even in a crisis	3. Paternalistic attitudes
4. Express empathy: Acknowledge harm and suffering created by the crisis. Address what people are feeling and the challenges being faced. This builds trust and rapport	4. Not countering rumors and myths in real time
5. Promote action: Give people meaningful things to do to calm anxiety, restore order, and promote a sense of control	5. Public power struggles and confusion
6. Show respect: Respectful communication promotes cooperation and rapport when people feel vulnerable	

Adapted from Office of Public Health Preparedness and Response (OPHPR). Crisis & Emergency Risk Communication (CERC). Centers for Disease Control and Prevention website. https://emergency.cdc.gov/cerc/. Accessed February 2021.

physicians and other subject matter experts, as well as administrators and managers, can share information.[36] Infectious disease physicians can contribute by creating content regarding the latest scientific information available. Disseminating scientific information in an easily accessible manner can provide necessary education and, importantly, reduce confusion and combat any online misinformation that may occur during a crisis or a pandemic.

Communication with facility leaders should be bidirectional, easy to access, and frequent. Feedback and questions must be welcomed, encouraged, and sought out on a continuous basis. To this end, a facility may elect to set up a unique e-mail address to which all questions, concerns, and issues can be sent. A method of giving anonymous feedback via phone or e-mail should be created to prevent staff from being afraid to offer negative feedback.[3] Daily or weekly open forums welcoming discussion should be arranged either in person or virtually.[37] In large group sessions, it is a good idea to devote some time to a positive experience or outcome and to find time to praise staff. This focus on good news, rather than letting any discussion simply devolve into talk about what is going poorly, can build morale and refocus efforts.[4]

ETHICAL CONSIDERATIONS

During pandemic conditions, many elements of health care are likely to be stretched to capacity, including hospital beds and ventilators; PPE; diagnostic, therapeutic, or preventative interventions; and health care workers themselves. Consideration must be given to how a hospital and its staff will respond when faced with a scarcity of resources.[38]

In times of austerity, a hospital may decide to shift their ethical framework from one of promoting and working toward the health of each individual patient to a plan to maximize benefits with limited resources. Maximizing public health benefit means taking into consideration a patient's ability to recover fully if treated and prioritizing scarce resources for these patients over those who are unlikely to survive if treated, as well as those who are likely to survive even without treatment.[39] This determination can be problematic and not clear-cut in many circumstances, because speculating about a patient's prognosis can be challenging even when resources are abundant. Undoubtedly, making these determinations would be complex, emotional, and potentially traumatic for all health care workers involved. In addition, there are legal considerations as the shift away from individual rights occurs, and as providers are faced with the unfortunate potential to make determinations based solely on discriminatory factors such as age.[40] Individuals with expertise in biomedical ethics and legal considerations in these determinations can be essential in providing guidance in decision-making. When surveyed about their ability and preparedness to make these determinations during a crisis situation, one group of physicians in Canada indicated feeling only partially prepared, with most reporting that this situation would be considerably difficult to experience.[41]

As such, it is imperative that hospitals create an ethical framework for the possible shift of resources during times of pandemic-associated scarcity. Clear, transparent, and consistent protocols for the use of resources must be drafted ahead of any pandemic, so that appropriate and sound stewardship of supplies can occur at the earliest onset of any shortage, to preempt physicians from having the difficult task of deciding which patients are offered life-saving measures during a crisis. Ideally, the triage of sick patients and determinations about the use of resources such as intensive care unit beds and ventilators would not be made by the treating team. These determinations should be made based on the framework already in place, and final decisions could be made by a team led by those with training in ethics, legal matters, and palliative care.[42]

Consideration may also need to be given to ethical questions regarding health care workers' obligations to continue to put themselves at risk for infection during a pandemic involving an infectious contagion. Doctors and nurses have a right to protect themselves and members of their family from illness. Shortages of PPE and staffing may lead to situations in which health care workers are potentially asked to care for patients without having all of the necessary equipment or support to do so while preventing disease transmission. Every effort should be made to ensure that health care workers, who have the specialized training to provide care and without whom operations would not be able to continue, are prioritized with regard to PPE distribution. An ethics team may consider having prepandemic discussions regarding a health care worker's right to discharge their duty in a situation in which resources are lacking. Collaboration with health care workers regarding expectations of duty during a pandemic should be undertaken before any such scenario.[43]

PREVENTING PSYCHOLOGICAL INJURY

Health care facilities have an obligation to make preparations to look out for the well-being of their staff during a pandemic. Health care workers will be asked to potentially put themselves in harm's way and to treat patients in times of medical uncertainty and scarcity of resources, during which poor outcomes are likely. Prevention of emotional distress and mitigation of its causative factors should be the goal, rather than only providing posttraumatic psychological services.[44] Preserving emotional wellness and resilience from the start of a pandemic achieves the goal of maintaining stable health care services and ideally preventing staff shortages from absenteeism.

Giving health care personnel the knowledge and tools to feel fully prepared to face pandemic conditions is the first and most essential step to preventing psychological and moral injury; this means keeping all staff well-informed and providing sufficient supplies of PPE. Staff who feel fully supported in their duties and properly prepared to face all challenges are less likely to suffer mental health problems after a crisis.[45]

Depending on the experiences of staff and the degree of moral injury or psychological damage that may occur during a pandemic, stress may manifest in different ways in health care workers, ranging from signs and symptoms of acute stress reactions to development of posttraumatic stress disorder.[46] Staff should be educated to recognize these symptoms in themselves, and leaders and managers should evaluate their staff regularly, as well. Regular counseling or debrief sessions held among health care worker cohorts with shared experiences can be one way to monitor staff for development of stress reactions, allow an outlet for emotions, and offer additional help when needed.[46]

Additional sources of stress during a pandemic include uncertainty about maintaining employment and income, as well as fear of bringing a contagion home from work and infecting family members. To whatever extent possible, income should be ideally guaranteed to frontline staff who are asked to put themselves at risk every day. For staff with significant exposures to infected individuals, testing should be offered quickly and free of charge. To allay fears of transmitting an infection to family, hospitals may make use of nearby hotels or other sites for quarantine accommodations for sick or isolated personnel.[47]

When a staff member presents with signs of mental health problems during or after a pandemic, hospitals should offer psychological support services in the form of counseling or even referral for psychiatric care. An organization's mental health providers could be redeployed to treat staff and provide counseling and therapy sessions. Required and regularly scheduled check-ins with peer support counselors or trained therapists for all frontline staff can help normalize the act of seeking psychological support.[48]

SUMMARY

The high likelihood of future pandemics from emerging or reemerging infectious pathogens is widely accepted.[49] The increasing interrelatedness of our world, the changing climate, antibiotic misuse, and animal exposures are all reasons why novel pathogens are likely to increasingly crossover to infect humans with pandemic potential. Despite diligent efforts in emergency preparedness, the COVID-19 pandemic found many health care facilities underprepared for several aspects of pandemic readiness. We must learn from this experience and use this time to better prepare for continued high-quality health care delivery and for the continued well-being and safety of health care personnel before the next pandemic.

REFERENCES

1. Cavallo JJ, Donoho DA, Forman HP. Hospital capacity and operations in the coronavirus disease 2019 (COVID-19) pandemic—planning for the Nth patient. JAMA Health Forum 2020;1(3):e200345.

2. Banach DB, Johnston BL, Al-Zubeidi D, et al. Outbreak response and incident management: SHEA guidance and resources for healthcare epidemiologists in United States acute-care hospitals. Infect Control Hosp Epidemiol 2017;38(12): 1393–419.
3. Federal Emergency Management Agency (FEMA). Emergency Management Institute (EMI). National Incident Management. System (NIMS) website. Available at: https://training.fema.gov/nims/. Accessed March 31, 2021.
4. Gupta S, Federman DG. Hospital preparedness for COVID-19 pandemic: experience from department of medicine at Veterans Affairs Connecticut Healthcare System. Postgrad Med 2020;132(6):489–94.
5. Orsini E, Mireles-Cabodevila E, Ashton R, et al. Lessons on outbreak preparedness from the cleveland clinic. Chest 2020;158(5):2090–6.
6. Zorn CK, Pascual JM, Bosch W, et al. Addressing the challenge of COVID-19: one health care site's leadership response to the pandemic. Mayo Clin Proc Innov Qual Outcomes 2021;5(1):151–60.
7. Varia M, Wilson S, Sarwal S, et al. Hospital Outbreak Investigation Team. Investigation of a nosocomial outbreak of severe acute respiratory syndrome (SARS) in Toronto, Canada. CMAJ 2003;169(4):285–92.
8. Centers for Disease Control and Prevention (CDC). Cluster of severe acute respiratory syndrome cases among protected health-care workers–Toronto, Canada, April 2003. MMWR Morb Mortal Wkly Rep 2003;52(19):433–6.
9. Galanis P, Vraka I, Fragkou D, et al. Seroprevalence of SARS-CoV-2 antibodies and associated factors in healthcare workers: a systematic review and meta-analysis. J Hosp Infect 2021;108:120–34.
10. Sahu AK, Amrithanand VT, Mathew R, et al. COVID-19 in health care workers - A systematic review and meta-analysis. Am J Emerg Med 2020;38(9):1727–31.
11. Selvaraj SA, Lee KE, Harrell M, et al. Infection rates and risk factors for infection among health workers during ebola and marburg virus outbreaks: a systematic review. J Infect Dis 2018;218(suppl_5):S679–89.
12. Thorne CD, Khozin S, McDiarmid MA. Using the hierarchy of control technologies to improve healthcare facility infection control: lessons from severe acute respiratory syndrome. J Occup Environ Med 2004;46(7):613–22.
13. Morawska L, Tang JW, Bahnfleth W, et al. How can airborne transmission of COVID-19 indoors be minimised? Environ Int 2020;142:105832.
14. United States Environmental Protection Agency. Indoor Air Quality: What is a HEPA Filter?. Available at: https://www.epa.gov/indoor-air-quality-iaq/what-hepa-filter-1. Accessed March 31, 2021.
15. Centers for Disease Control and Prevention (CDC). Ventilation in buildings. Available at: https://www.cdc.gov/coronavirus/2019-ncov/community/ventilation.html. Accessed March 31, 2021.
16. Centers for Disease Control and Prevention (CDC). Infection Control Guidance for Healthcare Professionals about Coronavirus (COVID-19). Available at: https://www.cdc.gov/coronavirus/2019-ncov/hcp/infection-control.html. Accessed March 31, 2021.
17. Chu DK, Akl EA, Duda S, et al. COVID-19 systematic urgent review group effort (SURGE) study authors. Physical distancing, face masks, and eye protection to prevent person-to-person transmission of SARS-CoV-2 and COVID-19: a systematic review and meta-analysis. Lancet 2020;395(10242):1973–87.
18. Whaley CM, Pera MF, Cantor J, et al. Changes in health services use among commercially insured US populations during the COVID-19 pandemic. JAMA Netw Open 2020;3(11):e2024984.

19. U.S. Department of Health and Human Services. Medical surge capacity and capability handbook, chapter 1, what is medical surge?. Available at: https://www.phe.gov/Preparedness/planning/mscc/handbook/chapter1/Pages/whatis medicalsurge.aspx. Accessed March 31, 2021.

20. Abate SM, Ahmed Ali S, Mantfardo B, et al. Rate of Intensive Care Unit admission and outcomes among patients with coronavirus: a systematic review and meta-analysis. PLoS One 2020;15(7):e0235653.

21. Griffin KM, Karas MG, Ivascu NS, et al. Hospital preparedness for COVID-19: a practical guide from a critical care perspective. Am J Respir Crit Care Med 2020;201(11):1337–44.

22. Chou R, Dana T, Buckley DI, et al. Epidemiology of and risk factors for coronavirus infection in health care workers: a living rapid review. Ann Intern Med 2020; 173(2):120–36.

23. Keeley C, Jimenez J, Jackson H, et al. Staffing up for the surge: expanding the New York city public hospital workforce during The COVID-19 Pandemic. Health Aff (Millwood) 2020;39(8):1426–30.

24. Rawaf S, Allen LN, Stigler FL, et al. Global forum on universal health coverage and primary health care. Lessons on the COVID-19 pandemic, for and by primary care professionals worldwide. Eur J Gen Pract 2020;26(1):129–33.

25. Lau J, Knudsen J, Jackson H, et al. Staying connected in the COVID-19 pandemic: telehealth at the largest safety-net system In The United States. Health Aff (Millwood) 2020;39(8):1437–42.

26. Lonergan PE, Washington SL Iii, Branagan L, et al. Rapid utilization of telehealth in a comprehensive cancer center as a response to COVID-19: cross-sectional analysis. J Med Internet Res 2020;22(7):e19322.

27. Krist AH, DeVoe JE, Cheng A, et al. Redesigning primary care to address the COVID-19 pandemic in the midst of the pandemic. Ann Fam Med 2020;18(4): 349–54.

28. Judson TJ, Odisho AY, Neinstein AB, et al. Rapid design and implementation of an integrated patient self-triage and self-scheduling tool for COVID-19. J Am Med Inform Assoc 2020;27(6):860–6.

29. Galmiche S, Rahbe E, Fontanet A, et al. Implementation of a self-triage web application for suspected COVID-19 and its impact on emergency call centers: observational study. J Med Internet Res 2020;22(11):e22924.

30. Schrager JD, Schuler K, Isakov AP, et al. Development and usability testing of a web-based COVID-19 self-triage Platform. West J Emerg Med 2020;21(5): 1054–8.

31. Ford D, Harvey JB, McElligott J, et al. Leveraging health system telehealth and informatics infrastructure to create a continuum of services for COVID-19 screening, testing, and treatment. J Am Med Inform Assoc 2020;27(12):1871–7.

32. Kwon KT, Ko JH, Shin H, et al. Drive-through screening center for COVID-19: a safe and efficient screening system against massive community outbreak. J Korean Med Sci 2020;35(11):e123.

33. Yaffee AQ, Peacock E, Seitz R, et al. Preparedness, adaptation, and innovation: approach to the COVID-19 pandemic at a decentralized, quaternary care department of emergency medicine. West J Emerg Med 2020;21(6):63–70.

34. Garg S, Basu S, Rustagi R, et al. Primary health care facility preparedness for outpatient service provision during the COVID-19 pandemic in india: cross-sectional study. JMIR Public Health Surveill 2020;6(2):e19927.

35. Office of Public Health Preparedness and Response (OPHPR). Crisis & Emergency Risk Communication (CERC). Centers for Disease Control and Prevention

website. Available at: https://emergency.cdc.gov/cerc/. Accessed March 31, 2021.

36. Anyanwu EC, Ward RP, Shah A, et al. A mobile app to facilitate socially-distanced hospital communication during the COVID-19 pandemic: implementation experience. JMIR Mhealth Uhealth 2021.

37. Chowdhury JM, Patel M, Zheng M, et al. Mobilization and preparation of a large urban academic center during the COVID-19 pandemic. Ann Am Thorac Soc 2020;17(8):922–5.

38. Leider JP, Debruin D, Reynolds N, et al. Ethical guidance for disaster response, specifically around crisis standards of care: a systematic review. Am J Public Health 2017;107(9):e1–9.

39. Sese D, Ahmad MU, Rajendram P. Ethical considerations during the COVID-19 pandemic. Cleve Clin J Med 2020.

40. Farrell TW, Francis L, Brown T, et al. Rationing limited healthcare resources in the COVID-19 era and beyond: ethical considerations regarding older adults. J Am Geriatr Soc 2020;68(6):1143–9.

41. Dewar B, Anderson JE, Kwok ESH, et al. Physician preparedness for resource allocation decisions under pandemic conditions: a cross-sectional survey of Canadian physicians, April 2020. PLoS One 2020;15(10):e0238842.

42. Emanuel EJ, Persad G, Upshur R, et al. Fair allocation of scarce medical resources in the time of covid-19. N Engl J Med 2020;382(21):2049–55.

43. Bakewell F, Pauls MA, Migneault D. Ethical considerations of the duty to care and physician safety in the COVID-19 pandemic. CJEM 2020;22(4):407–10.

44. Walton M, Murray E, Christian MD. Mental health care for medical staff and affiliated healthcare workers during the COVID-19 pandemic. Eur Heart J Acute Cardiovasc Care 2020;9(3):241–7.

45. Greenberg N, Docherty M, Gnanapragasam S, et al. Managing mental health challenges faced by healthcare workers during covid-19 pandemic. BMJ 2020;368:m1211.

46. Zaka A, Shamloo SE, Fiorente P, et al. COVID-19 pandemic as a watershed moment: a call for systematic psychological health care for frontline medical staff. J Health Psychol 2020;25(7):883–7.

47. Almaghrabi RH, Alfaraidi HA, Al Hebshi WA, et al. Healthcare workers experience in dealing with Coronavirus (COVID-19) pandemic. Saudi Med J 2020;41(6):657–60.

48. Carmassi C, Foghi C, Dell'Oste V, et al. PTSD symptoms in healthcare workers facing the three coronavirus outbreaks: what can we expect after the COVID-19 pandemic. Psychiatry Res 2020;292:113312.

49. Morens DM, Fauci AS. Emerging pandemic diseases: how we got to COVID-19. Cell 2020;182(5):1077–92.

UNITED STATES POSTAL SERVICE®

Statement of Ownership, Management, and Circulation (All Periodicals Publications Except Requester Publications)

1. Publication Title: INFECTIOUS DISEASE CLINICS OF NORTH AMERICA

2. Publication Number: 001 – 556

3. Filing Date: 9/18/2021

4. Issue Frequency: MAR, JUN, SEP, DEC

5. Number of Issues Published Annually: 4

6. Annual Subscription Price: $347.00

7. Complete Mailing Address of Known Office of Publication (Not printer) (Street, city, county, state, and ZIP+4®)
ELSEVIER INC.
230 Park Avenue, Suite 800
New York, NY 10169

Contact Person: Malathi Samayan
Telephone (Include area code): 91-44-4299-4507

8. Complete Mailing Address of Headquarters or General Business Office of Publisher (Not printer)
ELSEVIER INC.
230 Park Avenue, Suite 800
New York, NY 10169

9. Full Names and Complete Mailing Addresses of Publisher, Editor, and Managing Editor (Do not leave blank)

Publisher (Name and complete mailing address)
DOLORES MELONI, ELSEVIER INC.
1600 JOHN F KENNEDY BLVD. SUITE 1800
PHILADELPHIA, PA 19103-2899

Editor (Name and complete mailing address)
KERRY HOLLAND, ELSEVIER INC.
1600 JOHN F KENNEDY BLVD. SUITE 1800
PHILADELPHIA, PA 19103-2899

Managing Editor (Name and complete mailing address)
PATRICK MANLEY, ELSEVIER INC.
1600 JOHN F KENNEDY BLVD. SUITE 1800
PHILADELPHIA, PA 19103-2899

10. Owner (Do not leave blank. If the publication is owned by a corporation, give the name and address of the corporation immediately followed by the names and addresses of all stockholders owning or holding 1 percent or more of the total amount of stock. If not owned by a corporation, give the names and addresses of the individual owners. If owned by a partnership or other unincorporated firm, give its name and address as well as those of each individual owner. If the publication is published by a nonprofit organization, give its name and address.)

Full Name	Complete Mailing Address
WHOLLY OWNED SUBSIDIARY OF REED/ELSEVIER, US HOLDINGS	1600 JOHN F KENNEDY BLVD. SUITE 1800 PHILADELPHIA, PA 19103-2899

11. Known Bondholders, Mortgagees, and Other Security Holders Owning or Holding 1 Percent or More of Total Amount of Bonds, Mortgages, or Other Securities. If none, check box ▸ ☐ None

Full Name	Complete Mailing Address
N/A	

12. Tax Status (For completion by nonprofit organizations authorized to mail at nonprofit rates) (Check one)
The purpose, function, and nonprofit status of this organization and the exempt status for federal income tax purposes:
☒ Has Not Changed During Preceding 12 Months
☐ Has Changed During Preceding 12 Months (Publisher must submit explanation of change with this statement)

PS Form **3526**, July 2014 [Page 1 of 4 (see instructions page 4)] PSN: 7530-01-000-9931 PRIVACY NOTICE: See our privacy policy on www.usps.com.

---

13. Publication Title: INFECTIOUS DISEASE CLINICS OF NORTH AMERICA

14. Issue Date for Circulation Data Below: JUNE 2021

15. Extent and Nature of Circulation

		Average No. Copies Each Issue During Preceding 12 Months	No. Copies of Single Issue Published Nearest to Filing Date
a. Total Number of Copies (Net press run)		246	216
b. Paid Circulation (By Mail and Outside the Mail)	(1) Mailed Outside-County Paid Subscriptions Stated on PS Form 3541 (Include paid distribution above nominal rate, advertiser's proof copies, and exchange copies)	162	150
	(2) Mailed In-County Paid Subscriptions Stated on PS Form 3541 (Include paid distribution above nominal rate, advertiser's proof copies, and exchange copies)	0	0
	(3) Paid Distribution Outside the Mails Including Sales Through Dealers and Carriers, Street Vendors, Counter Sales, and Other Paid Distribution Outside USPS®	49	43
	(4) Paid Distribution by Other Classes of Mail Through the USPS (e.g., First-Class Mail®)	0	0
c. Total Paid Distribution (Sum of 15b (1), (2), (3), and (4))		211	193
d. Free or Nominal Rate Distribution (By Mail and Outside the Mail)	(1) Free or Nominal Rate Outside-County Copies included on PS Form 3541	19	8
	(2) Free or Nominal Rate In-County Copies Included on PS Form 3541	0	0
	(3) Free or Nominal Rate Copies Mailed at Other Classes Through the USPS (e.g., First-Class Mail)	0	0
	(4) Free or Nominal Rate Distribution Outside the Mail (Carriers or other means)	0	0
e. Total Free or Nominal Rate Distribution (Sum of 15d (1), (2), (3) and (4))		19	8
f. Total Distribution (Sum of 15c and 15e)		230	201
g. Copies not Distributed (See Instructions to Publishers #4 (page 3))		16	15
h. Total (Sum of 15f and g)		246	216
i. Percent Paid (15c divided by 15f times 100)		91.73%	96.01%

* If you are claiming electronic copies, go to line 16 on page 3. If you are not claiming electronic copies, skip to line 17 on page 3.

16. Electronic Copy Circulation

	Average No. Copies Each Issue During Preceding 12 Months	No. Copies of Single Issue Published Nearest to Filing Date
a. Paid Electronic Copies ▸		
b. Total Paid Print Copies (Line 15c) + Paid Electronic Copies (Line 16a) ▸		
c. Total Print Distribution (Line 15f) + Paid Electronic Copies (Line 16a) ▸		
d. Percent Paid (Both Print & Electronic Copies) (16b divided by 16c × 100) ▸		

☒ I certify that 50% of all my distributed copies (electronic and print) are paid above a nominal price.

17. Publication of Statement of Ownership
☒ If the publication is a general publication, publication of this statement is required. Will be printed in the DECEMBER 2021 issue of this publication.   ☐ Publication not required.

18. Signature and Title of Editor, Publisher, Business Manager, or Owner

Malathi Samayan *Malathi Samayan* - Distribution Controller

Date: 9/18/2021

I certify that all information furnished on this form is true and complete. I understand that anyone who furnishes false or misleading information on this form or who omits material or information requested on the form may be subject to criminal sanctions (including fines and imprisonment) and/or civil sanctions (including civil penalties).

PS Form **3526**, July 2014 (Page 3 of 4) PRIVACY NOTICE: See our privacy policy on www.usps.com

Moving?

Make sure your subscription moves with you!

To notify us of your new address, find your **Clinics Account Number** (located on your mailing label above your name), and contact customer service at:

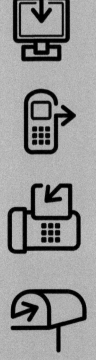

Email: **journalscustomerservice-usa@elsevier.com**

800-654-2452 (subscribers in the U.S. & Canada)
314-447-8871 (subscribers outside of the U.S. & Canada)

Fax number: 314-447-8029

Elsevier Health Sciences Division
Subscription Customer Service
3251 Riverport Lane
Maryland Heights, MO 63043

ELSEVIER